Mechanisms of
Gastrointestinal
Motility and Secretion

NATO ASI Series

Advanced Science Institutes Series

A series presenting the results of activities sponsored by the NATO Science Committee, which aims at the dissemination of advanced scientific and technological knowledge, with a view to strengthening links between scientific communities.

The series is published by an international board of publishers in conjunction with the NATO Scientific Affairs Division

A	Life Sciences	Plenum Publishing Corporation
B	Physics	New York and London
C	Mathematical and Physical Sciences	D. Reidel Publishing Company Dordrecht, Boston, and Lancaster
D	Behavioral and Social Sciences	Martinus Nijhoff Publishers
E	Engineering and Materials Sciences	The Hague, Boston, and Lancaster
F	Computer and Systems Sciences	Springer-Verlag
G	Ecological Sciences	Berlin, Heidelberg, New York, and Tokyo

Recent Volumes in this Series

Volume 73—Targets for the Design of Antiviral Agents
          edited by E. De Clercq and R. T. Walker

Volume 74—Photoreception and Vision in Invertebrates
          edited by M. A. Ali

Volume 75—Photoreceptors
          edited by A. Borsellino and L. Cervetto

Volume 76—Biomembranes: Dynamics and Biology
          edited by Robert M. Burton and Francisco Carvalho Guerra

Volume 77—The Role of Cell Interactions in Early Neurogenesis: Cargèse 1983
          edited by A.-M. Duprat, A. C. Kato, and M. Weber

Volume 78—Organizing Principles of Neural Development
          edited by S. C. Sharma

Volume 79—Regression of Atherosclerotic Lesions
          edited by M. Rene Malinow and Victor H. Blaton

Volume 80—Mechanisms of Gastrointestinal Motility and Secretion
          edited by Alan Bennett and Giampaolo Velo

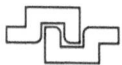

Series A: Life Sciences

Mechanisms of Gastrointestinal Motility and Secretion

Edited by

Alan Bennett

King's College
School of Medicine and Dentistry

and

Giampaolo Velo

University of Verona
Verona, Italy

Plenum Press
New York and London
Published in cooperation with NATO Scientific Affairs Division

Proceedings of a NATO Advanced Study Institute on
Mechanisms of Gastrointestinal Motility and Secretion,
held September 5–16, 1983,
in Erice, Sicily, Italy

Library of Congress Cataloging in Publication Data

NATO Advanced Study Institute on Mechanisms of Gastrointestinal Motility and Secretion (1983: Erice, Sicily)
  Mechanisms of gastrointestinal motility and secretion.

  (NATO ASI series. Series A, Life sciences; v. 80)
  "Proceedings of a NATO Advanced Study Institute on Mechanisms of
Gastrointestinal Motility and Secretion, held September 5–16, 1983, in
Erice, Sicily, Italy"—Verso t.p.
  "Published in cooperation with NATO Scientific Affairs Division."
  Includes bibliographical references and index.
  1. Gastrointestinal system—Motility—Congresses.
I. Bennett, Alan, 1936–   . II. Velo, G. P. III. North Atlantic Treaty
Organization. Scientific Affairs Division.   IV. Title.   V. Series.
QP180.N38   1983   612'.32   84-16045
ISBN 978-1-4684-4855-9   ISBN 978-1-4684-4853-5 (eBook)
DOI 10.1007/978-1-4684-4853-5

PREFACE

    Gastroenterology is a large and diverse topic, and because of
this scientists working in one area often know little of advances
in other areas.   This is particularly undesirable in a system with
different functions that interact and affect each other.   But to
discuss the many aspects and their interactions adequately requires
more time than is generally available at meetings.   A 10-day International School of Pharmacology on "Mechanisms of Gastrointestinal
Motility and Secretion" was therefore organised in Erice, Sicily,
September 1983, kindly supported by NATO.   This book combines the
chapters written by the internationally recognised authorities who
participated, and reflects the breadth and the depth of the subject matter.

                                          Alan Bennett
                                          Giampaolo Velo

CONTENTS

Anatomy of the gastrointestinal tract in relation to
    motility and secretion 1
    Jeremy R. Jass

Techniques for studying gastrointestinal motility in
    vitro 13
    Gareth J. Sanger and Alan Bennett

Motility: Methods for in vivo measurements 35
    Paul Bass and Deborah A. Fox

Smooth muscle electrophysiology 55
    Joseph H. Szurszewski

Electrophysiological studies of myenteric neurons in
    tissue culture 73
    Menachem Hanani

Gastrointestinal nerves, hormones and autacoids in
    relation to human gastrointestinal motility 87
    Alan Bennett

Distribution of gut peptides and their actions 109
    Susan M. Wood

Histamine and the digestive functions 117
    Giulio Bertaccini and Gabriella Coruzzi

Relationships of prostaglandins to gastrointestinal
    motility and secretion 129
    Alan Bennett and Gareth J. Sanger

Gallbladder motility and its regulation 159
    John R. Wood and David R. Jenkins

Histopathological findings relating to disordered
    motility and secretion 177
    Jeremy R. Jass

Neuro-hormonal control of gastric acid secretion:
The role of histamine 189
Stanislaw J. Konturek

Gastrointestinal mucus 205
A. Allen, N. Carroll, A. Garner, D.A. Hutton
and C.W. Venables

Intestinal absorption and secretion of fluid and
electrolytes 219
Henry J. Binder

Gallbladder fluid transport 229
John R. Wood and Joar Svanvik

Relationships among intestinal motility, transit
and absorption 239
Sidney F. Phillips

The entero-insular axis 259
Susan M. Wood

Neuro-hormonal control of exocrine pancreatic
secretion in humans and animals 277
Manfred V. Singer

Acute and chronic actions of alcohol on pancreatic
exocrine secretion in humans and animals 281
Manfred V. Singer

Dopamine antagonists as anti-emetics and as
stimulants of gastric motility 287
Brian McRitchie, Christine M. McClelland
Stephen M. Cooper, David H. Turner and
Gareth J. Sanger

Mechanisms by which metoclopramide can increase
gastrointestinal motility 303
Gareth J. Sanger

Laxatives: A review of their mechanisms of action 325
Paul Bass and Deborah A. Fox

Lectures 345

Participants 347

Index 349

ANATOMY OF THE GASTROINTESTINAL TRACT IN RELATION TO MOTILITY AND SECRETION

Jeremy R. Jass

Department of Histopathology
Westminster Medical School
London SW1P 2AR UK.

INTRODUCTION

A broad outline of the structure of the gut will be given, slanted towards the activities of motility and secretion. Emphasis will be placed on the functional divergence of epithelial secretory cell populations.

BASIC STRUCTURE OF GUT

The wall of the alimentary canal shows a similar structure throughout its length. Four layers are constantly present including the serosa, muscularis externa, submucosa and mucosa. The serosa (peritoneum) comprises a mesothelium and a connective tissue layer. The muscularis externa is arranged in an inner circular and an outer longitudinal layer of smooth muscle. Located between them is the myenteric (Auerbach's) plexus. In the stomach three somewhat indistinct muscle layers have been detailed. Striated muscle forms the upper third of the oesophageal muscularis externa. The submucosa is composed of loosely arranged connective tissue, which allows the mucosa to adopt its characteristic pattern of folds. Within it is the submucous (Meissner's) plexus, which is less conspicuous than the myenteric plexus. It is particularly poorly developed in the oesophagus. Submucosal glands are found in the oesophagus and duodenum (Brunner's). Conspicuous lymphoid aggregates (Peyer's patches) occur in the terminal ileum.

1

The mucosa includes the muscularis mucosae, lamina propria and lining epithelium. The lamina propria is composed of delicate connective tissue and within it are found fibroblasts, mast cells, macrophages, lymphocytes, plasma cells and eosinophils. The mucosal lining of the oesophagus and anal canal is a non-keratinised stratified squamous epithelium. The remainder of the gut is lined by a columnar epithelium. This varies according to the different regions and will be discussed in more detail below.

INNERVATION OF THE GUT

The nerve supply to the gut may be divided into extrinsic and intrinsic components. The extrinsic innervation of the gut is through the autonomic nervous system, which is divided into sympathetic and parasympathetic components. The parasympathetic supply to the oesophagus, stomach, small intestine and proximal colon is through the vagus nerve. The colon is also innervated through the sacral spinal nerves. The preganglionic fibres terminate in the myenteric plexus. An exception are the fibres supplying the striated muscle of the oesophagus which terminate as motor end plates. The vagus contains many afferent fibres to complete possible reflex loops. The sympathetic supply is through lower thoracic and lumbar spinal nerves. These end in prevertebral ganglia (coeliac, superior mesenteric, inferior mesenteric) which are closer to the spinal cord than the organs to be innervated. The postganglionic fibres terminate in either the myenteric or submucous plexus, or may supply sphincteric smooth muscle directly. The sympathetic nerves also contain afferent fibres whose cell bodies may reside either within the gut (eg. acting as mechanoreceptors) or within the dorsal root ganglia. These will complete short and long reflex circuits respectively. The intrinsic innervation is through the myenteric and submucosal plexuses. These are composed of intercommunicating ganglia in which are found nerve (ganglion) cell bodies, nerve processes and glia. Most of the direct innervation of smooth muscle is through the intrinsic neurons of the two plexuses (Baumgarten, 1982).

The intrinsic neurons which act directly on the smooth muscle of the gut wall are of two types. These are excitatory, mainly cholinergic neurons and inhibitory non-cholinergic neurons. The former are driven either by excitatory interneurons or extrinsic preganglionic cholinergic fibres. They are inhibited either directly by extrinsic postganglionic adrenergic fibres or indirectly through presynaptic inhibition of excitatory interneurons. The inhibitory, non-cholinergic fibres supplying smooth muscle are again driven either by excitatory interneurons or extrinsic, preganglionic cholinergic (parasympathetic) fibres. Some interneurons may also be inhibitory. It is clear that noradrenaline · and acetyl choline are not the only neurotransmitters released within the gut and a variety of alternatives have been proposed for the non-adrenergic, non-cholinergic neurons (Furness and Costa, 1982). 5 hydroxytryptamine is a likely candidate (Gershon and Erde, 1981) though no specific role for 5HT nerves has been identified. Vaso-active intestinal polypeptide may act as the neurotrans-mitter for the inhibitory neurons supplying smooth muscle whereas substance P may function as an excitatory neurotransmitter (Furness and Costa, 1982).

Before the advent of immunohistochemistry, the neurons of the myenteric plexus were classified accord-ing to whether or not they were argyrophil and cholin-esterase positive (Smith, 1970). Unfortunately these classical light microscopic techniques show no clear correlation with current functional classifications in which the neurotransmitter substances are identified histochemically and ultrastructurally (Burnstock,1981).

SMOOTH MUSCLE

The smooth muscle cells of the gut are spindle shaped and covered by a thin basement membrane. At the cell surface are caveolae or pinocytotic invaginations which may be associated with the smooth endoplasmic reticulum. These are possibly involved in Ca 2+ transport. Three types of cytoplasmic filament have been identified – thin (actin), intermediate (desmin) and thick (myosin). Dense bands are also present, but without the regular organization of striated muscle. Electrical coupling is achieved through the junctional complexes which are of three types – interdigitations, gap junctions (nexuses) and intermediate junctions (Gabella,1979). The electron dense material on the cytoplasmic side of the intermediate junction is anchored by intermediate filaments. Individual muscle cells are not necessarily supplied by nerve terminals. Nerve processes with bead-like varicosities surround groups of muscle fibres and neurotransmitters are released into tissue spaces to reach the target cells by diffusion.

CELL POPULATIONS WITHIN THE GASTROINTESTINAL COLUMNAR EPITHELIUM

The five main cell types include columnar, goblet, glandular, Paneth and endocrine cells. Cell kinetic and morphologic studies indicate that all arise from a single undifferentiated stem cell (Cheng and Leblond, 1974). Intermediate cells showing features of both Paneth and goblet cell or endocrine and goblet cell point to the common origin of these lines. Alternatively it is possible that the endocrine cells are of neural crest origin, in keeping with the APUD concept (Pearse, 1969). This topic remains controversial (Stevens and Moore, 1983). Columnar cells function as both secretory and absorptive units, though one or other activity may predominate within a particular cell type. However, all columnar cells reveal a secretory phase during their early maturation (Trier, 1964; Wetzel et al., 1966; Chang and Leblond, 1971). Transmission and scanning electron microscopy have helped to chararacterise special types of columnar cells including microfold (Owen, 1977) and tuft or caveolated cells (Nabeyama and Leblond, 1974). The glandular cell secretion may be serous or mucinous.

Oesophagus

The submucous glands resemble minor salivary glands in their fine structure (Al Yassin and Toner, 1977) and in secreting sulphomucins (Lambert et al., 1971). The mucosal or cardiac glands occurring near the gastro-oesophageal junction secrete a mixture of neutral mucins, sialomucins and sulphomucins (Filipe, 1979).

Stomach

The longitudinal axis of the stomach comprises three zones which are distinguished by their mucosal histology. Distal to the gastro-oesophageal junction is the macroscopically ill-defined cardiac zone. The body of the stomach is lined by fundic mucosa and the distal part or antrum by pyloric mucosa. The mucosa of each zone may be divided into an upper crypt compartment and a lower glandular compartment which are separated by a narrow neck zone (fig 1). The crypts are lined by columnar cells secreting neutral mucins and lacking a well developed microvillous brush border. The immature cells of the crypt base and neck region secrete small amounts of acid mucus (Filipe, 1979).

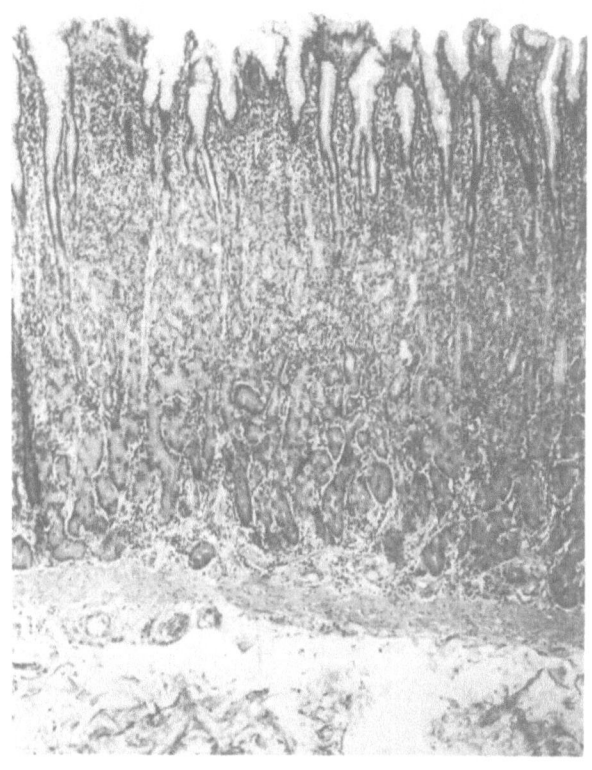

Fig. 1. Fundic mucosa of stomach stained with H & E (X40)

The fundic glands (fig. 1) include mucous gland (neck) cells and parietal cells in their upper portion, whereas the amphophilic principal (chief) cells are located in the lower third. Pepsinogen (types I and II) is secreted by the principal or zymogenic cells and to a lesser extent by the mucous gland cells (Samloff and Liebman, 1973). Type I pepsinogen is also secreted by the seromucinous pyloric and Brunner's glands. The parietal cells have a pale eosinophilic cytoplasm and ultrastructural studies reveal a complex canalicular system and numerous mitochondria. They secrete hydrochloric acid and intrinsic factor. The mucous gland cells secrete neutral mucins and possibly a trace of acid mucin. The pyloric and cardiac glands also elaborate a neutral mucosubstance.

Endocrine cells with small, eosinophilic subnuclear granules are scattered amongst the glandular tubules. Gastrin secreting cells (G cells) occur in the antrum

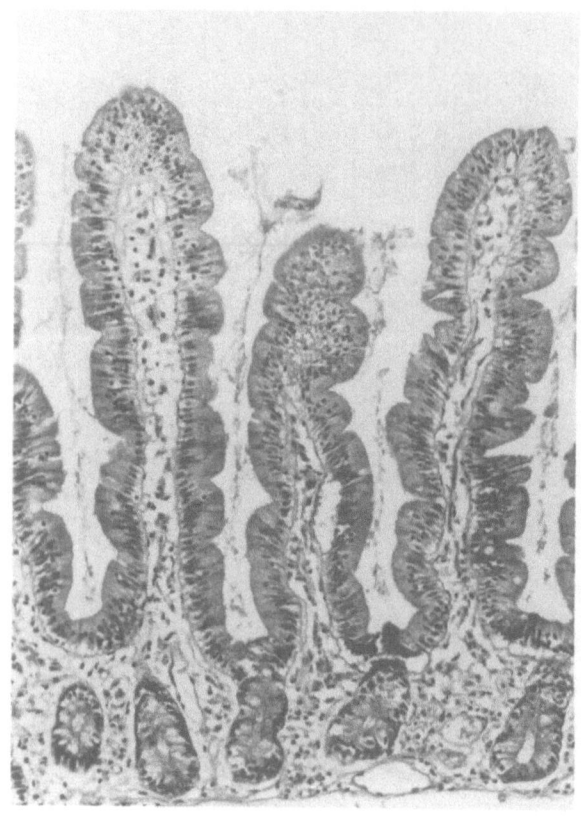

Fig. 2.   Mucosa of small intestine stained with H & E
          (X 160).

and other peptides have been identified (bombesin, somatostatin). The secretory granules may be characterised
both by their specific immunochemistry and ultrastructural appearance (Solcia et al., 1973 and 1982;
Bloom and Polak, 1981).

Small intestine

     The surface area of the small intestine is increased
by numerous finger-like villi covered by columnar cells
and scattered goblet cells (fig. 2). The latter secrete
mainly N-acetyl sialomucins (Filipe, 1979) and also small
amounts of carcinoembryonic antigen (Ahnen et al., 1982).
The columnar cells are specialised for absorption with
a well developed microvillous brush border containing a
a range of enzymes. The columnar cells located within the
crypts of Lieberkuhn show conspicuous secretory activity.
Small droplets staining as neutral mucins may be observed
in their apical cytoplasm (Trier, 1964). The crypt

columnar cells elaborate secretory component which is
involved in intracellular IgA and IgM transport (Jones,
1972). Paneth cells with large supranuclear, eosinophilic
droplets are sited in the crypt base. They secrete
lysozyme and may function as regulators of the bacterial
population (Erlandsen et al., 1974). They have also been
implicated in zinc metabolism in animal studies (Elmes,
1976) though contain relatively small amounts of zinc in
man (Jones and Elmes, 1982). Endocrine cells are scatter-
in the crypt base and secrete the range of peptides found
in the stomach and some additional ones (secretin,
cholecystokinin, enteroglucagon, gastric inhibitory
polypeptide, motilin, neurotensin) (Bloom and Polak,
1981; Solcia et al., 1982). 5HT containing cells are
most numerous in the ileum.

Colon and rectum

Colorectal mucosa is relatively simple, being
composed of crypts and surface epithelium. The goblet
cells secrete mainly acid mucins in which sulphate groups
and O-acylated sialomucins are well represented (Filipe,
1979). However the mucin histochemistry varies according
to the region of the colorectum. Also, mucins of the

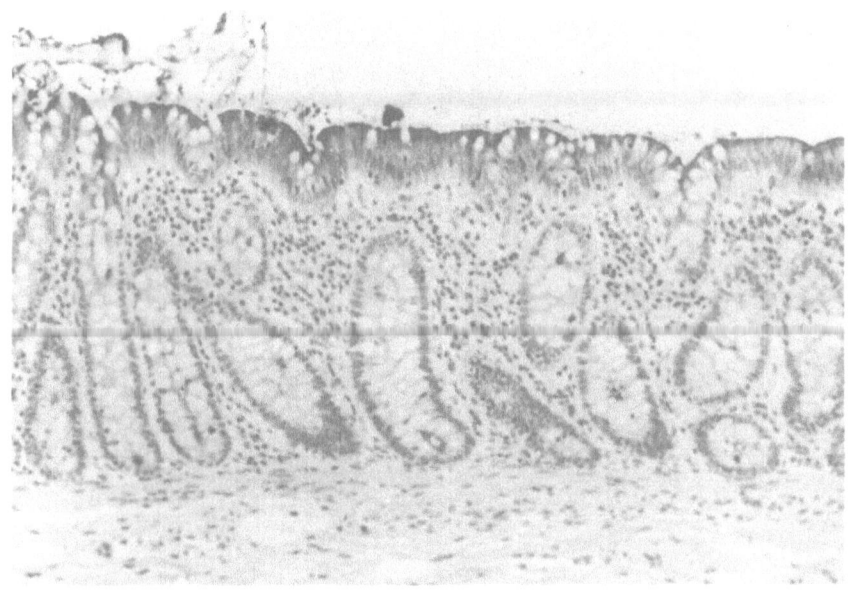

Fig. 3. Colonic mucosa stained for carcinoembryonic
         antigen by immunoperoxidase technique (X 160).

upper crypt and surface epithelium are more periodic
acid Schiff positive than those of the lower crypt.
The columnar cells bear microvilli which are less
developed than those of the small intestine and brush
border enzyme activities are reduced or absent. This
reflects the more limited absorptive specialization.
Mucin secretion has been described in both the columnar
cells of the crypts (Wetzel et al., 1966; Chang and
Leblond, 1971) and surface epithelium (Michaels, 1977).
When stained with diastase periodic acid Schiff the
apical cytoplasm of normal columnar cells shows a faint
diffuse reaction product. Vesicles containing glycoprotein
have been demonstrated at the EM level (Michaels, 1977;
Thomopoulos et al., 1983). This secretion contributes to
the formation of the glycocalyx or fuzzy coat. The
columnar cells also secrete carcinoembryonic antigen
(Ahnen et al., 1982 and this is especially conspicuous
along the lumenal border of the crypt base cells and
surface columnar cells (fig. 3). In addition, elaboration
of secretory component and transcellular movement of
IgA may be observed in the crypt columnar cells (fig. 4).
Paneth cells are occasionally found in the right colon.
Endocrine cells secreting enteroglucagon and neurotensin
are detected in the crypt bases (Bloom and Polak, 1981;
Solcia et al., 1982).

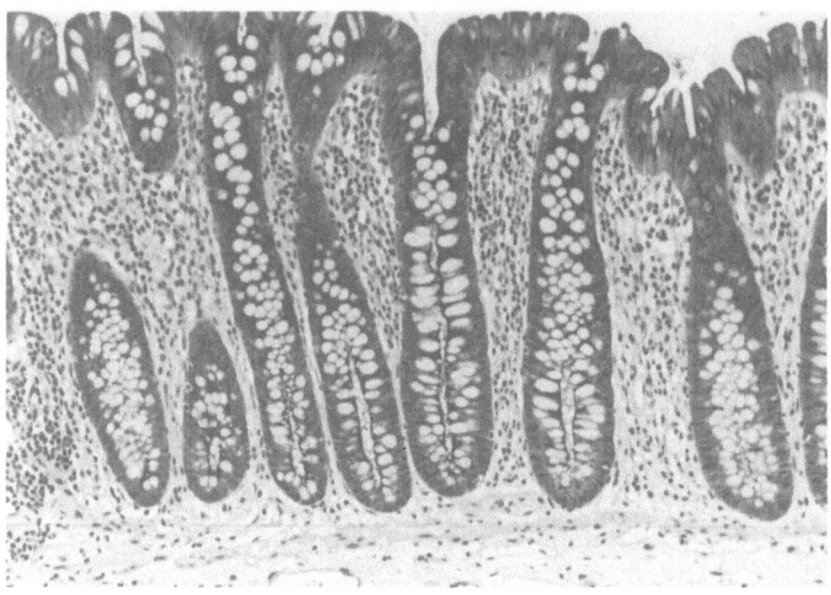

Fig. 4.   Colonic mucosa stained for secretory component
          by immunoperoxidase technique (X 160).

REFERENCES

Ahnen, D.J., Nakane, P.K., and Brown, W.R., 1982, Ultra-structural localization of carcinoembryonic antigen in normal intestine and colon cancer, Cancer, 49: 2077.

Al Yassin, T.M., and Toner, P.G., 1977, Fine structure of squamous epithelium and submucosal glands of human oesophagus, J. Anat., 123:705.

Baumgarten, H.G., 1982, Morphological basis of gastro-intestinal motility: structure and innervation of gastrointestinal tract, in: "Mediators and drugs in gastrointestinal motility I. Morphological basis and neurophysiological control," G. Bertaccini, ed., Springer-Verlag, Berlin Heidelberg New York.

Bloom, S.R., and Polak, J.M., 1981, in: "Gut hormones", Churchill livingstone, Edinburgh.

Burnstock, G., 1981, Ultrastructural identification of neurotransmitters, Scand. J. Gastroenterol., suppl. 70, 16:1.

Chang, W.W.L., and Leblond, C.P., 1971, Renewal of the epithelium in the descending colon of the mouse, Amer. J. Anat., 131:73.

Cheng, H., and Leblond, C.P., 1974, Origin, different-iation and renewal of the four main epithelial cell types in the mouse small intestine. Amer. J. Anat., 141:537.

Elmes, M., 1976, The Paneth cell population of the small intestine of the rat- effects of fasting and zinc deficiency on total count and on dithizone reactive count, J. Pathol.

Erlandsen, S.L., Parsons, J.A., and Taylor, T.D., 1974, Ultrastructural localization of lysozyme in the Paneth cells of man, J. Histochem. Cytochem., 22:401.

Fllipe, M.I., 1979, Mucins in the human gastrointestinal epithelium: a review, Invest. Cell Pathol., 2:195

Furness, J.B., Costa, M., 1982, Identification of gastro-intestinal neurotransmitters, in: "Mediators and drugs in gastrointestinal motility I. Morphological basis and neurophysiological control," G. Bertaccini, ed., Springer-Verlag, Berlin Heidelberg New York.

Gabella, G., 1979, Smooth muscle cell junctions and structural aspects of contraction, Br. Med. Bull., 35/3:213.

Gershon, M.D., and Erde, S.M., 1981, The nervous system
    of the gut, Gastroenterology, 80:1571.
Jones, E.A., 1972, Progress report: immunoglobulins and
    the gut, Gut, 13:825.
Jones, J.G., and Elmes, M.E., 1982, The quantitation of
    zinc in the mucosal cells of human small intestine
    using X-ray microanalysis, Scand. J. Gastroent-
    erol., suppl. 70, 16:37.
Lambert, R., Andre, C., and Berard, A., 1971, Origin of
    sulphated glycoproteins in human gastric
    secretions, Digestion, 4:234.
Michaels, J.E.,1977, Glycoprotein containing vesicles
    in the surface epithelial cells of the ascending
    colon of the rat, Anat. Rec., 188:525.
Nabeyama, A., and Leblond, C.P., 1974, Caveolated cells
    characterised by deep surface invaginations and
    abundant filaments in the mouse gastrointestinal
    epithelium, Amer. J. Anat., 140:147.
Owen, R.L. 1977, Sequential uptake of horseradish
    peroxidase by lymphoid follicle epithelium of
    Peyer's patches in the normal unobstructed
    mouse intestine: an ultrastructural study,
    Gastroenterology,72:440.
Pearse, A.G.E., 1969, The cytochemistry and ultra-
    structure of polypeptide hormone producing cells
    (the APUD series) and the embryologic, physio-
    logic and pathologic implications of the concept,
    J. Histochem. Cytochem., 17:303.
Samloff, I.M., and Leibman, W.M., 1973, Cellular
    localization of the group II pepsinogens in human
    stomach and duodenum by immunofluorescence,
    Gastroenterology, 65:36.
Smith, B., 1970, Disorders of the myenteric plexus,
    Gut, 11:271.
Solcia, E., Pearse, A.G.E., Grube, D., Kobayashi, S.,
    Bussolati, G., and Creutzfeldt, W., 1973,
    Revised Weisbaden classification of gut endocrine
    tumours, Rendiconti di gastro-enterologia, 5:13.
Solcia, E., Capella, C., Buffa, R., Usellini, L., and
    Tenti, P., 1982, Morphological basis of gastro-
    intestinal motility. Ultrastructure and histo-
    chemistry of endocrine-paracrine cells, in:
    "Mediators and drugs in gastrointestinal motility
    I. Morphological basis and neurophysiological
    control, " G. Bertaccini, ed., Springer-Verlag,
    Berlin Heidelberg New York.
Stevens, R.E., and Moore, G.E., 1983, Inadequacy of APUD
    concept in explaining production of peptide
    hormones by tumours, Lancet, 1:118.

Thomopoulos, G.N., Schulte, B.A., and Spicer, S.S., 1983, The influence of embedding media and fixation on the post-embedment ultrastructural demonstration of complex carbohydrates. I. Morphology and periodic acid-thiocarbohydrazide-silver proteinate staining of vicinal diols, Histochem. J., 15:763.

Trier, J.S., 1964, Studies on small intestinal crypt epithelium II., Gastroenterology, 47:480.

Wetzel, M.G., Wetzel, B.K., and Spicer, S.S., 1966, Ultrastructural localization of acid muco-substances in the mouse colon with iron containing stains, J. Cell. Biol., 30:299.

Wood, J.D., 1981, Physiology of the enteric nervous system, in: "Physiology of the gastrointestinal tract," L.R. Johnson, ed., Raven Press, New York.

TECHNIQUES FOR STUDYING GASTROINTESTINAL MOTILITY IN VITRO

Gareth J. Sanger and Alan Bennett

Beecham Pharmaceuticals, Medicinal Research Division
The Pinnacles, Harlow, Essex CM19 5AD and Department of
Surgery, King's College Hospital Medical School, The
Rayne Institute, London SE5 9NU

INTRODUCTION

Many different techniques are used for studying gastrointestinal
motility in vitro.   Muscle strips and whole segments of stomach or
intestine can be studied by adding drugs to the surrounding bathing
solution and/or through the vasculature, by electrical stimulation
of nerve activity, and during muscle stretch.   Responses are usually
consistent and reproducible, since the environment of the isolated
system is precisely controlled.

Isolated tissue experiments overcome many ethical and technical
problems often associated with experiments in vivo.   They may have
other advantages such as in the study of drug interactions with receptors, which are best carried out in the controlled environment
of an in vitro experiment (Furchgott, 1968).   However, in most
studies with isolated tissues, consideration must be given to the
way in which the responses reflect in vivo function.   Drugs usually
produce similar responses in human gastrointestinal muscle in vitro
and in vivo, but there are important exceptions (Bennett, 1968);
these aspects are discussed later.

We have previously described in detail the techniques which are
available for studying the motility of isolated gastrointestinal
preparations (Sanger & Bennett, 1982).   The following account is
therefore an updated discussion of these techniques, which are
described only briefly, with emphasis on the reasons for using
particular methods.

Aspects of general methodology

The basic techniques, types of tissue baths and bathing solutions, temperature and oxygenation required for maintaining viable
isolated gastrointestinal preparations have been described in detail
by Bennett (1973). Transducers used for detecting muscle activity,
and their advantages and disadvantages for individual experiments
are further discussed by Paton (1975a).

It is important to use the appropriate bathing solution in
isolated tissue work, since small changes can greatly affect smooth
muscle responses. For example, lowering the pH of the bathing
fluid for 30 min from 7.4 to 7.0 increased resting muscle tension
in strips of opossum oesophagus, lower oesophageal sphincter or
stomach muscle, and reduced the amplitude and/or frequency of spontaneous contractions and relaxations by approximately 15-50%, depending on the measurement. Lowering the pH from 7.4 to 7.2 caused
similar, but less marked changes (Schulze-Delrieu & Lepsien, 1982).

Preparations of smooth muscle are usually set up for study as
soon as possible after their removal from the animal, to avoid degenerative changes. Storage of different preparations of animal
intestine for 48 h at 4-6ºC in oxygenated bathing solution prevents
peristalsis (Ambache, 1946; Innes et al. 1957), and may reduce the
response to α-adrenoceptor stimulants (Lum et al. 1966). Cold,
anoxic storage of guinea-pig gastric fundus for 12-24 h prevented
the contraction caused by electrical stimulation of intrinsic excitatory nerves, but did not affect the relaxations caused by electrical stimulation of inhibitory nerves (Cook, 1982).

Fortunately, human gastrointestinal muscles do not change their
sensitivity to a variety of drugs after overnight storage, and they
do not lose their ability to respond to nerve stimulation (Bennett
& Whitney, 1966), even after 3 days of storage (Bucknell, 1966).
Human tissue resected at operation late on one day may therefore be
used after overnight storage.

Preparations of muscle segments and strips

Isolated gastrointestinal preparations are often segments of
intestine prepared with the lumen left open, or strips of muscle
cut parallel to the longitudinal or circular muscle fibres. These
types of preparation are usually suspended in a tissue bath under a
load of 0.5-1.5g, depending on the tissue (see Bennett, 1973).
Heavy loads are used with more robust preparations to facilitate
muscle relaxation between contractions and to reduce spontaneous
activity. Light loads are necessary for sensitivity and for delicate tissues. For example Miyazaki et al (1982) studied strips of
intestinal muscle obtained from rat fetuses. The strips were laid
in the groove between 2 capillary tubes, inclined at an angle and

superfused with bathing solution.   One end of the strip was fixed
at the top and the load was provided by the weight of the tissue.
Movements were detected by measuring light conductance through the
lower end of the muscle strip.

In some studies, length-tension curves have been constructed
for gastrointestinal tissues (Lipshutz & Cohen, 1971).   The length
(determined by the load placed on the tissue) which allowed the
optimum development of tension in response to acetylcholine differed
for circular muscle strips cut from different opossum oesophageal
and gastric tissues.   The loads required to obtain the length for
optimum tension development were approximately 1, 2 and 2.5g respectively for the lower oesophageal sphincter, the oesophagus and
stomach.   Loads which are too low or too high may mean that the
magnitude of the isometric response to a drug is greatly underesti-
mated (Lipshutz & Cohen, 1971).

Segments of intestine are convenient to prepare and require less
dissection (and therefore produce less damage) than muscle strips.
Preparations of muscle strips are especially useful for studying
particular regions such as sphincters, and for large preparations
(such as human gut) where there would be problems of handling whole
segments, and of oxygenation unless the vasculature is perfused.
In addition, cutting muscle strips minimises mechanical interaction
between longitudinal and circular muscle layers (Bortoff, 1976).
An advantage of large preparations is the ease of separating the longitudinal and circular muscle layers.

Strips to study the circular muscle fibres can be produced by
cutting spirals of intestine from small animals (eg guinea-pig intestine; Bennett & Fleshler, 1970), or by making a series of transverse
cuts (Harry, 1963).   In some tissues the longitudinal muscle has
been prepared as a flat sheet (Ambache, 1954), or gently rolled off
the circular muscle after tangential stroking through the longitudinal
muscle at its mesenteric attachment (the longitudinal muscle-myenteric
plexus preparation, Ambache & Freeman (1968). Human muscularis mucosa
has been prepared by tying strips of mucosa, containing the muscularis
mucosa, into cylinders with the mucosal surface inside (Walder, 1953).
Tying the upper and lower ends of the cylinder minimises contamination
of the bathing solution by mucus which, as Walder found, interfered
with the muscle sensitivity.   Angel et al.,(1983) prepared strips of
canine gastric muscularis mucosa by careful dissection of the muscle
from the mucosa and submucosa.

Isolated muscle preparations have been used to investigate the
interaction between the longitudinal and circular muscle layers of
rabbit intestine.   MacKenna & McKirdy (1970) removed the mucosa from
a 1cm square section of muscle with the longitudinal and circular
muscle fibres parallel to the respective cut edges.   Two adjacent
cut edges were fixed and the others were connected to separate iso-

metric transducers which therefore measured longitudinal and circular muscle activity.   Ozaki (1979) cut an L-shaped section, with each arm cut parallel to either the longitudinal or circular muscle fibres. The junction of the strips was fixed and the free ends connected to isotonic transducers.   Interferences between the longitudinal and circular muscle fibres was prevented by separating the muscle layers and removing the circular muscle from the strip cut parallel to the longitudinal muscle fibres.

Hayashi et al.,(1982) applied drugs or electrical stimulation to one part of a guinea-pig ileum longitudinal muscle-myenteric plexus preparation, and measured the response in another part of the tissue. The muscle was fixed in a V-shape by passing it through a polyethylene partition plate and both ends were attached to force transducers. The partition plate not only fixed the muscle in the tissue bath, but also separated the tissue bath into 2 compartments.   Drugs could therefore be added to the tissue in only one compartment.

In experiments with isolated gastrointestinal muscle strips or open segments, drugs are usually added to the bathing solution and reach their site of action by diffusion through the serosa and the mucosal or submucosal surfaces.   Diffusion into the muscle may mimic local endogenous release, but does not necessarily reflect the way in which drugs reach the tissue by diffusion from the blood circulation in vivo (Bennett, 1968).   Although studies on muscle strips generally reflect in vivo gastrointestinal motility (Bennett, 1968, 1974) this is not always so.   Thus morphine does not affect muscle strips of human or dog ileum, but stimulates small intestine motility in vivo or when perfused through the vasculature of dog isolated ileum (Daniel et al., 1959).   Although 5-hydroxytryptamine (5HT) bathing muscle strips or injected through the blood-perfused rat isolated ileum caused contraction, the contraction in the respective preparations was due to 5HT acting on receptors located on the smooth muscle or on the intrinsic neurones (Sakai et al., 1979a).   Similar differences in sites of drug action were also described for histamine and ATP in these two preparations of rat ileum (Sakai, 1979; Sakai et al., 1979b).

Some techniques for perfusing the vascular system of isolated gut have relied on blood from a donor animal which may be either anaesthetized (Daniel et al., 1959; Fisk et al., 1968; Sakai et al., 1979a,b) or conscious (Gill et al., 1981).   Other perfusates are (a) heparinized blood diluted with Ringer's solution (Salerno et al., 1966), (b) erythrocytes in artificial plasma containing albumin, dextran, dextrose and electrolytes without (Dubois et al. 1968) or with various added amino acids (Holst et al., 1981), or (c) Krebs solution containing dextran to minimise oedema (Weems & Seygal, 1981; Levine et al., 1982).   All these methods involve perfusion into an artery supplying the tissue, but only some experimenters collected the venous effluent.   If the effluent bathes the surface of the

preparation the injected drug may have another type of action.   In
addition, if closed-lumen gastrointestinal preparations are used
(discussed in the methods for measuring gastric and intestinal
motility), the drug may accumulate in the lumen.   Substances may
have different actions when added serosally or mucosally.

Gastric motility

Details of many of the older methods are described by Sanger &
Bennett (1982).   Generally in vitro methods for studying gastric
motility depend on a partial inflation of the stomach with bathing
solution.   Motility is then assessed by measuring intraluminal
pressure changes either at an approximately constant stomach volume
(Paton & Vane, 1963; Spedding, 1977; Cook, 1982) or by measuring
the expulsion of fluid through a cannula tied into (a) a hole cut
into the body wall (Paton & Vane, 1963), (b) into the pylorus and
extending into the antrum (Armitage & Dean, 1966; Campbell, 1966)
or (c) into the duodenum (Armitage & Dean, 1962, 1966, see later;
Van Nueten et al. 1978).   Fluid expelled into a closed system can
be measured with a pressure manometer or an ultrasonic transit time
device which relies on the Doppler principle (Van Nueten et al. 1978).
In some methods the stomach is divided surgically into "fundic",
"antral" and "pyloric" sections.   The cut opening is tied over a
cannula and the stomach section partially inflated with bathing
solution (Paton & Vane, 1963) or a flaccid, water-filled balloon
(Gerner et al. 1976).   Others have treated the stomach as if it were
a muscle strip, by fixing the fundus and suspending the pyloric
opening from a force transducer (Greeff & Holtz, 1956; Greeff et
al. 1962).

In the method of Armitage & Dean (1962, 1966), a rat stomach is
suspended in a tissue bath by two cannulae, one tied into a hole cut
in the fundus the other tied into the duodenum (Fig 1).   Pressure
in the body of the stomach is measured by a transducer connected
through the side arm of the fundic cannula, and pressure in the
antrum is measured by a fine cannula passed through the antral wall.
Intraluminal pressure can be increased by raising a fluid filled
Marriotte bottle connected to the fundic cannula, and the fuid propelled by the stomach through the pylorus is collected and measured.
Hukuhara & Neya (1966) used a similar "open" preparation of rat
stomach, but measured stomach motility via strain-gauge transducers
fixed to the greater curvature of the stomach.

Scheurer et al.(1983) measured intraluminal pressure changes
simultaneously in different areas of rat stomach and duodenum, using
an intraluminal pressure-sensor device consisting of a gastroduodenal acrylic cast with water-filled perfusion catheters connected
to pressur transducers.   The sensor device was passed into the
stomach through a 5mm incision which was then loosely sutured over

17

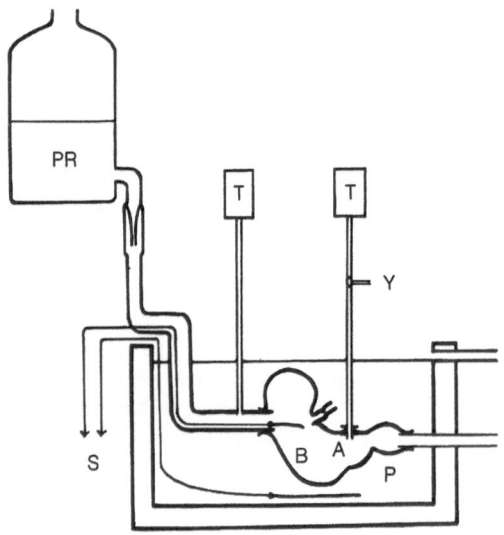

Fig. 1.   Apparatus for measuring rat gastric motility and propulsion.
The pylorus P, gastric antrum A and body B were cannulated.   Pressures
in the body and antrum were measured with the transducers T connected
to the respective cannulas via air-filled and saline-filled tubes.
Intragastric pressure was increased by raising the pressure resevoir
PR.   For gastric transmural stimulation, coaxial platinum wires were
connected to a stimulator S.   Slow injections of saline through a
3-way tap Y prevented blockage of the antral cannula by mucus produced
during stimulation.   (Adapted from Armitage & Dean, 1966).

a tube containing the perfusion catheters. The stomach was placed in an organ bath containing bathing solution which was allowed to pass between the sensor head and the mucosal surface of the stomach and duodenum. Despite the restrictions of muscle movement by the sensor device, pressure changes caused by cholecystokinin octapeptide added to the bathing solution were approximately comparable to the effects of cholecystokinin in isolated muscle strips.

Increased intraluminal pressure alone does not satisfactorily stimulate peristalsis in rat isolated stomach (Armitage & Dean, 1962, 1966; Paton & Vane, 1963), although it can produce irregular spontaneous activity (Hukuhara & Neya, 1966; Van Nueten & Janssen, 1978) and "receptive relaxation" (Paton & Vane, 1963; Schulze-Delrieu & Wall, 1982). Motility is therefore usually evoked by vagal or transmural electrical stimulation (Paton, 1955; see section on electrical stimulation) or pharmacologically.

One advantage of the "open" system of measuring gastric motility is that intraluminally added or naturally produced substances do not accumulate. This may also be important if drugs reach the lumen after injection into the arterial system, but without collection of the venous effluent. Another advantage is that drugs can easily be administered to either the serosal or mucosal surfaces of the stomach, where the effects may differ. For example, metoclopramide added to the serosal surface of rat stomach had no effect or caused inhibition of the electrically evoked motility, but intraluminal metoclopramide caused stimulation (G. J. Sanger, unpublished).

Intestinal peristalsis

Peristalsis is the co-ordinated movement of alimentary muscle, resulting in the propulsion of contents. The peristaltic reflex is evoked in vitro by a radial distension of the gut wall (Trendelburg, 1917; Kosterlitz & Robinson, 1959). Stimulation of sensory receptors in either the mucosal or submucosal layer (Bülbring et al, 1958; Ginzel, 1959; Diament et al. 1961; Frigo & Lecchini, 1970), activates intrinsic neurones mediating the reflex action (Bayliss & Starling, 1899; Kosterlitz et al. 1956). Since the most appropriate type of stimulus to elicit peristalsis may vary in different parts of the intestine, methods for evoking peristalsis in ileum and colon are described separately.

Ileum. Trendelburg (1917) first described a method for studying peristalsis in a segment of guinea-pig ileum tied distally to a tube connected to a reservoir and pressure transducer, and attached proximally to an isotonic recording system. Raising the reservoir to increase the intraluminal pressure elicits a peristaltic response, measured as longitudinal muscle contractions and increased intraluminal pressure (corresponding to the circular muscle contractions which begin proximally and move along the intestine).

Assessment of muscle activity changes in peristalsis are often made by eye. Quantitation of the number and amplitude of contractions (Bennett et al. 1968; Van Nueten et al. 1973; Sanger & Watt, 1978), are laborious and do not greatly improve on visual assessment. It is better to quantify peristalsis by measuring the amount of fluid propelled. Using techniques which also measure longitudinal and circular muscle activity (see Sanger & Bennett, 1982), propulsion can be assessed by collecting fluid expelled by the intestine (method of Bülbring et al. 1958 and its adaptation by Bennett et al. 1968 and Tonini et al. 1981), or by recording the movement of an air bubble in the tubing leading from the distal end of the ileum (Van Nueten et al. 1973).

"Open" systems (Bülbring et al. 1958; Bennett et al. 1968) have certain advantages over a "closed" system in which the intraluminal fluid is trapped (Trendelburg, 1917). These include the measurement of propelled fluid, lack of intraluminal accumulation, better mucosal oxygenation since the intraluminal fluid is continually renewed, ease of adding drugs intraluminally, and the ability to remove them from the lumen. Intraluminal injection is important for studying substances such as 5-hydroxytryptamine which increase peristaltic activity when in contact with the mucosal surface of guinea-pig ileum, but causes inhibition when added serosally (Bülbring & Lin, 1958). Furthermore, in a "closed" system the fluid cannot escape, so that the muscle contractions may generate greater intraluminal pressure, which in turn may affect muscle activity (Eley et al. 1977; Weems & Seygal, 1980; Sanger & Bennett, 1982). Eley et al., (1977) suggested that differences with "open" and "closed" peristaltic systems might affect the response of guinea-pig ileum to prostaglandins. In vivo there will be some resistance to propulsion of fluid, and the conditions will presumably be somewhere between those in "open" and "closed" systems. It may therefore be desirable to modify an "open" system to give distal resistance to propulsion.

In a different approach, Weems & Seygal (1981) evaluated the ability of segments of cat proximal duodenum, midjejunum and terminal ileum to propel fluid along the intestine in the absence of an artificial pressure applied proximally. The technique measures compressional work in an intestinal segment, connected at each end to separate Krebs solution reservoirs of constant capacitance and negligible input resistance. An intraluminal pressure of 5 and/or 10cm H_2O was established by injecting bathing solution into the intestine, causing spontaneous repetitive fluid propulsion in both oral and aboral directions, or just aborally. Under the same conditions, the duodenum and jejunum did not propel fluid.

Colon. Trendelenburg's method (1917), and adaptations of it, have been used to elicit and measure guinea-pig and rabbit colonic peristalsis (Lee, 1960; MacKenna & McKirdy, 1972; Eley et al. 1977;

Pescatori et al. 1980).   Results are generally satisfactory, but in
guinea-pig colon, co-ordinated muscle activity is often difficult
to obtain (K.G.Eley, personal communication), and intraluminal pressures necessary to evoke peristalsis may be 3 to 6 times greater than
in the small intestine (Weems & Szurszewski, 1977).

     Frigo & Lecchini (1970) concluded that in distal colon a solid
bolus is a more physiological stimulus than diffuse distension with
fluid.   They fixed guinea-pig or cat colon horizontally in a tissue
bath, pushed a thin rubber balloon proximally into the lumen, and
induced peristalsis by rapidly inflating the balloon with warm water.
This induced a reflex distal propulsion of the balloon, measured by
an isotonic transducer connected to the balloon through the proximal
end of the colon.   Some of the results with this method differed
from those of Lee (1960) who distended the whole colon with fluid.

     Ishizawa & Miyazaki (1973a, b, 1975) measured the propulsion of
a plastic ball through guinea-pig isolated colon, using a technique
similar to that of Frigo & Lecchini (1970).   Costa & Furness (1976)
monitored the speed of propulsion of faecal pellets already present
in segments of colon after the intestine was removed from the animal.
They also used dried pellets of faeces coated with thin layers of
epoxy resin.   The pellets were introduced into the proximal end of
the intestine and their progress monitored visually and photographi-
cally.   Tension changes in the circular muscle were recorded with
transducers attached to clips on small areas of the intestine;   the
tissue opposite each clip was fixed.   These procedures for measuring
tension changes did not appear to modify the propulsion of the
pellets.

Effects of distension

     Radial distension of the intact small intestine activates
stretch receptors, and initiates co-ordinated peristaltic activity
which depends largely on the propagation of intrinsic nerve activity
along the intestine.   To study the pathways involved in this reflex,
Costa & Furness (1976) distended one area of the intestine and
studied the mechanical response distally.   Segments of guinea-pig
colon or rectum 4-10cm long were fixed horizontally in a tissue bath
by an intraluminal stainless steel rod, and radial tension applied
as shown in Fig 2.   Circular muscle activity can be recorded at
various points either side of the stretched area by force transducers attached to small clips.   Distension of the colon caused
the circular muscle to contract proximally and relax distally;
both responses were blocked by tetrodotoxin, suggesting a dependence
on nerve activity.   Tonini et al.(1982) used a similar technique,
but they distended rabbit colon with a water-filled stationary intraluminal rubber balloon.

     Costa & Furness (1976) also studied the effects of stretch on

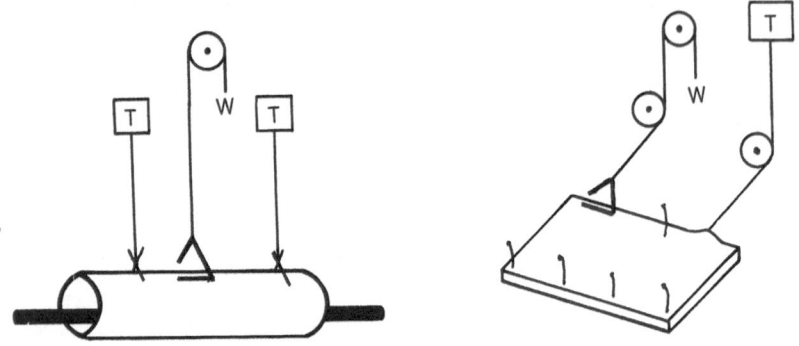

Fig. 2.   Arrangements for recording intestinal reflexes in response to distension.   The intestine on the left-hand side is fixed
by a horizontal bar passed through the lumen.   Increasing the load
W distends the intestine and initiates reflex nerve activity either
side of the area of distension.   Muscle activity is detected by
the transducers T.   In the right-hand arrangement, segments of
intestine were opened along the mesenteric border and pinned flat.
The transducer records circular muscle activity.   (Adapted from
Costa & Furness, 1976).

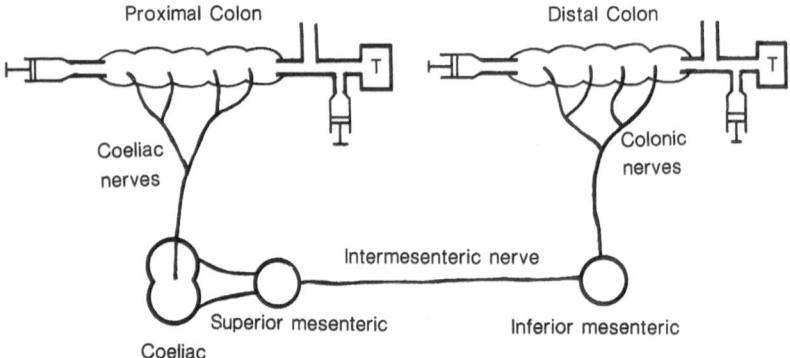

Fig. 3.   Preparation of guinea-pig colon connected to the prevertebral ganglia.   The circles represent the right and left coeliac ganglia (coeliac), the superior and the inferior mesenteric
ganglia.   Each ganglion is pinned to the floor of a tissue bath
for intracellular recording.   The colon is suspended in a separate
tissue bath.   Colonic motility is evoked and measured by a modification of the Trendelenburg (1917) technique.   (Adapted from
Kreulen & Szurszewski, 1979).

a flat preparation of colon, cut along the mesenteric border.   One
cut edge was fixed, and muscle stretch and recordings were made from
connections to the other cut edge (Fig 2).   With this arrangement,
different muscle layers of colon could be removed or severed during
the experiment, to determine the origins and pathways of the stretch-
induced reflex.

Kreulen & Szurszewski (1979) used a guinea-pig colon prevertebral ganglia preparation to study the colon-colonic inhibitory reflex
evoked by local intraluminal distension.   The colon and attached
prevertebral ganglia were placed in a 2-compartment tissue bath,
with the ganglia in one compartment and the colon in the other.
The interconnecting nerves were laid across the interconnecting wall
and kept moist with bathing solution, and the colon divided into a
proximal and a distal segment (respectively comprising about 60%
and 40% of the preparation) (Fig 3).   Intraluminal pressure was
controlled and measured by a modification of Trendelenburg's (1917)
method.   Catheters were tied into each end of the intestine, the
proximal one being connected to a 12ml syringe and the distal one to
a cylindrical reservoir and a 12ml syringe.   The pressure and volume
in each segment could therefore be altered by changing the amount of
bathing solution.   Distension of either segment of colon by intraluminal pressures of up to 10cm H_2O inhibited motility in the other
segment.   This reflex was abolished by sectioning the intermesenteric nerves which connect the proximal prevertebral ganglion to
the distal ganglion.

The response of an area at which distension is applied can also
be modified by intrinsic nerve activity.   Furness & Costa (1977)
and Davison & Pearson (1979) fixed whole segments of guinea-pig colon
(as described earlier; Costa & Furness, 1976; Fig 2) so that circular muscle activity could be measured at the point of stretch.
The colonic distension to the application of a series of weights
(4-24g) partially involved non-adrenergic, non-cholinergic inhibitory
nerves.   These nerves may mediate the relaxations of intestinal circular muscle around and distal to a distending bolus.

Muscle strips which are stretched can also show an increase in
tension, due at least partly to membrane depolarisation (Bülbring,
1955; Burnstock & Prosser, 1960; Gillespie, 1962).   However, certain preparations and types of stretch do not elicit a response
(Meiss, 1971).   Examples are that a quick stretch along the longitudinal axis does not elicit a response in guinea-pig ileum (Kosterlitz & Robinson, 1959), and that gastrin is released from human
isolated antrum (mucosa and attached muscle) by phasic but not tonic
distension (Strunz et al, 1980).   Methods for applying stretch to
strips of smooth muscle have been well reviewed by Kosterlitz & Watt
(1975) and Stephens (1975).

Electrical stimulation of autonomic nerves

A nerve bundle or plexus may contain various types of neurone, including fibres which are cholinergic, adrenergic, non-adrenergic, non-cholinergic (NANC) inhibitory (Burnstock, 1972; Furness & Costa, 1973), NANC excitatory (Ambache & Freeman, 1968; Bennett & Fleshler, 1969; Furness & Costa, 1973), serotoninergic (Gershon, 1982), and nerves which release peptides or other substances (Furness & Costa, 1982). The effect of autonomic nerve stimulation therefore depends on the types and relative importance of the neurones present, in addition to other factors such as the state of the muscle and its type of response and sensitivity to the substances which may be released. Distinction between the different types of nerve-induced responses may sometimes be achieved by using selective inhibitory drugs and/or by varying the stimulation parameters. In other cases there are no satisfactory antagonists (eg to many peptides, or to 5-hydroxytryptamine acting as a modulator of neurotransmitter release).

In general, muscle responses to activation of noradrenergic nerves are detected using frequencies of approximately 2 Hz or above (pulse duration 0.1-0.5ms), whereas lower frequencies may preferentially stimulate cholinergic nerves (Garry & Gillespie, 1955). Responses to NANC excitatory nerves were elicited in muscle strips from some areas of the human gastrointestinal tract at pulse frequencies below 1Hz (pulse duration 1ms), whereas contractions above this frequency may be due only to cholinergic nerve stimulation (Stockley & Bennett, 1974; Bennett & Stockley, 1975). Frequencies of 1-10 Hz caused inhibition of human taenia coli due to activation of NANC inhibitory neurones; higher frequencies caused relaxations due to stimulation of adrenergic neurones (see Stockley & Bennett, 1977 for references). In addition, an increased pulse width may reduce the adrenergic contribution to the overall inhibitory response (Stockley & Bennett, 1977). Houghton & Bennett (1977) found in studies using labelled noradrenaline that in human isolated colon an adrenergic-mediated response may be masked by the effects of the NANC nerves, since substantial amounts of label may be released at the frequencies which caused muscle relaxations apparently by NANC activation.

Bennett & Stockley (1975) also detected a fast after-contraction following inhibitory nerve stimulation in human gastrointestinal muscle strips. These contractions were due mainly to cholinergic nerve stimulation, and partly to a hyosine-resistant pathway. However, a slow after-contraction induced by NANC nerve activity occurred in ascending colonic circular muscle at stimulation frequencies of 8-32 Hz. Bennett & Fleshler (1969), and Furness & Costa (1973) reported similar slow after-contractions in guinea-pig colon. In the latter work these were detected at frequencies as low as 5 Hz and were maximal at 20-50 Hz, with pulse durations of 0.2-0.5 ms.

Some experiments question the physiological meaning of the contractions which occur following inhibitory nerve stimulation. In those by Andrews & Grundy (1981) with anaesthetized ferrets, electrical stimulation of the vagus activated intrinsic inhibitory neurones in the gastric corpus, followed by a contraction when the stimulus was stopped.   However, when the intrinsic inhibitory neurones were reflexly activated by rapid antral distension, there was no after-contraction.   If the same inhibitory neurones are activated similarly by both methods, the after-contractions may be due merely to the abrupt cessation of the electrical stimulus.

Gastrointestinal nerves.   The gut contains intrinsic nerve plexuses, and also receives extrinsic nerve fibres which mainly innervate the plexuses.   Techniques for stimulating intrinsic and extrinsic nerve fibres are now considered separately.

Intrinsic nerves.   In general, intrinsic nerves are electrically stimulated either by producing a voltage gradient across the gastrointestinal wall ("transmural stimulation") or by short-circuiting an electric current across two electrodes positioned in the bathing solution either side of a muscle strip ("field stimulation").

Paton (1955) first described the method of transmural stimulation for guinea-pig ileum and it has since been used mainly on intestinal tissues (see Paton, 1975b).   However, Armitage & Dean (1962, 1966) and Paton & Vane (1963) adapted the technique for use with whole stomach preparations.   Basically an intraluminal platinum electrode is insulated from the external bathing solution which contains a second platinum electrode, usually made the cathode.   Stimulation with a single rectangular pulse elicits a muscle contraction which, at a constant pulse duration (usually 0.2-1 ms), is dependent on voltage strength.   With pulses of 0.5 ms duration the threshold voltage for stimulation is approximately 1V, and about 5-25V are required for a maximum contraction (Paton, 1955).

There is considerable evidence that these parameters of transmural stimulation cause contraction of guinea-pig ileum by stimulating post-ganglionic cholinergic nerves (see Paton, 1975b).   However, particularly with frequencies of electrical stimulation at or above 2 Hz, other types of neurone can be stimulated and locally produced substances released (noradrenergic nerve terminals, and the release of prostaglandin-like material and enkephalins; see Sanger & Bennett, 1982).   Direct muscle stimulation may also occur with low pulse widths, since part of the contraction, particularly at higher frequencies, is resistant to tetrodotoxin (Bennett & Stockley, 1973, 1974).

Transmural stimulation can produce consistent twitch or tetanic muscle responses, and is widely used to study the ways in which drugs affect the contractions of guinea-pig ileum evoked by electrical stimulation of the cholinergic nerves.   The disadvantages of this method are that secreted products accumulate in the lumen, electrolysis may cause changes in pH (for this reason it is better to use pulses of alternating polarity, Bennett & Stockley 1973) and only changes in longitudinal muscle activity can be satisfactorily recorded (see Sanger & Bennett, 1982).

Field stimulation is used in muscle strips to study the responses to electrical stimulation of nerves.   Bennett & Stockley (1974) examined different electrode arrangements for selective stimulation of nerves.   The best was found to be electrodes fixed either side of the tissue, but insulated on entry to the bath;   electrodes above and below the tissue gave least selectivity for stimulation of the intrinsic nerves (ie most direct muscle stimulation).   Electrodes opposite only a part of the tissue may stimulate only a localised area, and cause a response which involves propagation of the induced stimulus (Burnstock et al. 1966).   This technique has been used to study rectoanal reflexes in the cat (Penninckx et al. 1982).

Since field stimulation involves passing current through a bathing solution of low resistance, the power requirements of the stimulator can be high.   The current may heat the solution (Sperelakis, 1962) and cause electrolysis or oxidise compounds such as noradrenaline (Wyse, 1977).   The use of bipolar pulses or alternate pulses of opposite polarity (Bennett & Stockley, 1973) largely circumvents the problems of electrolysis.   Stimulators may not be able to provide the high power required for field stimulation, and may give maximum output at a voltage below the maximum indicated by the stimulator dial.   Electrical output for field stimulation should therefore always be checked using an oscilloscope.

Extrinsic nerves.   Finkleman (1930) described a technique for stimulating the sympathetic nerve fibres running alongside the mesenteric blood vessels of rabbit isolated ileum.   Other in vitro techniques have been described for rat isolated stomach (Paton & Vane, 1963;   Armitage & Dean, 1966), longitudinal (taenia) or circular muscle of guinea-pig caecum (Akubue, 1966, 1977), rabbit rectum-pelvic nerve preparations (Garry & Gillespie, 1954, 1955) and rat anococcygeus muscle (Gillespie, 1972).   Weems & Szurszewski (1977) studied guinea-pig isolated colon, attached to the inferior mesenteric ganglion via the lumbar colonic nerves (see the section on muscle stretch).   They recorded the nervous input into the ganglion following intraluminal distension of the colon and the resultant peristaltic activity.   Colonic motility was inhibited by electrical stimulation of preganglionic nerves, (the inferior splanchnic nerve from the central nervous system, and the colonic intermesenteric and hypogastric nerves from the abdominal viscera). Krier & Szurszewski (1982) later used the preparation to examine the effects of adding substance P to the solution bathing either the colon or the mesenteric ganglion.

REFERENCES

Akubue, P.I., 1966, A periarterial nerve - circular muscle preparation from the caecum of the guinea-pig, J Pharm. Pharmacol., 18:390.

Akubue, P.I., 1977, A periarterial nerve - longitudinal muscle (taenia) preparation from the guinea-pig caecum, J. Pharm. Pharmacol., 29:122.

Ambache, N., 1946, Interaction of drugs and the effect of cooling on the isolated mammalian tissue, J. Physiol., 104:266.

Ambache, N., 1954, Separation of the longitudinal muscle of the rabbits ileum as a broad sheet, J. Physiol., 125:53P.

Ambache, N., and Freeman, M.A., 1968, Atropine-resistant longitudinal muscle spasm due to excitation of non-cholinergic neurones in Auerbach's plexus, J. Physiol., 199:705.

Andrews, P.L.R., and Grundy, D., 1981, The effect of stimulus characteristics on the rebound contraction in the gastric corpus, J. Physiol., 313:24P.

Angel, F., Go. V.L.W., Schmalz, P.F., and Szurszewski, J.H., 1983, Vasoactive intestinal polypeptide: A putative neurotransmitter in the canine gastric muscularis mucosa, J. Physiol., 341:641.

Armitage, A.K., and Dean, A.C.B., 1962, A new technique for studying gastric peristalsis in small animals, World Med. Electron., 1:17.

Armitage, A.K., and Dean, A.C.B., 1966, The effects of pressure and pharmacologically active substances on gastric peristalsis in transmurally stimulated rat stomach-duodenum preparation, J.Physiol., 182:42.

Bayliss, W.B., and Starling, E.H., 1899, The movements and innervation of the small intestine, J. Physiol., 24:99.

Bennett, A., 1968, Relationship between in vitro studies of gastrointestinal muscle and motility of the alimentary tract in vivo, Am. J. Dig. Dis., 13:410.

Bennett, A., 1973, The pharmacology of isolated gastrointestinal muscle, in: "Encyclopedia of pharmacology, Vol 39A", P. Holton, ed., Pergamon, Oxford, New York.

Bennett, A., 1974, Relation between gut motility and innervation in man, Digestion, 11:392.

Bennett, A., Eley, K.G., and Scholes, G.B., 1968, Effect of prostaglandins E, and E$_2$ on intestinal motility in the guinea-pig and rat. Br J Pharmacol., 34:639.

Bennett, A., and Fleshler, B., 1969, A hyoscine-resistant excitatory nerve pathway in guinea-pig colon, J Physiol., 203:62P.

Bennett, A., and Fleshler, B., 1970, Prostaglandins and the gastrointestinal tract, Gastroenterol., 59:790.

Bennett, A., and Stockley, H.L., 1973, Electrically-induced contractions of guinea-pig isolated ileum resistant to tetrodotoxin,
Br. J. Pharmacol., 48:357P.

Bennett, A., and Stockley, H.L., 1974, Effect of electrode positions
on contractions of guinea-pig isolated ileum to electrical stimulation, Br. J. Pharmac., 50:453P.

Bennett, A., and Stockley, H.L., 1975, The intrinsic innervation of
the human alimentary tract and its relation to function, Gut,
16:443.

Bennett, A., and Whitney, B., 1966, A pharmacological investigation
of the human isolated stomach, Br. J. Pharmacol. Chemother.,
27:286.

Bortoff, A., 1976, Myogenic control of intestinal motility, Physiol.,
Rev., 56:418.

Bucknell, A., 1966, Studies on the physiology and pharmacology of
the colon of man and other animals, PhD thesis, University of
London, U.K.

Bülbring, E., 1955, Correlation between membrane potential spike
discharge and tension in smooth muscle, J. Physiol., 128:200

Bülbring, E., Crema, A., and Saxby, O.B. 1958, A method for recording
peristalsis in isolated intestine, Br. J. Pharmac. Chemother.,
13:440.

Bülbring, E., and Lin, R.C.Y., 1958, The effects of luminal application of 5-hydroxytryptamine and 5-hydroxytryptophan on peristalsis: The local production of 5-HT and its release in relation to intraluminal pressure and propulsive activity, J. Physiol.,
140:381.

Burnstock, G., 1972, Purinergic nerves, Pharmacol. Rev., 24:509.

Burnstock, G., Campbell, G., and Rand, M.T., 1966, The inhibitory
innervation of the taenia of the guinea-pig caecum, J. Physiol.,
182:504.

Burnstock, G., and Prosser, C.L., 1960, Responses of smooth muscle
to quick stretch: relation of stretch to conduction, Am. J.
Physiol., 198:921.

Campbell, G., 1966, The inhibitory nerve fibres in the vagal supply
to the guinea-pig stomach, J. Physiol., 185:600.

Cook, M.A., 1982, Pharmacological analysis of non-adrenergic inhibitory responses of the guinea-pig stomach in vitro, in: "Motility
of the digestive tract", M. Wienbeck, ed., Raven Press, New York.

Costa, M., and Furness, J.B., 1976, The peristaltic reflex: An
analysis of the nerve pathways and their pharmacology, Naunyn-
Schmiedeberg's Arch. Pharmacol., 294:47.

Daniel, E.E., Sutherland, W.H., and Bogoch, A., 1959, Effects of
morphine and other drugs on motility of the terminal ileum,
Gastroenterol., 36;510.

Davison, J.S., and Pearson, G.J., 1979, The role of intrinsic non-
adrenergic non-cholinergic inhibitory nerves in the regulation
of distensibility of the guinea-pig colon, Pflugers Arch., 381:75.

Diament, M.L., Kosterlitz, H.W., and McKenzie, J., 1961, Role of the mucous membrane in the peristaltic reflex in the isolated ileum of the guinea-pig, Nature, 190: 1205.

Dubois, R.S., Vaughan, G.D., and Roy, C.C., 1968, Isolated rat small intestine with intact circulation, in: "Organ perfusion and pre-servation", J.C. Norman, ed., Appleton-Century Crofts, New York.

Eley, K.G., Bennett, A., and Stockley, H.L., 1977, The effect of prostaglandins E_1, E_2, $F_{1\alpha}$ and $F_{2\alpha}$ on guinea-pig ileal and colonic peristalsis, J. Pharm. Pharmacol., 29: 276.

Finkleman, B., 1930, On the nature of inhibition of the intestine, J Physiol., 70: 185.

Fisk, R.L., Browlee, R.T., Brown, D.R., McFarlane, D.F., Budney, D., Dritsas, K.G., Kowalewski, K., and Couves, C.M., 1968, Perfusion of isolated organs for prolonged functional preservation, in: "Organ perfusion and preservation", J.C. Norman, ed., Appleton-Century Crofts, New York.

Frigo, G.M., and Lecchini, S., 1970, An improved method for studying the peristaltic reflex in the isolated colon, Br. J. Pharmac., 39: 346.

Furchgott, R.F., 1968, A critical appraisal of the use of isolated organ systems for the assessment of drug action at the receptor level, in: "Importance of fundamental principles in drug evaluation", D.M. Ledeschi and R.R. Tedeschi, ed., Raven Press

Furness, J.B., and Costa, M., 1973, The nervous release and the action of substances which affect intestinal muscle through neither adrenoceptors nor cholinoreceptors, Philos. Trans. R. Soc. Lond. (Biol)., 265: 123.

Furness, J.B., and Costa, M., 1977, The participation of enteric in-hibitory nerves in accommodation of the intestine to distention, Clin. Exp. Pharmacol. Physiol. 4: 37.

Furness, J.B., and Costa, M., 1982, Identification of gastrointesti-nal neurotransmitters, in: "Handb. Exp. Pharmacol, 59, Mediators and drugs in gastrointestinal motility I", G Bertaccini, ed. Springer-Verlag, Berlin, Heidelberg, New York.

Garry, R.C., and Gillespie, T.S, 1954, An in vitro preparation of the distal colon of the rabbit with orthosympathetic and parasympa-thetic innervation, J. Physiol. 123: 60P.

Garry, R.C., and Gillespie, J.S., 1955, The response of the muscula-ture of the colon of the rabbit to nerve stimulation in vitro of the parasympathetic and sympathetic outflows. J. Physiol. 128: 557.

Gerner, T., Maehlumshagen, P., and Haffner, J.F., 1976, Pressure-responses to cholecystokinin in the fundus and antrum of isolated guinea-pig stomachs, Scand. J. Gastroénterol., 11: 823.

Gershon, M.D., 1982, Serotonergic neurotransmission in the gut, Scand. J. Gastroenterol., 17 (Suppl 71): 27.

Gill, R., Knight, M., Pilot, M-A., and Thomas, P.A., 1981, Cross-perfusion of an isolated canine stomach using a conscious donor dog; a model for the study of the hormonal control of gastric motility, J Physiol., 313: 9P.

Gillespie, J.S., 1962, Spontaneous mechanical and electrical activity of stretched and unstretched intestinal smooth muscle cells and their response to sympathetic-nerve stimulation, J Physiol, 162: 54.

Gillespie, J.S., 1972, The rat anococcygeus muscle and its response to nerve stimulation and some drugs, Br J Pharmac, 45: 404.

Ginzel, K.H., 1959, Are mucosal nerve fibres essential for the peristaltic reflex? Nature, 184: 1235.

Greeff, K., and Holtz, P., 1956, Untersuchuhgen am isolierten Vagus-Magenpraparat, Arch exp Path Pharmakol, 227: 427.

Greeff, K., Kasperat, H., and Osswald, W., 1962, Paradoxe wirkungen der Elektrischen Vagusreizung am isolierten Magen-und Hersvorhofpraparat des Meerschweinchens Sowie deren Beeinflussung durch Ganglien-blocker, Sympatholytica, Reserpin und Cocain, Arch exp Path Pharmakol, 243: 528.

Harry, J., 1963, The action of drugs on the circular muscle strip from the guinea-pig isolated ileum, Br J Pharmac Chemother, 20: 399.

Hayashi, E., Maeda, T., and Shinozuka, K., 1982, Sites of actions of adenosine in intrinsic cholinergic nerves of ileal longitudinal muscle from guinea-pig, Eur J Pharmac, 84: 99.

Holst, J.J., Lauritsen, K., Jensen, S.L., Nielsen, O.V., and Schaffalitzky de Muckadell, O.B., 1981, Secretin release from the isolated, vascularly perfused pig duodenum, J Physiol, 318: 327.

Houghton, J., and Bennett, A., 1977, Release of (^{3}H) noradrenaline by electrical stimulation of human isolated taenia coli, in: "Gastrointestinal motility in health and disease, Proc 6th Int Sym Gastrointestinal Motility", MTP Press, Lancaster.

Hukuhara, T., and Neya, T., 1966, On the rat gastric motility, Jap J Physiol, 16: 497.

Innes, I.R., Kosterlitz, H.W., and Robinson, J.A., 1957, The effects of lowering the bath temperature on the responses of the isolated guinea-pig ileum, J Physiol, 137: 396.

Ishizawa, M., and Miyazaki, E., 1973a, Action of prostaglandins on gastrointestinal motility, Sapporo Med J, 42: 366.

Ishizawa, M., and Miyazaki, E., 1973b, Effect of prostaglandins on the movement of guinea-pig isolated intestine, Jpn J Smooth Muscle Res, 9: 235.

Ishizawa, M., and Miyazaki, E., 1975, Effect of prostaglandin $F_{2\alpha}$ on propulsive activity of the isolated segmental colon of the guinea-pig, Prostaglandins, 10: 759.

Kosterlitz, H.W., and Robinson, J.A., 1959, Reflex contractions of the longitduinal muscle coat of the isolated guinea-pig ileum, J Physiol, 146: 369.

Kosterlitz, H.W., and Watt, A.J., 1975, Stimulation by stretch in: "Methods in pharmacology, Vol 3", E.E. Daniel and D.M. Paton, ed., Plenum Press, New York.

Kosterlitz, H.W., Pirie, V.W., and Robinson, J.A., 1956, The mechanism of the peristaltic reflex in the isolated guinea-pig ileum. J. Physiol., 133: 681.

Krier, J., and Szurszewski, J.H., 1982, Effect of substance P on colonic mechanoreceptors, motility and sympathetic neurones, Am. J. Physiol., 243: G259.

Kreulen, D.L., and Szurszewski, J.H., 1979, Reflex pathways in the abdominal prevertebal ganglia: Evidence for a colon-colonic inhibitory reflex, J. Physiol., 295: 21.

Lee, C.Y., 1960, The effect of stimulation of extrinsic nerves on peristalsis and on the release of 5-hydroxytryptamine in the large intestine of the guinea-pig and of the rabbit, J Physiol., 152: 405.

Levine, D.F., Burleigh, D.E. and Motson, R., 1982, A method for studying the actions of drugs on vascularly perfused segments of human colon, Scand. J. Gastroenterol., 17 (Suppl 71): 163.

Lipshutz, W., and Chohen, S., 1971, Physiological determinants of lower esophageal sphincter function, Gastroenterol., 61: 16.

Lum, B.K.B., Kermani, M.H., and Heilman, R.D., 1966, Intestinal relaxation produced by sympathomimetic amines in the isolated rabbit jejunum: Selective inhibition by adrenergic blocking agents and by cold storage, J. Pharmacol. Exp Ther., 154: 463.

MacKenna, B.R., and McKirdy, H.C., 1972, Peristalsis in the rabbit distal colon, J. Physiol., 220: 33.

Meiss, R.A., 1971, Some mechanical properties of cat intestinal muscle, Am. J. Physiol., 220:2000.

Miyazaki, H., Ohga, A., and Saito, K., 1982, Development of motor response to intramural nerve stimulation and to drugs in rat small intestine, Br. J. Pharmac., 76: 531.

Ozaki, T., 1979, Effects of stimulation of Auerbach's plexus on both longitudinal and circular muscles, Jpn. J. Physiol., 29: 195.

Paton, W.D.M., 1955, The response of the guinea-pig ileum to electrical stimulation by coaxial electrodes, J. Physiol., 127: 40P.

Paton, W.D.M., 1975a, The recording of mechanical responses of smooth muscle, in: "Methods in pharmacology, Vol 3", E.E. Daniel and D.M. Paton, ed., Plenum Press, New York.

Paton, W.D.M., 1975b, Transmural and field stimulation of nerve-smooth muscle preparations, in: "Methods in pharmacology, Vol 3", E.E. Daniel and D.M. Paton, ed., Plenum Press, New York.

Paton, W.D.M., and Vane, J.R., 1963, An analysis of the responses of the isolated stomach to electrical stimulation and to drugs, J. Physiol., 165: 10.

Penninckx, F.M., Mebis, J.H., and Kerremans, R.P., 1982, The recto-anal reflex in cats analysed in vitro, Scand. J. Gastroenterol., 17 (Suppl 71): 147.

Pescatori, M., Marsicano, B., Mancinelli, R., Salinari, S., and Bertuzzi, A., 1980, Control of peristalsis in the isolated rabbit colon, in: "Gastrointestinal motility", J. Christensen, ed., Raven Press, New York.

Sakai, K., 1979, A pharmacological analysis of the contractile action of histamine upon the ileal region of the isolated blood-perfused small intestine of the rat, Br J Pharmacol, 67: 587.

Sakai, K., Akima, M., and Shiraki, Y., 1979a, Comparative studies
with 5-hydroxytryptamine and its derivatives in isolated blood
perfused small intestine and ileum of the rat, Jpn. J. Pharmacol.
29: 223.

Sakai, K., Akima, M., and Matsushita, H., 1979b, Analysis of the
contractile responses of the ileal segment of the isolated
blood-perfused small intestine of rats to adenosine triphosphate and related compounds, Eur. J. Pharmac., 58: 157.

Salerno, R.A., Iijima, K., and Healey, W.V., 1966, Extra-corporeal
circulation of excised sigmoid colon segments, Surg. Gynecol.
Obstet., 122: 767.

Sanger, G.J., and Bennett, A., 1982, In vitro techniques for the
study of gastrointestinal motility, in: "Handb. Exp. Pharmacol.,
59, Mediators and drugs in gastrointestinal motility, I", G.
Bertaccini, ed., Springer-Verlag, Berlin, Heidelberg, New York.

Sanger, G.J., and Watt, A.J., 1978, The effect of PGE, on peristalsis and on perivascular nerve inhibition of peristaltic activity in guinea-pig isolated ileum, J. Pharm. Pharmacol., 30: 762.

Scheurer, U., Varga, L., Drack, E., Burki, H-R., and Halter, F.,
1983, Measurement of cholecystokinin octapeptide-induced motility of rat antrum, pylorus and duodenum in vitro, Am. J.
Physiol., 244: G261.

Schulze-Delrieu, K., and Lepsien, G., 1982, Depression of mechanical
and electrical activity in muscle strips of opossum stomach and
esophagus by acidosis, Gastroenterol., 82: 720.

Schulze-Delrieu, K., and Wall, J.P., 1982, Gastric tone, Dig. Dis.
Sci., 27: 665.

Spedding, M., 1977, A modified guinea-pig stomach preparation,
Br.J. Pharmac., 61: 155P.

Sperelakis, N., 1962, Contraction of depolarised smooth muscle by
electric fields, Am. J. Physiol., 202: 731.

Stephens, N.J., 1975, Physical properties of contractile systems,
in: "Methods in pharmacology, Vol 3", E.E. Daniel and D.M.
Paton, ed., Plenum Press, New York.

Stockley, H.L., and Bennett, A., 1974, The intrinsic innervation of
human sigmoid colonic muscle, in: "Proc. 4th Int. Sym. Gastrointestinal motility", E.E. Daniel, ed., Mitchell, Vancouver.

Stockley, H.L., and Bennett, A., 1977, Relaxations mediated by
adrenergic and nonadrenergic nerves in human isolated taenia
coli, J. Pharm. Pharmacol., 29: 533.

Strunz, U.T., Neeb, S., Lux, G., and Domschke, W., 1980, Does antral
motility stimulate gastrin release? An in vitro study, in:
"Gastrointestinal motility", J. Christensen, ed., Raven Press,
New York.

Trendelenburg, P., 1917, Physiologische und pharmakologische
Versuche uber die Dunndarmperistaltik, Naunyn-Schmiedeberg's
Arch. Exp. Pathol. Pharmakol., 81: 55.

Tonini, M., Frigo, G., Lecchini, S., D'Angelo, L., and Crema, A.,
1981, Hyoscine-resistant peristalsis in guinea-pig ileum,

Eur. J. Pharmac., 71: 375.

Tonini, M., Onori, L., Lecchini, S., Frigo, G., Perucca, E., and Crema, A., 1982, Mode of action of ATP on propulsive activity in rabbit colon, Eur. J. Pharmac., 82: 21.

Van Nueten, J.M., Ennis, C., Helsen, L., Laduron, P.M., and Janssen, P.A.J., 1978, Inhibition of dopamine receptors in the stomach: An explanation of the gastrokinetic properties of domperidone, Life Sci., 23: 453.

Van Nueten, J.M., Geivers, H., Fontaine, J., and Janssen, P.A.J., 1973, An improved method for studying peristalsis in the isolated guinea-pig ileum, Arch. Int. Pharmacodyn. Ther., 203: 411.

Van Nueten, J.M., and Janssen, P.A.J., 1978, Is dopamine an endogenous inhibitor of gastric emptying? in: "Proc 6th Int.Sym. Gastrointestinal motility", H.L. Duthie, ed., MTP, Lancaster.

Walder, D.N., 1953, The muscularis mucosae of the human stomach, J Physiol., 120: 365.

Weems, W.A., and Seygal, G.E., 1980, Intestinal propulsion: Studies employing a method for its quantitative evaluation, in: "Gastrointestinal motility", J. Christensen, ed., Raven Press, New York.

Weems, W.A., and Seygal, G.E., 1981, Fluid propulsion by cat intestinal segments under conditions requiring hydrostatic work, Am. J. Physiol., 240: G147.

Weems, W.A., and Szurszewski, J.H., 1977, Modulation of colonic motility by peripheral neural inputs to neurons of the inferior mesenteric ganglion, Gastroenterol., 73: 273.

Wyse, D.G., 1977, Alteration of exogenous noradrenaline caused by electrical "field" stimulation and its role in post-stimulant relaxation, Can. J. Physiol. Pharmacol., 55: 990.

MOTILITY: METHODS FOR <u>IN VIVO</u> MEASUREMENTS

Paul Bass and Deborah A. Fox

School of Pharmacy
Center for Health Sciences
University of Wisconsin-Madison
Madison, Wisconsin

INTRODUCTION

The absorption from, and transport down the gastrointestinal tract is an important, integrated function. It is accomplished in spite of the heterogeneous motor functions of various portions of the tract; every region within the tract is unique in its relationship to lumenal content. For example, the esophagus is essentially a transport organ, carrying a bolus in a caudad fashion through the closed chest cavity into the stomach in approximately 9.5 sec. The stomach is really two organs: a "hopper" or body and a "grinder" or antrum. Both storage, reduction of particle size and approach to isoosmolarity of content occur in this organ. The prime function of the small intestine is absorption of nutrients. The integration of nutrient absorption and caudad propagation of non-absorbable material defies explanation. We do not have a clear idea or even a working hypothesis for the systematic mechanisms of such a multiple meter-length of tubing. The colon, permits us to be civilized. Again, final absorption of water and electrolytes (a spin-drying effect), as well as higher nervous system control, permit us to empty the colon at our convenience. The above general activities of the various areas of the gastrointestinal tract have been known for years.

Modern recording devices have permitted us to quantify and predict some of the integrative functions of the various organs which make up the gastrointestinal tract. Several groups have begun to evaluate the role and relationships of consecutive contractile wave forms. Engstrom et al.,(1979) demonstrated that all contractions are not propagated down the duodenum. A serious, systematic approach is being made by Macagno and Christiansen at the University of Iowa (1980,1982). Their modeling of intestinal contractions, based on principals developed in fluid mechanics, should lead to new insights into the role of individual wall movement in absorption and transport. At the present time, such studies are in their infancy. The current ideas concerning integration of contractions with fluid movement have been reviewed (Weems, 1982).

The present review shall relate the methods of recording contractions to the functions of the GI tract which are presently known. As seen with a propagative peristaltic wave of the esophagus, the bolus is "swept" through the organ. In contrast, dysrhythmic, simultaneous "giant" contractions, characteristic of esophageal spasm, retard bolus passage. In the area of pharmacology, morphine can retard transport by stimulating rhythmic segmentation; atropine can also alter transport by total relaxation of the bowel. Thus, physiological patterns and pharmacological responses do not always reveal the function of individual contractions or contractile patterns in various portions of the bowel. This has been reviewed by Bass, 1971; Bass and Weisbrodt, 1971; Corazziari, 1982; and Bass and Russell, 1983.

HISTORICAL

The earliest data on gut motility was derived from direct observations, x-ray or large recording balloons placed in the lumen. The opening of an animal's abdomen in a saline bath and observing the writhing movements of the gut in response to castor oil, narcotics, or cotton swabs, led Bayliss and Starling to formulate the law of the intestine. Radiographic methods yielded extensive qualitative information. However, the contrast luminal material utilized in radiography, covers only the mucosal layer of the gut. Therefore, movement of the material may be due to several integrated muscle areas: the villi, submucosal muscle, as well as the circular and longitudinal outer muscle layers. Thus, detailed relationships of the various muscles to luminal content are speculative. In addition, quantification of this system is not with normal nutrient but with artificial contrast media of high specific gravity. However, the addition of image intensifiers associated with cineflurography has advanced our knowledge of integrated wave forms and luminal flow.

Large balloons filled with air or water have essentially been abandoned. Such units cover large areas within the intestine and integrate several areas of activity. The resulting output is a markedly dampened signal. Data are further confounded by the elastic properties of the balloon, obstructive nature and possible stimulation of the gut. Exceptions to the use of large balloons may be the recording of pressure-volume relationships of certain select areas. The "tonal" changes of the body of the stomach may be observed using a large balloon system that fills the entire cavity. Similar studies may be made on the colon and rectal ampulla.

INTRALUMINAL PRESSURE RECORDINGS: SMALL BALLOONS, OPEN-TIP CATHETERS, PRESSURE RECORDING PROBES AND RADIOTELEMETERING CAPSULES

Measurement of intraluminal pressure with small balloons or open-tip catheters requires an external strain gage force transducer coupled with the respective luminal devices. This permits the transduction of mechanical pressure to high fidelity electric systems, permitting the recording of true pressure signals.

A small balloon, for example, 7 x 10 mm, mitigates most of the disadvantages of a large balloon described previously. Small balloons are still popular in the colon, where material may obstruct open catheters, and other larger cavities such as the orad antrum of the stomach. Balloons are also desirable for characterizing junctional zones and sphincters. For example, two small balloons placed in the anal canal may demonstrate reflex contraction and simultaneous relaxation of the external and internal sphincters, respectively, to intrarectal pressures (Schuster et al., 1963).

The perfused open-tip catheter is popular for recording intraluminal pressures from various portions of the gut, especially the body and lower sphincter of the esophagus. The perfusion unit was developed by Harris and Pope (1964) and its physical properties characterized by the group of workers in Milwaukee (Dodds, 1976; Arndorfer et al., 1977; Stef et al., 1977). The early work with catheters was performed with air and static water filled systems. The latter tend to compress or leak, leaving a tube with variable compressibility and inaccurate sensing of the intraluminal pressures. Catheters perfused with a continuous flow of distilled water transmit intraluminal pressure when recording from the open lumen of closed segments, or wall occluding forces when squeezed by a narrow lumen or sphincter area. Rates of fluid infusion, tube or orafice size, system compliance, elasticity and thickness of catheters may alter system fidelity. Experimentation has led to a certain amount of standardization in this area.

It should be emphasized that either balloon or open-tip catheters will not record pressures if "compartments" are open at one end permitting the pressure to dissipate. Such units "see" no pressure in the body of the stomach. They also tend to underread antral and gastroduodenal junction pressures because of the lack of adequate segmental closure. The pressure is recorded by open-tip units as long as the orafice is in the high pressure zone. This can be a problem in a narrow area like the lower esophageal sphincter in man. This problem was resolved by John Dent who developed a catheter "sleeve" that would sense the continuous pressure as the sphincter moved up or down (Dent, 1976). Such a unit has permitted 24 hr recording of the sphincter. The sleeve consists of 5-6 cm long, thin sheets of silicone located at the

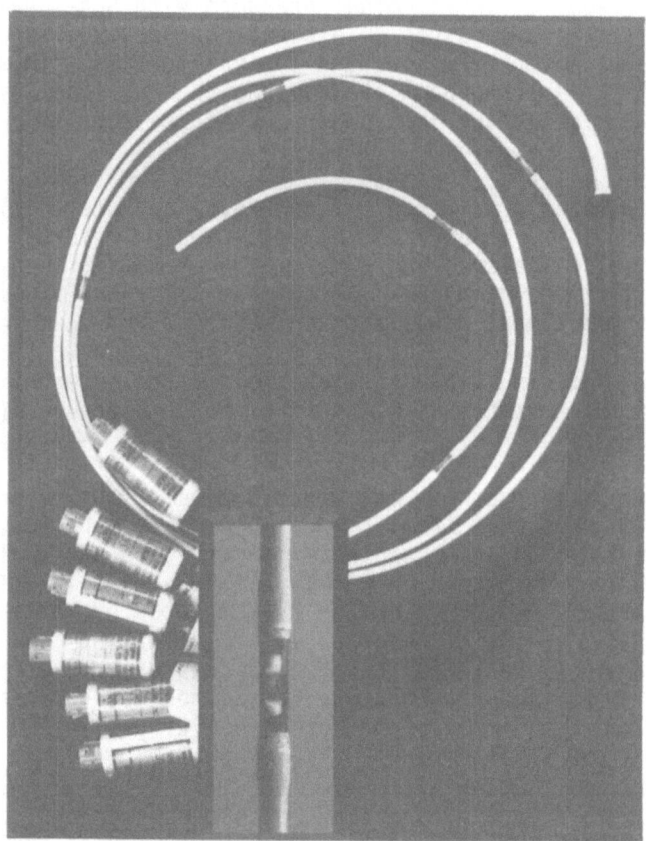

Figure 1. Pressure recording probe with six microforce transducers 10 cm apart. The probe is 2.67 mm in outside diameter. Inset shows a magnification of a single transducer which is a Millar MT-10, an ultraminiature silicon strain gage. This unit is manufactured by Millar Instruments, Inc., Houston, Texas (courtesy of J. R. Mathias, University of Florida, Gainesville).

terminal end of the catheter. Water is infused at a constant rate at the sealed proximal end of the sleeve and flows into the catheter lumen from the open distal end.

A direct sensing unit for recording pressure, described by Sninsky et al., 1982, is available which may replace the perfusion type of catheter. This unit is less bulky, requires no perfusion fluid and has a high fidelity response. However, it is clearly more costly and may not have the durability of a perfusion system. Technically, the pressure recording probe consists of six micro-pressure transducers enclosed in a flexible tube for intranasal passage into the gastrointestinal tract (see Figure 1). Each pressure transducer is connected to a pressure transducer control unit which represents a passive interface between the pressure sensor and the physiologic recorder. Recently, Sninsky et al., have utilized this pressure recording probe in the diagnosis and treatment of patients with chronic, unexplained abdominal pain, nausea and vomiting.

A final method of intraluminal recording is the radiotele-metering capsule. Such a unit transmits a radio signal at a frequency modulated by changes in intraluminal pressures. It has the advantage of being devoid of outside attachments, which confine the subject to a recording machine. The disadvantages of these units are that they lack permanent location in the GI tract, and their specific locus cannnot be identified. These problems can be overcome by tethering the unit for a period of time to a portion of the tract. Foster et al., (1983) have linked two radiotelemetry capsules with various lengths of string, and have been able to simultaneously assess phases of the migrating motor complex (mmc) in both the gastric antrum and jejunum. This group has been able to detect differences in the MMC in patients with various disease states.

For clinical trials, intraluminal devices appear to be the instruments of choice in monitoring GI activity. This is likely to continue in the future.

SEROSAL RECORDINGS: ELECTRODES, TRANSDUCERS AND OPAQUE MARKERS

GI muscle contractile activity can be assessed by recording either electrical or mechanical activity with serosal implants. The chronic recording of both of these activities from the serosal surface of the bowel of unanesthetized animals was developed by myself and my associates. These techniques will be discussed below.

Several types of electric signals are generated from the gas-trointestinal tract. They are: 1) transmucosal potentials - which

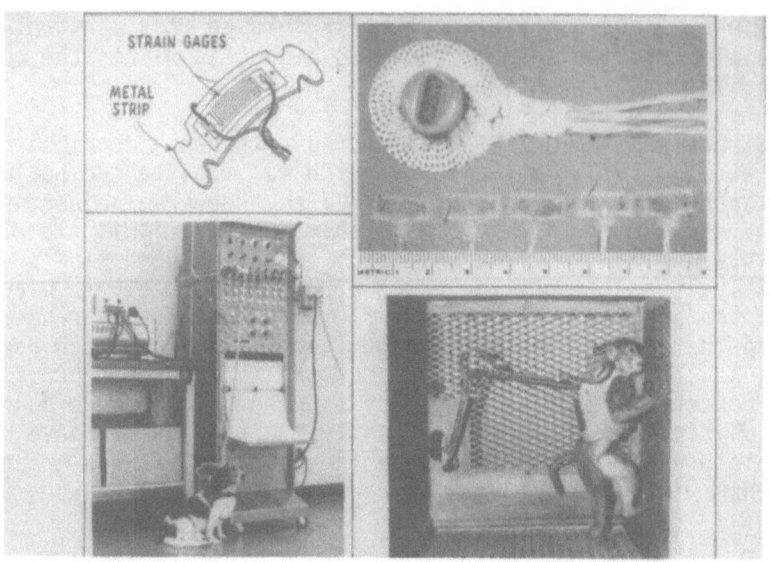

Figure 2. Techniques of recording gastrointestinal motility with extraluminal strain gage force transducer. Upper left - schematic of strain gage bonded to clip and wired, upper right - encapsulatd strain gages connected to encapsulated electrical conductor, lower left - unanesthetized dog and recorder in recording situation, lower right - unanesthetized monkey in recording situation (adapted from Bass and Weisbrodt, 1971).

are voltage changes across the mucosa due to secretory function; 2) transmembrane potentials - voltage changes across the membrane of a single muscle cell, which can be recorded from microelectrodes in vitro. This same type of signal can be obtained from many cells by using the sucrose gap technique. 3) Surface (extracellular) potentials - voltage changes recorded with electrodes placed on the surface of tissue or in the extracellular fluid of the organ or both. These recordings register the mean of potentials generated by the organ. The electrocardiogram, electroencephalogram, and in the gut, the electrogastrogram and electroenterogram are examples of the type of signals which can be recorded with surface electrodes.

Two types of surface potentials have been recorded from the muscle of the gastrointestinal tract in several species. One type, the basic electric rhythm (BER) or "slow wave", is an omnipresent, cyclic potential. The other type of electric activity, spike potentials, may occur as single or multiple rapid oscillations (Figure 7). Since extracellular electrodes register the mean potential generated by many cells, this type of recording cannot be used to explain membrane phenomena of single cells. The technique of monitoring electric activity has the advantage of recording from a localized area. This area is defined by the diameter of the electrode tip which can be as small as a few millimeters or less. Thus the method is particularly useful for exploring junctional zones, for example, the gastroduodenal junction, as well as the entire organ system. The technique of construction and chronic electric recording has been described (McCoy and Bass, 1963). Also, the information obtained by recording the electrical activity has been reviewed (Bass, 1968). These electrical signals generated from the smooth muscle of the GI tract are useful in developing concepts of motor function, and can compliment data obtained from manometry, radiology and other methods.

The extraluminal strain gage force transducers were developed to record muscle activity from various hollow organs. They have been useful on various portions of the gut (Jacoby et al., 1963; Reinke et al., 1967; Anderson et al., 1968), gallbladder (Ludwick and Bass, 1967), and uterus (Bass and Callantine, 1964). These transducers have also been applicable for both acute experiments or studies in the chronic unanesthetized animal. The construction and uniqueness of the units have been described (Bass and Weisbrodt, 1971 and Bass and Wiley, 1972). Briefly, each unit consists of two foil strain gages, bonded back-to-back. The electrical wiring is attached so that two arms of a wheatstone bridge are contained within the unit. The units are then waterproofed and encapsulated in silicone rubber. Several of these units can be connected to an encapsulated electrical connector and the entire unit sterilized for implantation. During surgery, the units are sewn on the serosal surface of the gastrointestinal tract segment to be monitored. The wires soldered to the connector, are led out of the abdominal cavity and are tunneled subcutaneously where they emerge from the midscapular region for connection to a recorder. The units are adaptable to many of the common laboratory animals (see Figure 2).

Miniaturization of the extraluminal transducer was undertaken by Dr. Pascaud to facilitate recording from smaller laboratory animals (Pascaud et al., 1978a,b). A semiconductor serosal unit has also been described (Nelson and Angell, 1979). The later units are extremely delicate and we await their use by other researchers.

The standard strain gage transducers are rather rigid and probably record isometric activity. A 4 cm flexible silicone rubber tubing filled with mercury and "sealed" with copper electrodes has been constructed for recording isotonic activity of the antrum of the dog (Kelly, 1974). Duplication of this device has not been successful by us; nor has data been presented by other workers. In our hands, the mercury leakage rendered the device inoperable.

41

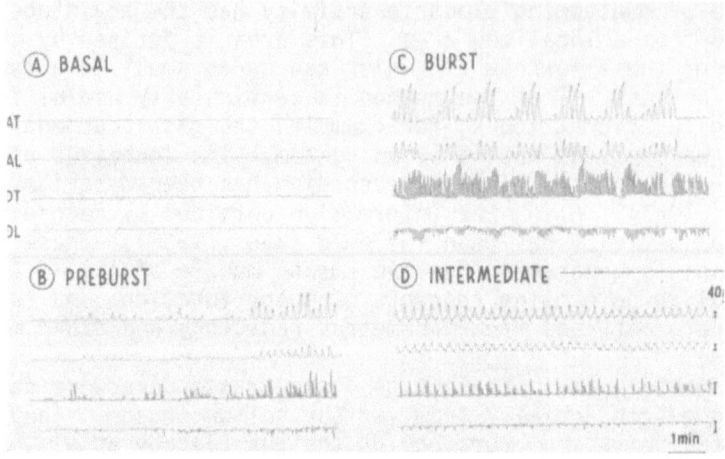

Figure 3. Canine gastric and duodenal contractile activity during interdigestive (A-basal, B-preburst, and C-burst) and digestive (D-intermediate) states. Interdigestive activity was obtained by fasting the animal for 20 hours before the recording session. Digestive activity was obtained by feeding a can of dog food (440 gm) at the beginning of the recording session. AT-antrum transverse (circular), AL-antrum longitudinal, DT-duodenum transverse (circular), DL-duodenum longitudinal. Calibration of the transducers to 40 gm is shown by the vertical bars in D (adapted from Carlson et al., 1970).

Strain gage force transducers have enabled us to characterize the two physiological states of the gastrointestinal tract. As has been amply verified, a distinctive motor pattern exists for the fasted (interdigestive) and fed (digestive) states of most mammals. This is seen in Figure 3.

The transducers offer several advantages over other methods of recording gastrointestinal motility: 1) the units record the contractile activity of the smooth muscle directly; 2) they are sewn on the serosal surface of the gastrointestinal tract. Thus, their use avoids any interference with flow of intraluminal contents and avoids stimulation of mucosal receptors. Since they are permanently fixed in position, the same site can be monitored repeatedly without using elaborate procedures to place the sensors in the desired position. 3) The units can be used in combination to monitor multiple sites of the gastrointestinal tract. 4) They can be used to monitor separately the activity of the circular and longitudinal muscle layers of the intestine. 5) There is no need to prepare fistulae or isolated loops of bowel.

There are some disadvantages of these units which limit their usefulness: 1) an electrical connection is needed between the animal and the recording unit. This necessity removes the animal from his normal environment and could influence the motor patterns. This limitation can be overcome through the use of radiotelemetry currently in development. 2) A major limitation of the transducer, as with any method of monitoring a single parameter, is that only the contractions and not the physiological function of the contractions are monitored. It is difficult to determine if a given sequence of contractions results in mixing or propulsion of intraluminal contents. 3) So far, these units have been applied to use in animals only. It may prove difficult to adapt them for chronic human studies.

A third type of serosal monitoring of GI muscle activity is through the use of opaque markers. Tasaka and Farrar (1969) were able to study the role of both muscle layers in the small intestine by simultaneously recording intraluminal pressure while utilizing cinefluorography to follow the movement of opaque markers (silver and tantalum chips bent into a circular shape of round tantalum discs, 2 cm in diameter) sutured to the serosa of the bowel. Basically this is a tedious technique. With the advent of computers for analysis of cinefluorography, novel information about muscle layer movement should be possible.

GASTRIC ELECTROGRAMS: CUTANEOUS ABDOMINAL VS. MUCOSAL SUCTION ELECTRODES

One of the earliest electrogastrograms in man was recorded from the abdominal surface by Alvarez, 1922. He clearly reported a 3 per minute cyclic wave that presumably reflected the basic electric rhythm of the stomach. Since then, several investigators have recorded gastric myoelectric activity in conscious humans using electrodes placed in the lumen through the peroral route (Garrett et al., 1963; Monges and Salducci, 1970; Waterfall et al., 1973; and You et al., 1980). In addition, Brown et al. (1975) have utilized both transcutaneous electrodes on the abdominal surface in conjunction with a gastric suction electrode. They have proven that the signal recorded from the skin effectively originated from the stomach. However, their transcutaneous recordings contained a significant amount of noise. Recently, Hamilton et al. (1983) have described a method to perform transcutaneous recordings with a highly improved signal to noise ratio. They have also confirmed the origin of the signal using gastric suction electrodes. The construction of the electrodes and methods of recording will be described below.

The abdominal surface electrodes utilized were standard Beckman 17 mm Ag/AgCl sintered bipotential electrodes filled with electrolyte cream. Myers et al. determined that the optimal site for recording the clearest reproducible signal is on the midline,

43

Suction Electrode

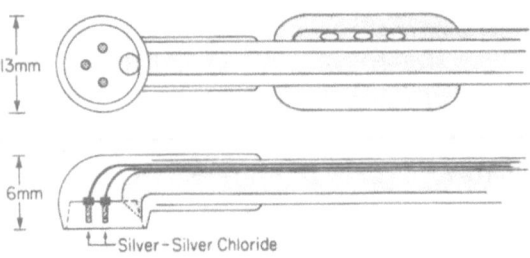

13mm

6mm

Silver-Silver Chloride

Figure 4. The gastric mucosal suction electrode with a suction
tube (shown stippled), stainless steel wires, and three Ag/AgCl
electrodes cast into a silicone rubber cup.

approximately 5 cm below the xiphoid process. Prior to placement
of the abdominal electrodes, the skin is lightly punctured with a
needle to minimize variations in skin potential.

The internal suction electrode was a modification of that
developed by Monges and Salducci, 1970. Three Ag/AgCl sintered
electrode pellets forming a triangle were cast into a silicone
rubber cup. The cup was connected to a silicone rubber tube containing another tube which provides the suction channel and three
electrically insulated steel wires (see Figure 4). A balloon can
also be attached to the suction electrode to detect pressure waves
in the stomach. The interal probe is passed into the stomach
through the mouth and positioned fluoroscopically.

An example of simultaneous skin and mucosal electrograms
recorded from a normal subject is shown in Figure 5. The 3/min
wave initially described by Alvarez is depicted. The abdominal
surface electrode should prove to be a useful noninvasive
technique for investigating patients with putative gastric
electric disturbances.

RELATIONSHIP OF MOTILITY MEASUREMENTS TO TRANSIT

This portion of the review will emphasize the relationship of

44

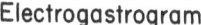

Electrogastrogram

Mucosa

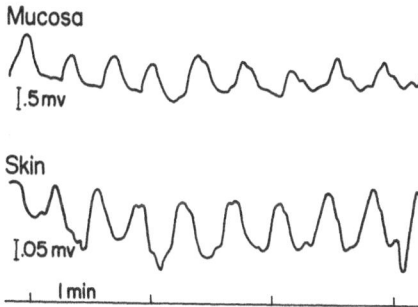

[.5mv

Skin

[.05mv

I min

Figure 5. Typical mucosal and transcutaneous electrogastrograms
show normal 3/min waves. The top tracing was obtained with an
electrode system shown in figure 4; the bottom tracing was
obtained with an abdominal surface electrode.

muscle activity to transit, with an emphasis on the control of
stomach emptying. Ingested substances may be absorbed or transported through the GI tract. The motor correlate of these activities may mix, propel, or retropulse the material. The direction
of flow is influenced by intraluminal pressure gradients, resistance caused by contraction or closure of the lumen, and possibly,
the composition and viscosity of the contents. The mean transport
time also varies with the organ, being fastest in the esophagus
and slowest in the colon.

The various techniques for measuring transit consist of
marking the contents with a nonabsorbable marker, radiographic
material, isotopic substance, discrete particle or a substance
converted to absorbable material by bacteria in the colon. Total
oral-anal transit time is the easiest though probably the least
informative of regional muscle function (Cummings et al., 1976;
Marlett et al., 1981). This has been well described in man
(Hansky and Connell, 1962) and animals (Purdon and Bass, 1973)
using various markers. Though these methods give us an estimate

of transit through the GI tract, the relationship of individual contractions to transit has not been established.

To study gastric retention and small intestinal transit of solid dosage forms in relation to motility patterns, enteric coated drug formulations have been utilized (Fara, 1983). Azulfidine EN-TABS, sulfasalazine, administered orally can give an index of mouth-to-colon transit time. This enteric coated formulation is designed to remain intact in the stomach. Then, upon arrival in the colon, the molecule is split by bacteria into 5-aminosalicylic acid and sulfapyridine. The sulfapyridine is rapidly absorbed and secreted into the saliva, where it can then be assayed.

Another method for measuring oral to colon transit time is obtained by administering an oral dose of lactulose. The lactulose is not absorbed, and is metabolized by the bacterial flora in the colon. The fermentation process releases hydrogen ions which are rapidly absorbed by the mucosa and appear in the expired air where they can be detected (Bond and Levitt, 1975).

Extensive studies have been done in quantitating gastric emptying and relating this emptying to antral-duodenal motor coordination. Gastric emptying involves the body and antrum of the stomach and the duodenum. Each area may play a different role in the emptying of liquids and solids. In the case of liquids, the rate of emptying is influenced by meal composition, osmolarity, and pH, as well as duodenal motor resistance (Hunt, 1968; Bass and Russell, 1983).

Both in animals and man, gastric emptying studies are performed with meals labeled with isotopes or nonabsorbable markers. Samples are then taken either serially or totally after a given time period. In the dog, the use of chronic implanted electrodes or force transducers facilitates the monitoring of muscle activity while simultaneously examining various test meals. This allows results of organ-organ integrative relationships while under the normal hormonal and neurological influences.

Liquids and the greatest part of solid meals ultimately leave the stomach in fluid form (as chyme or a solution). Therefore, we have employed liquid meals whose emptying rates could be precisely controlled by adjustments of its chemical or osmotic nature in our studies of motility-gastric emptying relationships. For example, the emptying rate of a water meal containing citrate can be slowed by the addition of oleic acid (a fatty acid). Weisbrodt's comparison of antral and duodenal contractile activity in response to equiosmolar meals of citrate (fast emptying) and citrate plus fat (slow emptying) demonstrates Hunt's concept of the intestinal control of emptying (Figure 6). Half of the citrate meal was emptied

TRISODIUM CITRATE

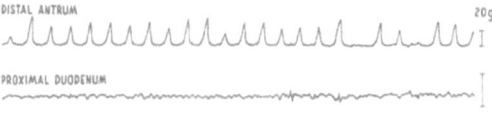

TRISODIUM CITRATE c̄ 10mN OLEIC ACID

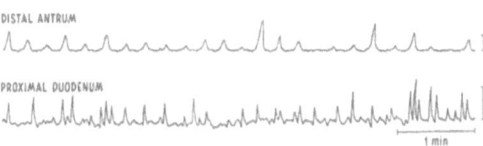

Figure 6. Force transducer recording of antral and duodenal
contractile activity after rapid (trisodium citrate) and slowly
emptying (citrate-fat) test meals. Note the lessening of the
antroduodenal force gradient after the addition of fat (adapted
from Weisbrodt et al., 1969).

from the stomach within 7 min, accompanied by antral contractile
activity (the pump) but almost no duodenal activity. After addition of fatty acid, the antrum to duodenum contractile gradient
was lessened, and the half emptying time of the meal increased to
32 min. Although the exact mechanism by which the fat was detected
by the intestine is obscure, the result is not: duodenal contractions delayed emptying of the fatty meal.

The terminal antrum ("sphincter", "ring") alone probably does
not actively participate in the control of liquid emptying. Specifically: a) chronic implantation of a noncompressible tube to prop
open the terminal antrum and pyloric canal does not affect the
emptying of a variety of liquid meals (Stemper and Cooke, 1976);
b) terminal or complete antrectomy does not greatly affect the
emptying of liquid meals (Dozois and Kelly, 1971; Russell et al.,
1982); and, c) removal of the terminal antrum, pyloric canal, and
the proximal duodenum (to the point of entry of the biliary duct)
does not alter the emptying of the citrate-fat meal (Gullikson,
1978). Terminal antral control of liquid emptying is further dis-
counted by examining the effects of pyloroplasty (sectioning of

the "sphincter") on the emptying of a citrate-fat meal. Creation of either a slightly enlarged (Heineke-Mikulicz) or greatly enlarged (Finney) gastroduodenal passage does not change the half emptying time of the citrate-fat meal (Ludwick et al., 1970; Ormsbee and Bass, 1976). Thus, the antrum or a "pyloric sphincter" is not required for the controlled delivery of liquid to the small intestine.

Distinct motor patterns are associated with the emptying of solid meals. Figure 7 demonstrates the electric relationships of the antrum to the duodenum during the emptying of solids. During the emptying of solids, most of the antral and about half of the duodenal BER are each superimposed with spike potentials. In a temporal sense, each antral spike potential is followed by one or two duodenal spike potentials (McCoy and Bass, 1963; Allen et al., 1964). A quiescent or nonspiking interval (N) on the duodenum immediately follows. These electric events correlate with the cineradiographic descriptions where: a) portions of the barium enter the duodenum while it is relaxed (nonspiking interval); and b) this delivery is completed by first a terminal antrum and then a duodenal contraction (antrum and then duodenal spike potentials). This organized pattern of antral and duodenal electric activity is dependent on a myo-neurally intact gastroduodenal junction (Bedi and Code, 1972). The postprandial antral and duodenal electric and motor activities are well coordinated, and the terminal antrum helps to regulate, break down, and empty solids (Kelly, 1980). In contrast, surgical alterations of the antral-duodenal area demonstrates that strict maintenance of antral-duodenal motor coordination is not requisite to unimpaired emptying of liquid meals. After certain gastrojejunostomies and antrectomies, where this

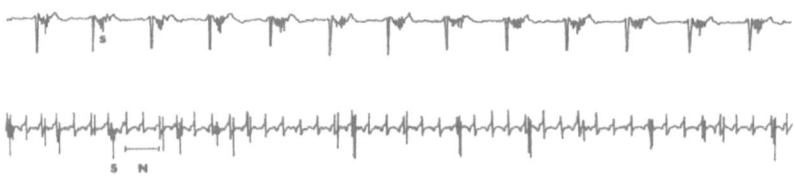

Figure 7. Recording of postprandial myoelectric activity of the antrum (top) and duodenum (bottom). S = spike potentials. N = nonspiking interval. BER frequencies of the antrum and duodenum are 4.75 and 18 cpm, respectively. Note that the mechanical counterpart to the spike potentials are muscle contractions. Gastric effluent is delivered to the relaxed duodenum (N), and this delivery is completed by antral and then duodenal contraction (adapted from Russell et al., 1982).

terminal relationship is lost, the emptying of liquids is
unaltered but solid emptying is impaired.

IN VIVO VS. IN VITRO MONITORING OF GI MOTILITY

Thus far in this review, the methods for recording motility
in vivo, and the advantages and disadvantages of these methods
have been elucidated. Our intent now is to discuss the information obtainable with in vitro techniques and compare it with that
of in vivo monitoring.

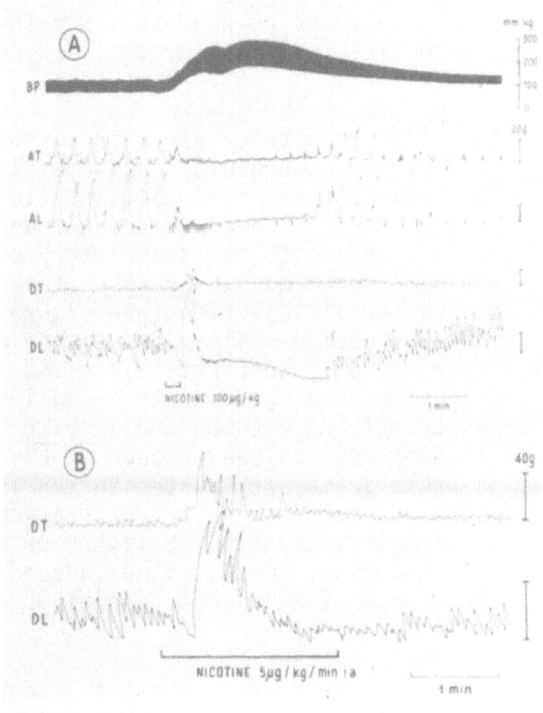

Figure 8. Comparison of the effects of intravenous (A) and intra-
arterial (B) administration of nicotine on the contractile activity of circular (T) or longitudinal (L) muscle of an anesthetized
dog. The left side of the records are typical motor patterns from
animals under phenobarbital anesthesia. Note the higher amplitude
of activity of the longitudinal muscle compared to the circular
muscle. Both areas of the gastrointestinal tract are inhibited by
systemic administration of nicotine. (The initial duodenal high
amplitude baseine shift was seen in only 50% of the experiments.
In contrast, intra-arterial (i.a.) administration of nicotine
always initiated a high amplitude rhythmic activity. B.P. = blood
pressure recording, A = antrum, D = duodenum, T = circular, and L
= longitudinal axis. (Adapted from Carlson et al., 1970).

In vitro preparations are widely used to study drug effects and to bioassay agents affecting smooth muscle. In vitro preparations offer several advantages over in vivo preparations: 1) only direct effects on the muscle or intrinsic nerves are measured. The influence of extrinsic nerves and reflexes as well as extrinsic hormonal effects are eliminated. This facilitates investigations of direct actions of a drug on the organ or tissue. 2) Certain measurements are easier to make, e.g., the measurements of membrane potential and oxygen consumption. 3) Many test procedures are more easily executed, e.g., the influence of changes in temperature or ionic environment on a drug response. 4) In vitro studies are usually easier to perform than experiments in vivo. Thus, in vitro preparations can be used to study the direct effects of drugs on the intrinsic and myogenic structures of the gastrointestinal tract.

The extrapolation of results obtained in vitro to explain the actions of drugs on the intact organism can be misleading. For example, intravenous administration of nicotine (10-100 µg/kg) causes a dose dependent inhibition of gastroduodenal contractile activity. This is in contrast to the stimulatory effect of nicotine on most intestinal smooth muscle in vitro (Day and Vane, 1963) and upon intra-arterial injection (see Figure 8). The relaxation in the unanesthetized animal is neither preceded nor followed by increased rhythmic contractile activity, and the relaxation is seen during both the digestive and interdigestive studies. The opposite effects between the in vivo and in vitro preparations are probably due to the absence of the major components of the sympathetic inhibitory system in the in vitro preparation. Since reserpine pretreatment or pretreatment of the unanesthetized animal with tolazoline abolishes or reduces the inhibitory effect of nicotine, the nicotine-induced relaxation is probably due to activation of adrenergic inhibitory systems (Carlson et al., 1970).

In summary, when designing experiments to study GI motility, the use of unanesthetized animals establishes normal physiological states and net effects of drugs on the motor patterns of various portions of the GI tract. In vitro gut preparations on the other hand are usually needed to better characterize the site and mechanism of drug action.

REFERENCES

Allen, G. L., Poole, E. W., and Code, C. F., 1964, Relationships between electrical activities of antrum and duodenum. Am. J. Physiol., 207:906-910.
Alvarez, W. C., 1922, The electrogastrogram and what it shows. J. Am. Med. Assoc., 78:1116-1119.

Anderson, J. J., Bolt, R. J., Ullman, B. M., and Bass, P., 1968, Differential response to various stimulants in the body and antrum of the canine stomach. Am. J. Dig. Dis., 13:147-156.

Arndorfer, R. C., Stef, J. J., Dodds, W. J., Linchan, J. H., and Hogan, W. J., 1977, Improved infusion system for intraluminal esphageal manometry. Gastroenterology, 73:23-27.

Bass, P. and Callantine, M. R., 1964, Simultaneous recording of electrical and mechanical activity of the uterus in the unanesthetized animal. Nature, 203:1367-1368.

Bass, P., 1968, In vivo electrical activity of the small bowel, p. 2051-2074, in: "Handbook of Physiology," Vol. 4, American Physiological Society, C. F. Code, ed., Washington, D.C.

Bass, P., 1971, The relationship of electric activity to contraction, p. 59-72, in: "Gastrointestinal Motility," L. Demling and R. Ottenjann, eds., Academic Press, New York.

Bass, P. and Weisbrodt, N. W., 1971, Current concepts on pharmacology of gastrointestinal motility, p. 149-167, in: "Gastrointestinal Motility," L. Demling and R. Ottenjann, eds., Academic Press, New York.

Bass, P. and Wiley, J. N., 1972, Contractile force transducer for recording muscle activity in unanesthetized animals. J. Appl. Physiol., 32:567-570.

Bass, P. and Russell, J., 1983, Gastric emptying of liquids: role of the small intestine, p. 157-165, in: "Functional Disorders of the Digestive Tract," W. Y. Chey, ed., Raven Press, New York.

Bayliss, W. M. and Starling, E. H., 1899, The movements and innervation of the small intestine. J. Physiol. (London), 24:99-143.

Bedi, B. S. and Code, C. F., 1972, Pathway of coordination of postprandial, antral and duodenal action potentials. Am. J. Physiol., 222:1295-1298.

Bond, J. H. and Levitt, M. D., 1975, Investigation of small bowel transit time in man utilizing pulmonary hydrogen (H_2) measurement. J. Lab. Clin. Med., 85:546-555.

Brown, B. H., Smallwood, R. H., Duthie, H. L., and Stoddard, C. J., 1975, Intestinal smooth muscle electrical potentials recorded from surface electrodes. Med. Biol. Eng., 13:97-102.

Carlson, G. M., Ruddon, R. W., Hug, C. C., Jr., and Bass, P., 1970, Effects of nicotine on gastric antral and duodenal contractile activity in the dog. J. Pharmacol. Exp. Ther., 172:369-376.

Corazziari, E., 1982, In vivo techniques for the study of gastrointestinal motility, p. 181-204, in: "Mediators and Drugs in Gastrointestinal Motility, II," G. Bertaccini, ed., Springer-Verlag, Berlin, Heidelberg, New York.

Cummings, J. H., Jenkins, D. J. A., and Wiggins, H. S., 1976, Measurement of the mean transit time of dietary residue through the human gut. Gut., 17:210-218.

Day, M. and Vane, J. R., 1963, An analysis of the direct and indirect action of drugs on the isolated guinea-pig ileum. Brit. J. Pharmacol., 20:150-170.

Dent, J., 1976, A new technique for continuous sphincter pressure measurements. Gastroenterology., 71:263-267.

Dodds, W. J., 1976, Instrumentation and methods for intraluminal esophageal manometry. Arch. Intern. Med., 136:515-523.

Dozois, R. R. and Kelly, K. A., 1971, Effect of a gastrin pentapeptide on canine gastric emptying of liquids. Am. J. Physiol., 221:113-117.

Engstrom, E. R., Webster, J. G., and Bass, P., 1979, Analysis of duodenal contractility in the unanesthetized dog. IEEE. Trans. Bio. ENG., BME-26:517-523.

Fara, J. W., 1983, Gastrointestinal transit of solid dosage forms, p. 23-26, in: "Drug Delivery Systems," Pharmaceutical Technology - Special Issue.

Foster, G. E., Arden-Jones, J. R., Beatie, A., Evans, D. F., and Hardcastle, J. D., 1983, Abnormal gastrointestinal motility in diabetics and after vagotomy. Gastro. Clin. Biol., 7:727.

Garrett, J. M., Schlegel, J. F., and Hoffman, H. N., 1963, Intraluminal detection of intestinal electrical activity. Fed. Proc., 22:225.

Gullikson, G. W., 1978, Changes in the physiology and pharmacological response of the electric and motor activity at the gastroduodenal junction following section and reanastomosis of the duodenum or orad jejunum to the antrum. Doctoral dissertation, University of Wisconsin.

Hamilton, J. W., Bellahsene, B. E., Reichelderfer, M., Webster, J. G., and Bass, P., 1983, Human cutaneous electrogastrography: comparison with internal recordings. Gastroenterology, 84, pt. 2:1180.

Hansky, Y. J. and Connell, A. M., 1962, Measurement of gastrointestinal transit using radioactive chromium. Gut, 3:187-188.

Harris, L. D. and Pope C. E., II., 1964, "Squeeze" vs. resistance, an evaluation of the mechanism of sphincter competence. J. Clin. Invest., 43:2272-2278.

Hunt, J. N., 1968, Regulation of gastric emptying, in: "Handbook of Physiology," Vol. 4, C. F. Code, ed., Amer. Physiol. Soc., Washington, D.C., p. 1917-1937.

Jacoby, H. I., Bass, P., and Bennett, D. R., 1963, In vivo extraluminal contractile force transducer for gastrointestinal muscle. J. Appl. Physiol., 18:658-665.

Kelly, M. A., 1974, The use of miniaturized mercury strain gauges to record gastric motility, in: "Proceedings of the 5th International Symposium on Gastrointestinal Motility," E. E. Daniel, ed., Mitchell, Vancouver, 323-329.

Kelly, K. A., 1980, Gastric emptying of liquids and solids: roles of proximal and distal stomach. Am. J. Physiol., 239:G71-G76.

Ludwick, J. R. and Bass, P., 1967, Contractile and electric
    activity of the extra hepatic biliary tract and duodenum.
    Surg., Gynecol. & Obstet., 124:536-546.
Ludwick, J. R., Wiley, J. N., and Bass, P., 1970, Gastric emptying
    following Finney pyloroplasty and vagotomy. Am. J. Dig. Dis.,
    15:347-352.
Macagno, E. O. and Christensen, J., 1980, Fluid mechanics of the
    duodenum, p. 139-158, in: Ann. Rev. Fluid. Mech., Vol. 12.
Macagno, E. O., Christensen, J., and Lee, C. L., 1982, Modeling
    the effect of wall movement on absorption in the intestine.
    Am. J. Physiol., 243:G541-G550.
Marlett, J. A., Slavin, J. L., and Brauer, P. M., 1981, Comparison
    of dye and pellet gastrointestinal transit time during con-
    trolled diets differing in protein and fiber levels. Dig. Dis.
    Sci., 26:208-213.
McCoy, E. J. and Bass, P., 1963, Chronic electrical activity of
    gastroduodenal area: effects of food and certain catechol-
    amines. Am. J. Physiol., 205:439-445.
Monges, H. and Salducci, H., 1970, A method of recording the gas-
    tric electrical activity in man. Am. J. Dig. Dis., 15:271-276.
Myers, T. J., Bass, P., Webster, J. G., Fontaine, A. B., and
    Miyauchi, A. Human surface electrogastrograms: ac and dc
    measurements, submitted for publication.
Nelsen, T. S. and Angell, J. B., 1979, Microminiature force
    transducers for chronic in vivo use. Abstracts 7th Inter-
    national Symposium on Gastrointestinal Motility. University of
    Iowa, Iowa City, p. 55.
Ormsbee, H. S., III and Bass, P., 1976, Gastroduodenal motor
    gradients in the dog after pyloroplasty. Am. J. Physiol.,
    230:389-397.
Pascaud, X. B., Genton, M. J. H., and Bass, P., 1978a, A miniature
    transducer for recording intestinal motility in unrestrained
    chronic rats. Am. J. Physiol., 235:E532-E538.
Pascaud, X. B., Genton, M. J. H., and Bass, P., 1978b, Gastroduo-
    denal contractile activity in fed and fasted unrestrained rats,
    p. 637-645, in: "Gastrointestinal Motility in Health and
    Disease," H. L. Duthie, ed., MTP Press Limited, Lancaster,
    England.
Purdon, R. A. and Bass, P., 1973, Gastric and intestinal transit
    in rats measured by a radioactive test meal. Gastroenterology,
    64:968-976.
Reinke, D. A., Rosenbaum, A. H., and Bennet, D. R., 1967, Patterns
    of dog gastrointestinal contractile activity monitored in vivo
    with extraluminal force transducers. Am. J. Dig. Dis., 12:113-
    141.
Russell, J., Miyauchi, A., and Bass, P., 1982, Myoelectric
    activity of the diverted antro-duodenum in the dog. Proc. Soc.
    Exp. Biol. Med., 171:201-206.

Schuster, M. M., Hendrix, T. R., and Mendeloff, A. I., 1963, The internal anal sphincter response. <u>J. Clin. Invest.</u>, 42:196-207.

Sninsky, C. A., Cottrell, C. R., Martin, J. L., Fernandez, A., and Mathias, J. R., 1982, Recording probe adds new dimension to the investigation of small bowel motility in humans. <u>Clin. Res.</u>, 30:290A.

Stef, J. J., Dodds, W. J., Hogan, W. J., Linehan, J. J., and Stewart, E. T., 1977, Intraluminal esophageal manometry: an analysis of variables affecting recording fidelity of peristaltic pressures. <u>Gastroenterology.</u>, 73:23-27.

Stemper, T. J. and Cooke, A. R., 1976, Effect of a fixed pyloric opening on gastric emptying in the cat and dog. <u>Am. J. Physiol.</u>, 230:813-817.

Tasaka, K. and Farrar, J. T., 1969, Mechanics of small intestinal muscle function in the dog. <u>Am. J. Physiol.</u>, 217:1224-1229.

Waterfall, W. E., Duthie, H. L., and Brown, B. H., 1973, The electrical and motor actions of gastrointestinal hormones on the duodenum in man. <u>Gut</u>, 14:689-696.

Weems, W. A., 1982, Intestinal wall motion, propulsion, and fluid movement: trends toward a unified theory. <u>Am. J. Physiol.</u>, 243:G177-G188.

Weisbrodt, N. W., Wiley, J. N., Overholt, B. F., and Bass, P., 1969, A relation between gastroduodenal muscle contractions and gastric emptying. <u>Gut</u>, 10:543-548.

You, C. H., Lee, K. Y., Chey, W. Y., and Menguy, R., 1980, Electrogastrographic study of patients with unexplained nausea, bloating, and vomiting. <u>Gastroenterology</u>, 76:311-314.

SMOOTH MUSCLE ELECTROPHYSIOLOGY

Joseph H. Szurszewski

Department of Physiology and Biophysics
Mayo Foundation and Clinic
Rochester, Minnesota 55905

STRUCTURE OF GASTROINTESTINAL SMOOTH MUSCLE

Individual smooth muscle cells are tapered structures. The average diameter of a smooth muscle cell at its widest point is about 3μm[1]. The average length in the gastrointestinal tract ranges from 200 to 400 μm[1]. The cells are packed into bundles; within a bundle each cell has a polyhedral profile and is surrounded by neighboring cells[1]. Each cell in the bundle is surrounded by about 12 other cells at any point along its length and approximately equal numbers of cells overlap either end of any given cell[1]. The geometrical packing of these bundles determines the shape of the muscle. If the bundles weave a three dimensional pattern, the shape will be rod-like as in the taenia of the human colon. If the weaving is planar, the shape will be a sheet-like structure.

The smooth muscle cells within a bundle are connected to each other at points along their length by areas of fusion of the outer lamellae of the muscle cells (nexus) or by areas of very close apposition (gap junctions)[1]. The nexus provides a low resistance pathway between cells. It is thought that gap junctions also provide pathways for electrical communication between cells. Changes in membrane potential in any one cell are shared by the adjacent cells through the nexus and gap junction. The tissue behaves electrically as if all cell interiors were in direct contact with one another. Both arrangements allow the tissue to behave as a functional syncytium.

The muscular effector unit in the gastrointestinal tract is not a single smooth muscle cell. The effector unit is a muscle bundle. Within a bundle, cells are electrically coupled. Separate bundles are electrically coupled by regions of anastomoses between bundles and by small bundles which join larger bundles together. Through such connecting bundles, slow waves and action potentials can propagate along gastric and intestinal muscle.

Smooth muscle in the digestive tract is arranged in layers. In the lower third of the human esophagus, there is an inner circular layer running around the circumference of the tube and an outer longitudinal layer running along the length of the tube. In the stomach, there are three or more layers with various distinct orientations: an inner circular, outer longitudinal and an oblique layer in between the two. In the small intestine, there is an outer longitudinal and an inner circular. In the colon, the outer longitudinal in some species including man is gathered into three bundles referred to as taenia coli; the inner circular layer is complete. In the colorectal area, the taenia give way to a complete longitudinal muscle layer covering the inner circular which thickens to form the internal sphincter.

IONIC BASIS FOR ELECTRICAL ACTIVITY

It is likely that diffusion potentials of Na, K and Cl ions influence the resting membrane potential of smooth muscle cells[2,3]. Recent evidence suggests that an electrogenic sodium pump also may contribute to the resting membrane potential[2,3,4,5]. The existence of an inwardly directed electrogenic chloride pump may also contribute to the cell's resting potential[4,5,6]. The active and passive ion movements and ion pumps that are considered to determine the resting membrane potential in smooth muscle are summarized in Figure 1. The unequal distribution of ions on either side of the membrane depends upon active ion transport and membrane permeability to the ions. The steady state resting membrane potential depends upon the diffusion potential of the ions and on the electrogenic potential. Hence, $E_M = E_{diff} + i_p R_m$ where E_{diff} = diffusion potential, i_p = pump current of the various electrogenic pumping mechanisms and R_m = specific membrane resistance. This equation provides only a rough estimate of the steady state membrane potential because of the many assumptions involved in its derivation.

The membrane potential of gastrointestinal smooth muscle is seldom at rest. Spontaneous, transmitter and hormonally induced changes in the membrane permeability to one or more ionic species cause fast and/or slow fluctuations in membrane potential. During these voltage changes, the muscle cell takes up and loses ions. If nothing was done about the efflux and influx of ions, the membrane potential would in time deteriorate and there would be equal

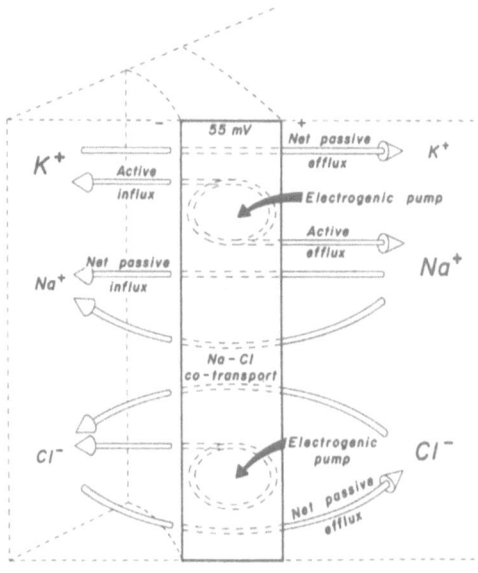

Figure 1 Summary of active and passive movements of Na, K, and Cl in
resting smooth muscle cell (From Ref 7).

concentrations of ions on both sides of the membrane. Simple diffusion, active transport and exchange diffusion or linked transport of
ions are three mechanisms which regulate the movement of ions
thereby preventing voltage run down[7].

Activation of the contractile proteins requires calcium. There
is considerable evidence supporting the hypothesis that spike-shaped
potentials and gastric action potentials result from an inward
calcium current[8]. Recent observations suggest that dc-shifts in
membrane potential of tonically active muscle as in the fundus of

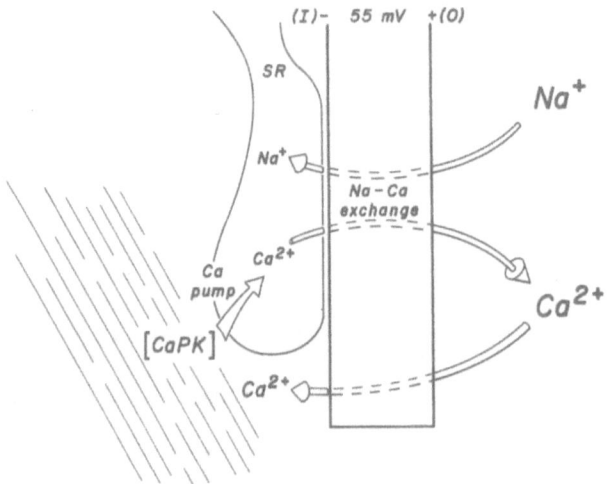

Figure 2 Summary of mechanisms that help maintain low intracellular
concentrations of calcium. I, inside, O, outside of cell
(From Refs 7 and 12).

the stomach also results from an inward calcium current[9]. In addition to inward calcium current, release of calcium from intracellular compartments such as the sarcoplasmic reticulum may also
contribute to increases in intracellular calcium during
contraction[10,11]. During relaxation, free intracellular calcium is
lowered by a calcium pump located in the sarcoplasmic reticulum and
by extrusion of calcium out of the cell by a Na-Ca exchange mechanism between the sarcoplasmic reticulum and extracellular space[12].
Mechanisms that help maintain low levels of intracellular ionic
calcium are summarized diagrammatically in Figure 2.

ELECTRICAL CORRELATES OF MOTOR ACTIVITY IN SMOOTH MUSCLE OF THE GASTROINTESTINAL TRACT

Smooth muscle potentials can be measured in one of two ways. The simpler way is to place one electrode in contact with the external surface of many cells and another electrode at a remote site. The recorded electromyogram results from local current flow from thousands of cells in the region of the muscle electrode. Smooth muscle potentials recorded in this manner are extracellular recordings. The more difficult way is to place one electrode inside a single smooth muscle cell and another outside the cell. The recorded potential is a measure of the resting membrane potential and a measure of variations in it if any occur. Potentials recorded in this manner are intracellularly recorded potentials which reflect voltage changes across the smooth muscle cell membrane. The hand drawn traces in Figure 3 illustrate the electrical potentials obtained from three regions of the gastrointestinal tract using extracellular and intracellular recording techniques. The mechanical activity associated with the potentials is also shown.

It should be kept in mind that contraction of smooth muscle is a mechanical manifestation of an electrical process at the surface membrane of the cells. Each contraction in the bowel is associated with electrical currents flowing through the affected muscle. These currents are not incidental to contraction, they in fact cause the muscle to contract.

Electrical Activity in Vivo. Smooth Muscle of the Fundus. Muscle in this region of the stomach is not autorhythmic. Fundus muscle does not usually generate slow waves, spikes or action potentials. Intracellular recordings indicate that the basis for excitation-contraction coupling is a graded change in the membrane potential (Figure 3) and that there is almost a linear relationship between depolarization and tension[9]. Sustained depolarization brought about by nervous activity, hormones and distension produces a proportionate and sustained increase in tension. Changes in tension are slow and sustained. The small changes in membrane potential which are involved usually cannot be recorded with extracellular electrodes in vivo. Thus when recordings are made in vivo, the electrical trace remains unaltered in the face of changes in tension in the fundus (Figure 3).

Smooth Muscle of the Corpus and Antrum. These muscles are autorhythmic. They generate spontaneous, regularly occurring action potentials. The occurrence of the action potential is a property of the muscle[13]. Occurrence of the action potential does not depend upon nervous activity. When recorded intracellularly, the spontaneous action potential has the shape sketched in Figure 3

A. FUNDUS MUSCLE

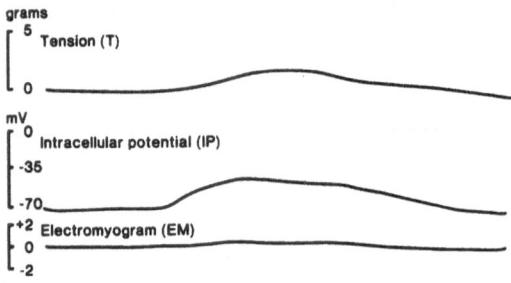

B. GASTRIC ANTRUM

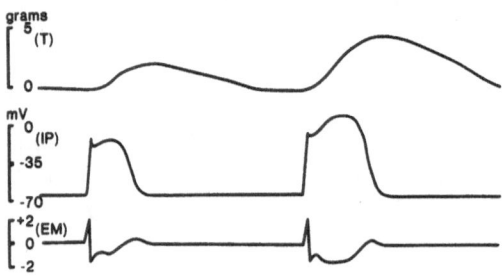

C. SMALL INTESTINE

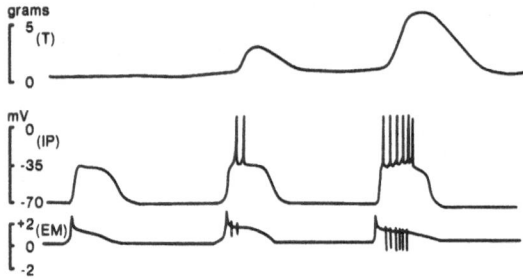

Figure 3 Schematic representation (hand drawn sketch) of electrical
and mechanical activity in three regions of the gastrointestinal tract. In each panel: top trace tension; middle
trace intracellular potential; lower trace extracellularly
recorded potentials. Note in gastric antrum increase in
amplitude of contraction due to increased amplitude of
intracellularly recorded action potential. Extracellular
representation is increase in amplitude of the negative dip
which follows triphasic potential. T, tension; IP, intracellular potential; EM, electromyogram.

(cf. Figures 4 and 5). It can last for as long as 8 seconds in the terminal antrum. Both circular and longitudinal muscle layers in the corpus and antrum generate gastric action potentials[14].

The pacemaker for the action potential is located high on the greater curvature somewhere in the proximal corpus[15,16,17]. From this region, the action potential spreads or migrates to the pylorus with an apparent velocity that increases as the action potential reaches the pylorus. The frequency is 3/min in man and is uniform throughout the corpus and antrum.

Except for the very terminal antrum, antral muscle does not generate spike potentials[14]. The basis for excitation-contraction coupling is the plateau potential of the intracellularly recorded gastric action potential[18,19]. Extracellularly, the plateau potential looks like a "dip" or "depression" on the electromyogram (Figure 3). The contractile response during the plateau potential is a twitch.

Since the muscle only contracts during the gastric action potential, the frequency of contraction is set by the frequency of the action potential. Since the action potential originates in the corpus and spreads to the pylorus, the associated contraction will also spread as a moving ring of contraction in peristaltic fashion from the corpus to the pylorus. The frequency, amplitude and direction of contraction is absolutely determined by the action potential.

Smooth Muscle of the Small Intestine. Slow wave potentials occur throughout the length of the small intestine. The shape of the slow wave recorded intracellularly and extracellularly is shown in Figure 3. The slow wave lasts for about 3.5 seconds. Recently, it has been suggested that the slow wave is not generated by the longitudinal muscle[20]. When recorded extracellularly, the slow wave has a complex wave form probably because of the complex geometry of current flow in volume conductor conditions.

The pacemaker for the intestinal slow wave is in the first few centimeters of the duodenum. It dominates and pulls to higher frequencies more distal pacemaking regions. Transection of the intestine irreversibly reduces the frequency at all points distal to the transection[21].

Unlike the stomach, there is an aboral decreasing frequency gradient in the small intestine[22,23]. In man, the frequency in the duodenum is 12/min, in the ileum it is 8/min. In the dog, the frequency gradient is 20 to 12.

Spike potentials superimposed on slow waves produce contraction (Figure 3). The greater the number of spikes, the greater the amplitude of contraction (Figure 3). The presence or absence of spikes depends upon the hormonal and neurogenic influences. Stimulatory agents increase spike activity; inhibitory stimuli reduce or block their occurrence. Recent electrophysiological data suggest that slow waves may also trigger phasic contractions[24].

The function of the slow wave is to provide the basic timing mechanism for short bursts of spikes and hence for rhythmic contraction. The frequency of the slow wave sets the maximum frequency of contraction.

Smooth Muscle of the Large Intestine. Our understanding of smooth muscle potentials in the large intestine is not nearly as complete as in the small intestine and stomach.

It does appear certain that these muscles are autorhythmic. Excitation-contraction coupling occurs by way of spike potentials timed by the occurrence of the slow wave and through the slow wave itself[25,26]. It has been recognized for some time that the slow wave potential originates in the circular muscle layer[25].

The large intestine of the cat has been studied most extensively. The slow wave frequency is about 5/min in the proximal colon and rises to about 5.8/min in the distal colon[27]. The slow wave frequency gradient and hence the gradient of contractile activity is much more labile than that of the stomach and small intestine. The dominant pacemaker in the large intestine can wander. At times the gradient reverses so that the frequency in the proximal colon is greater than the frequency in the distal colon. If the direction of fecal movement is dictated by the slow wave frequency gradient, than an aboral increasing gradient favors retention of contents, while a reversal to an aboral decreasing gradient might promote colon emptying.

Unlike the small intestine, the apparent velocity of the slow wave is greater in the circular axis than in the longitudinal axis[28]. This may help to establish ring contractions which help establish the haustral pattern in the colon.

Electrical Activity in Vitro. Measurements of electrical activity of smooth muscle from the gastrointestinal tract were made with large extracellular electrodes nearly seventy-five years ago[29] and continue to the present day. Our understanding of the qualitative relationship between electrical and mechanical activities and of the type of rhythmic electrical patterns normally occurring in the bowel derives from observations made with the extracellular electrode. The notions that an electrical pacemaker for the stomach

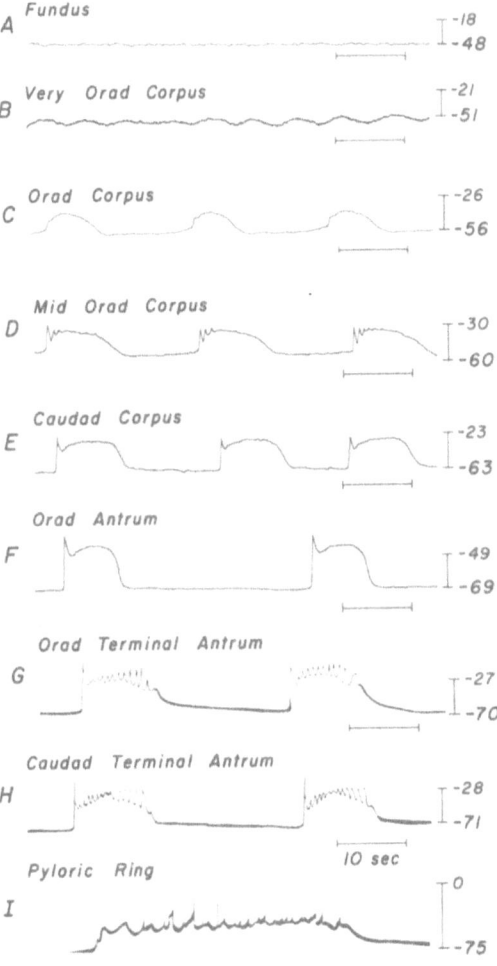

Figure 4 Regional differences in intracellularly electrical activity in different regions of the canine stomach (From Ref 7).

exists in the upper corpus and that functionally distinct regions of the stomach exhibit electrical differences were first defined through extracellular recordings. Furthermore, the definition of the slow wave frequency gradient in the small intestine and the absence of such a gradient in the large intestine similarly are based on data obtained from extracellular recordings made in vivo. The extracellular method, although easy to use yields in fact data often too complicated to be analyzed mechanistically. Intracellular recording with microelectrodes, although difficult to achieve, yields data which are in fact simpler to analyze. The taenia coli has been an often used preparation for intracellular recordings from smooth muscle cells as has been the circular smooth muscle of the cat small intestine. Recently, quantitative electrophysiological analysis has been applied to smooth muscle of the stomach. What follows is a brief review of the salient observations made in the canine stomach. A more detailed handling of the subject has been published[7].

The range of intracellularly recorded activity in different regions of the stomach is shown in Figure 4. Several regional differences are apparent. First, there are two opposing gradients in resting membrane potential. Orad to the mid-corpus, the potential becomes less negative whereas moving away distally from it, the potential becomes more negative. Second, although muscle from the mid-corpus to the gastroduodenal junction has the capacity for generating spontaneous activity, only muscle in orad and mid-corpus generates a spontaneous diastolic depolarization prior to each action potential. Such a diastolic depolarization is characteristic of pacemaker tissue. Third, except for the very orad corpus, spontaneous activity consists of an action potential which has a fast, initial, spike-like depolarization followed by a prolonged and sustained, positive potential. These two potentials have been referred to as the upstroke potential and plateau potential, respectivley[14]. And fourth, beginning in the orad terminal antrum, small oscillations in potential occur on top the plateau potential. Distally, these oscillations can give rise to spike-like potentials. Thus, throughout most of the stomach, spontaneous electrical activity is spike-free.

The relationship between the different types of electrical activity and contraction of the muscle is best understood when recordings are made simultaneously of both. When done under in vitro conditions, each upstroke potential produces a weak twitch-like contraction (Figure 5). When a second contraction follows, it occurs in time with the plateau potential in the corpus and with spike-like potentials in the caudad terminal antrum. The reason for absence of a second contraction in the antrum during spontaneous activity will be made clear later.

64

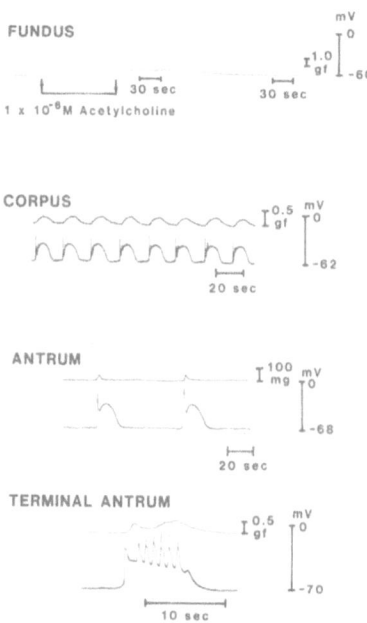

Figure 5 Simultaneously recorded spontaneous mechanical and intracellular electrical activity of circular muscle taken from
fundus, corpus, antrum and terminal antrum of canine
stomach. In each panel, top trace, contraction; bottom
trace, intracellular potential.

In the spike-free region of the stomach, excitatory neurotransmitters and hormones increase the force of contraction of the second
contraction by increasing the amplitude and prolonging the duration
of the plateau potential (Figure 6)[9,13,18,19]. Although the
increase in amplitude of the plateau potential is only a few millivolts, the contraction force can be increased several times[9]. Ion

substitution studies suggest that an inward calcium current flows during the plateau potential and that excitatory substances increase this calcium current[7],[14].

The observations made in vitro on mechanical and electrical activities have in vivo correlates. The in vivo correlate of the first twitch-like contraction may be the type I contraction[7]. The in vivo correlate of the second contraction, which is variable in

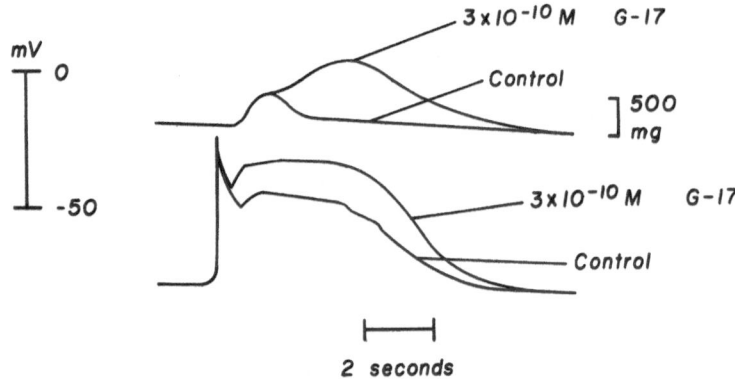

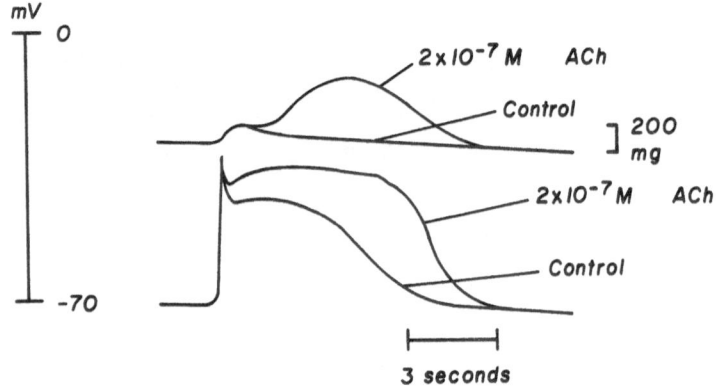

Figure 6 Effects of gastrin (G_{17}) and acetylcholine (ACh) on electromechanical coupling of circular muscle of canine orad antrum. In each panel, top trace, contraction; bottom trace, intracellularly recorded action potential (From Ref. 7).

amplitude and duration, may be the ring-like contraction seen during cineradiographic studies of gastric motility. This second contraction in all probability is responsible for movement and trituration of gastric content. The in vivo correlate of the upstroke potential is a triphasic or biphasic change observed with extracellular electrodes. The in vivo correlate of the plateau potential is the negative dip which follows the triphasic wave of the extracellularly recorded gastric action potential (Figure 3). The spike-like potentials which occur on top of the plateau potential in the caudad terminal antrum is represented in the extracellular trace as small negatively oriented spike potentials.

Both extracellular and intracellular recordings clearly show that smooth muscle from the fundus is electrically silent. It is interesting this should be so, particularly because the orad corpus is the site of the pacemaker. Recent studies have suggested that the decreasing gradient in potential between the mid-corpus and fundus may account for the absence of spontaneous electrical activity in the fundus. It has been suggested that the lower resting membrane potential inactivates the ionic mechanisms responsible for the gastric action potential[9]. Thus, spread of the action potential away from the pacemaker is decremental. In contrast, the increasing gradient in potential between the mid-corpus and gastroduodenal region may account for the faster rate of change in potential, and the larger voltage excursion[7] (Figure 4).

The electrical observations described above raise interesting questions. What is the basis of excitation-contraction coupling in fundus smooth muscle? Why is the amplitude of second contraction so sensitive to small changes in the amplitude of the plateau potential? Some insight into these issues can be obtained by considering the voltage-tension relationship of each region of the stomach.

Voltage-Tension Relationship of Gastric Smooth Muscle

A comparison of the voltage-tension relationship for the circular muscle of the fundus, corpus and antrum obtained by graded increases in external potassium concentration is shown in Figure 7. For each, there is a voltage (mechanical threshold) beyond which further depolarization produces a sharp increase in the force of contracton[7]. In the steep portion of the curve, small changes in potential produce significantly large increases in the force of contraction, either tonic or phasic. Except for the fundus, the resting membrane potential is more negative than the mechanical threshold. Thus, only fundus muscle should have active tone at rest. The location of the resting potential for fundus muscle on its voltage-tension relationship means that this region of the

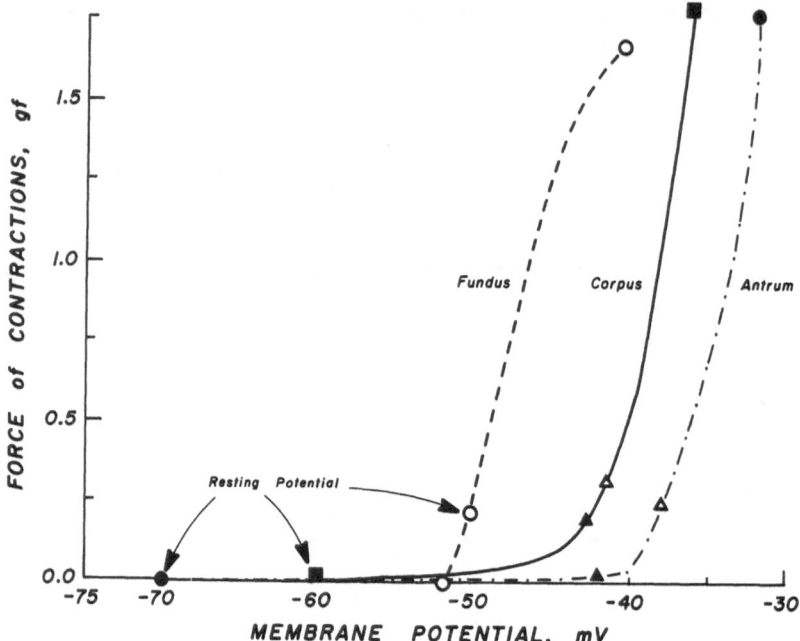

Figure 7 Comparison of voltage-tension curves of fundus, corpus and antrum of circular muscle of canine stomach. Mechanical threshold for corpus and antrum at approximately -45 mV and -40 mV, respectively. For fundus muscle, resting potential less negative than mechanical threshold. For corpus and antrum, ▲ marks peak amplitude of upstroke potential; △ marks location of peak amplitude of plateau potential of spontaneously occurring action potentials.

stomach is predisposed to contract in response to depolarization or to relax in response to hyperpolarization. The voltage-tension relationship precisely explains why in vivo, fundus muscle is well suited to perform its physiological role. Because of the relationship, fundus muscle operates truly as a tonic muscle.

The voltage-tension curve of antral muscle reveals that the resting membrane potential is at least 30 mV away from mechanical threshold (Figure 7). In consequence, antral muscle is not a tonic muscle under normal conditions. During the occurrence of an action potential, the voltage excursion caused by the initial upstroke depolarization briefly moves the membrane potential through the mechanical threshold thereby accounting for the brief twitch. Since the voltage of the plateau potential in unstimulated conditions settles below the mechanical threshold, the muscle relaxes (Figure 7). However, the membrane potential of the plateau potential is located only a few millivolts more negative than the mechanical threshold. Thus, the voltage of the membrane is poised at the base of the steeply rising portion of the curve. A small increase in peak voltage of the plateau as might be caused by an excitatory neurotransmitter will lead to a contraction. Because of the steepness of the relationship, small changes in voltage caused by excitatory or inhibitory substances will lead to substantial changes in the force of the phasic contraction.

The voltage-tension relationship for corpus smooth muscle reveals that the resting membrane potential is not far removed from its mechanical threshold (Figure 7). Since the entire voltage swing of the corpus action potential occurs above the mechanical threshold, a contraction is associated with both the upstroke and plateau potentials. Indeed, it can be seen in Figure 5, that a first and second contraction occurs during the upstroke and plateau potentials, respectively. Since the resting potential of corpus smooth muscle is slightly less than 10 mV away from the mechanical threshold, corpus muscle can generate tone provided the stimulus is capable of moving the resting potential beyond the mechanical threshold.

The electromechanical analysis described above provides the basis for understanding the in vivo function of the three regions of the stomach. By virtue of its voltage-tension characteristics, fundus muscle is well suited to regulate volume of the upper stomach. By virtue of the close proximity of its resting potential and mechanical threshold, corpus muscle is well suited to regulate capacity and to gently mix content. By virtue of the great difference between the resting potential and mechanical threshold of antral muscle, the antrum is well suited to resist changes in volume and to function virtually as a truly phasic muscle mixing and grinding gastric content.

SUMMARY

The quantitative analysis described above for gastric smooth muscle needs to be extended to all other regions of the gastrointestinal tract. In doing so, it may be possible to arrive at a better understanding of the cellular electrical events which operate under normal circumstances and perhaps also provide an understanding of the mechanisms responsible for gastrointestinal motor disturbances.

ACKNOWLEDGEMENTS

I am grateful to the National Institutes of Health for supporting some of the work described through Grant AM 17238.

Acknowledgment is made of Jan Applequist for her skilled assistance in the preparation of this manuscript.

REFERENCES

1. G. Burnstock, Structure of smooth muscle and its innervation, in: Smooth Muscle, E. Bülbring, A. F. Brading, A. W. Jones and T. Tomita, eds., pp 1-69, Williams and Wilkins, Baltimore (1970).

2. A. W. Jones, Content and fluxes of electrolytes, in: Handbook of Physiology, The Cardiovascular System, D. F. Bohr, A. P. Somlyo, and H. V. Sparks, eds., pp 253-299, Waverly Press, Baltimore (1980).

3. R. Casteels, The relation between the membrane potential and the ion distribution in smooth muscle cells, in: Smooth Muscle, E. Bülbring, A. F. Brading, A. W. Jones, and T. Tomita, eds., pp 70-99, Williams and Wilkins, Baltimore (1970).

4. R. Casteels, G. Droogmans, and H. Hendrickx, Electrogenic sodium pump in smooth muscle cells of the guinea pig taenia coli, Philos. Trans. R. Soc. Lond. (Biol.) 265:47-56 (1973).

5. J. H. Widdicombe, Ouabain-sensitive ion fluxes in the smooth muscle of the guinea-pig's taenia coli, J. Physiol. (Lond.) 266:235-254 (1977).

6. J. H. Widdicombe, and A. F. Brading, A possible role of linked Na and Cl movement in active Cl uptake in smooth muscle, Pfluegers Arch. 386:35-37 (1980).

7. J. H. Szurszewski, Electrical basis for gastrointestinal motility, in: Physiology the Gastrointestinal Tract, L. R. Johnson, ed., pp 1435-1466, Raven Press, New York (1981).

8. B. Johansson, and A. P. Somlyo, Electrophysiology and excitation-contraction coupling, in: Handbook of Physiology, The Cardiovascular System, D. F. Bohr, A. P. Somlyo, and H. V. Sparks, eds., pp 301-323, Waverly Press, Baltimore (1980).

9. K. G. Morgan, T. C. Muir, and J. H. Szurszewski, The electrical basis for contraction and relaxation in canine fundal smooth muscle, J. Physiol. (Lond.) 311:475-488 (1981).

10. T. B. Bolton, Mechanisms of action of transmitters and other substances on smooth muscle, Physiol. Rev. 59:606-718 (1979).

11. A. F. Brading, and P. Sneddon, Evidence for multiple sources of calcium for activation of the contractile mechanism of guinea-pig taenia coli on stimulation with carbachol, Br. J. Pharmacol. 70:229-240 (1980).

12. A. F. Brading, Maintenance of ionic composition, Br. Med. Bull. 35:227-234 (1979).

13. K. G. Morgan, and J. H. Szurszewski, Mechanisms of phasic and tonic actions of pentagastrin on canine gastric smooth muscle, J. Physiol. (Lond.) 301:229-242 (1980).

14. T. Y. El-Sharkawy, K. G. Morgan, and J. H. Szurszewski, Intracellular electrical activity of canine and human gastric smooth muscle, J. Physiol. (Lond.) 279:291-307 (1978).

15. K. A. Kelly, C. F. Code, and L. R. Elveback, Patterns of canine gastric electric activity, Am. J. Physiol. 217:461-470 (1969).

16. K. Milenov, On the rhythm of the electrical and motor activities in intact stomachs and after transverse resections, Izv. Inst. Fiziol. (Sofia) 11:79-86 (1968).

17. K. Sugawara, An electromyographic study on the motility of canine stomach after transection and end-to-end anastomosis, Tohoku J. Exp. Med. 84:113-124 (1964).

18. K. G. Morgan, P. F. Schmalz, V. L. W. Go, and J. H. Szurszewski, Effects of pentagastrin, G_{17} and G_{34} on the electrical and mechanical activities of canine antral smooth muscle, Gastroenterology 75:405-412 (1978).

19. K. G. Morgan, P. F. Schmalz, V. L. W. Go, and J. H. Szurszewski, Electrical and mechanical effects of molecular variants of CCK on antral smooth muscle, Am. J. Physiol. 235:E324-E329 (1978).

20. Y. Hara, and J. H. Szurszewski, Mechanical and intracellular electrical activity of smooth muscle of the canine jejunum, Gastroenterology 80:1169 (1981).

21. C. F. Code, and J. H. Szurszewski, The effect of duodenal and mid small bowel transection on the frequency gradient of the pacesetter potential in the canine small intestine, J. Physiol. (Lond.) 207:281-289 (1970).

22. C. E. Bunker, L. P. Johnson, and T. S. Nelsen, Chronic in situ studies of the electrical activity of the small intestine, Arch. Surg. 95:259-268 (1967).

23. J. Christensen, H. P. Schedl, and J. A. Clifton, The small intestinal basic electrical rhythm (slow wave) frequency gradient in normal men and in patients with a variety of diseases, Gastroenterology 50:309-315 (1966).

24. K. M. Sanders, Excitation-contraction coupling without Ca^{2+} action potentials in smooth muscle, Am. J. Physiol. C356-C361 (1983).

25. J. Christensen, R. Caprilli, and G. F. Lund, Electric slow waves in circular muscle of cat colon, Am. J. Physiol. 217:771-776 (1969).

26. M. Kocylowski, K. L. Bowes, and Y. J. Kingma, Electrical and mechanical activity in the ex vivo perfused total canine colon, Gastroenterology 77:1021-1026 (1979).

27. M. Wienbeck, J. Christensen, and N. W. Weisbrodt, Electro-myography of the colon in the unanesthetized cat, Dig. Dis. Sci. 17:356-362 (1972).

28. J. Christensen, and R. L. Hauser, Longitudinal axial coupling of slow waves in proximal cat colon, Am. J. Physiol. 221:246-250 (1971).

29. J. Marimon, Biträge zur Kenntnis der Darmbewegungen, Inaugural dissertation, Gschade, Berlin (1907)

ELECTROPHYSIOLOGICAL STUDIES OF MYENTERIC NEURONS IN TISSUE CULTURE

Menachem Hanani

Laboratory of Experimental Surgery
Hadassah University Hospital, Mt. Scopus
Jerusalem 91240, Israel

INTRODUCTION

The enteric nervous system (ENS) has been the subject of many studies in recent years, and it is now evident that it is highly developed morphologically, pharmacologically and physiologically. Many kinds of neuron have been identified in the ENS with both the light- and the electron- microscope[1],[2], some 10 putative neurotransmitters have been found by various histochemical methods[3],[4],[5], and up to 8 categories of cells were found by electrophysiological methods[6-9].

The introduction of intracellular recording techniques has greatly contributed to the recent progress in ENS research[6],[7]. This method provides information on the physiology of single neurons and on drug effects at the cellular level. Such information cannot be obtained using the classical methods of organ bath and in vivo pharmacology. The results of the intracellular studies have been described in several recent reviews[8],[9],[10].

Although the individual elements of the ENS are well characterized, little is known about the connectivity of the neurons and their physiological functions. As noted by Furness and Costa[3] a major obstacle for the understanding of the ENS is the lack of correlation between nerve types defined by different criteria - morphological, histochemical and physiological. This situation may be explained by the great complexity of the ENS and also by the experimental difficulties which are encountered in the electrophysiological work.

ENTERIC NEURONS IN TISSUE CULTURE

The tissue culture preparation of enteric neurons[12,13] appears
to be a promising model for studying the ENS. This preparation offers
certain distinct advantages over the conventional in situ preparation
which consists of the longitudinal intestinal muscle with the attached myenteric plexus. In culture the cells are free of muscle and
connective tissue, which facilitates biochemical measurements. The
cells can be observed in great detail with the light microscope for
immunocytochemical and autoradiographic studies. The myenteric and
submucous plexuses are denervated both from each other and from the
extrinsic innervation and thus can be studied in isolation. The neurons are accessible to recording microelectrodes, and as the muscle
is absent, movement problems are eliminated. As the cell surface is
exposed, microinjection of drugs is greatly facilitated.

Jessen and co-workers have shown in a series of recent articles
that enteric neurons in tissue culture retain most of the properties
observed in situ. The cells contain putative neurotransmitters such
as gamma-amino butyric acid (GABA)[13], substance P, VIP and enkephalin [14]. The activity of nerve-associated enzymes such as acetylcholine esterase and monamine oxidase is retained, as well as certain
biochemical properties of the glial cells[15]. The neurons exhibit
many of the ultrastructural features of the in situ preparation, as
observed by light- and electron- microscopy[16,17]. Intracellular
recordings show that myenteric neurons express many of the physiological characteristics found in situ[16].

Enteric neurons in culture undergo several developmental stages.
After 10-12 days in culture the neurons, which had initially formed
a monolayer, migrate and form discrete aggregates, which also contain
glial cells. This has been termed Stage 4 [12]. The aggregates are
interconnected by bundles of nerve fibers and this resembles the
normal organization of the enteric ganglia. Stage 4 cultures offer
a significant experimental advantage over younger cultures as the
fiber bundles can be stimulated electrically in order to elicit synaptic potentials in the neurons. The results described below are from
myenteric neurons dissected from the taenia caeci of the guinea pig
(for details on the preparation see refs 11,12). Most of the cultures
were at stage 4.

THE ORGANIZATION OF STAGE 4 CULTURES

Fig. 1 shows the organization of a typical Stage 4 culture (23
days). Each aggregate contains several neurons whose processes form
the fiber bundles radiating from the aggregates. One cell was injected with horseradish peroxidase (HRP). This neuron sends a single
long process (an axon?) towards a neighboring aggregate and a few
short ones which do not leave the aggregate. A similar arrangement

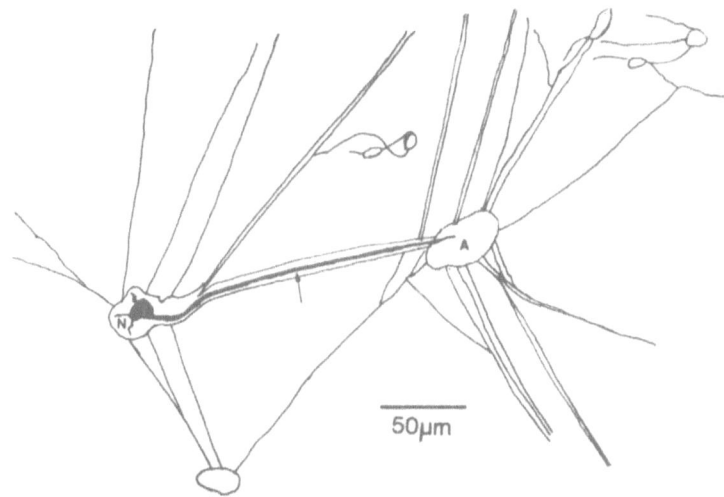

Fig. 1.   Structure of Stage 4 in the development of the myenteric
           plexus from the guinea-pig taenia caeci in culture. Only
           a small part of the culture is shown in this schematic
           drawing. The neurons are grouped in aggregates (A) which
           are connected with bundles of nerve fibers. One neuron (N)
           was stained with HRP. It sends short neurites within the
           aggregate and a long process (arrow) extends into another
           aggregate. The aggregates are associated with large areas
           of fibroblasts which are not shown in the drawing.

is seen in the in situ preparation, where dye injections have shown
that neurons send processes both out of the ganglia and within
them[18]. The aggregates are associated with large areas of fibroblasts
which appear to be important for the development of Stage 4 cultures[12].

ELECTROPHYSIOLOGICAL CHARACTERIZATION OF THE NEURONS

     Glass micropipettes were used to record the electrical activity
of neurons in culture (see ref 16 for experimental details). Four
neuron types were identified. The most common type resembles the
neurons which were defined as type S by Hirst et al.[6] (type 1 according to Nishi and North[7]). These neurons responded with long trains
of action potentials to depolarizing currents delivered from the
recording electrode. The current threshold was quite low (< 0.1 nA).
The spike frequency increased with the current intensity (Fig. 2A,B).
S-type cells responded with several spikes at the offset of a hyperpolarizing pulse - anode break excitation (Fig. 2C). Spontaneous

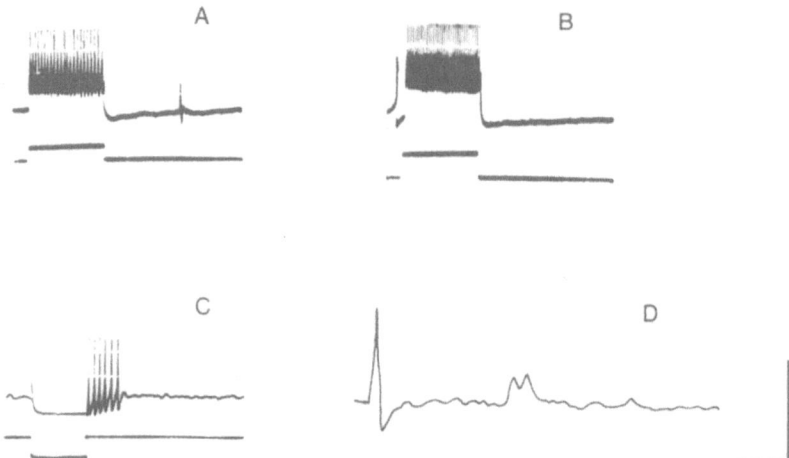

Fig. 2. Intracellular recordings from S-type myenteric neurons in
culture. A depolarizing current (lower trace) caused prolonged discharge of action potentials (A). The spike frequency increased when the current was raised (B). C, an
off-response at the offset of a hyperpolarizing current
pulse. D, spontaneous potentials in an S cell, these potentials appear to be synaptic and one evoked an action potential. Time calibration: 0.8 s for A-C, 60 ms for D; vertical
calibration: 80 mV and 0.4 nA for A and B, 80 mV and 2 nA
for C, 30 mV for D.

activity was observed in most of the S-type cells, consisting of
depolarizing potentials 5–15 mV in amplitude and 10–20 ms in duration.
These potentials occasionally reached threshold and triggered action
potentials (Fig. 2D). The subthreshold potentials resembled the excitatory post-synaptic potentials (epsp's) recorded from S-type neurons
in situ[7,19]. S-type cells responded to electrical stimulation of the
fibers with fast epsp's (hence the designation "S"). These potentials
are caused by acetylcholine acting on nicotinic receptors[6,7]. Similar
responses were obtained in culture (see below). Action potentials in
S-type cells in situ are blocked by tetrodotoxin[6,7], but this has
not been tested in culture.

A second kind of neuron found in culture resembles the AH-type
described by Hirst et al.[6] (type 2 according to Nishi and North[7])
These cells were less excitable than the S cells and required higher
currents to elicit an action potential (about 0.5 nA). Long depolarizing currents evoked only 1–4 spikes (Fig. 3) and there was no anode
break excitation. Other distinguishing characteristics of AH neurons

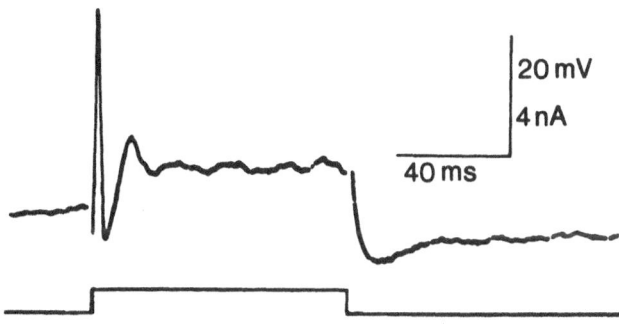

Fig. 3. Response of an AH neuron to a depolarizing current. A relatively high current (0.5 nA) was required to elicit a single
spike, which was followed by prolonged hyperpolarization.

are: a prolonged after-hyperpolarization associated with action potential discharge (Fig. 3) and tetrodotoxin-resistant action potential[6],[7].
It should be mentioned, however, that after-hyperpolarizations were
also observed in S-type cells (Fig. 2A,B). According to North[8] this
potential is recorded in both cell types but is less prominent in
S cells. According to the earlier reports[6],[7] AH cells do not receive
synaptic inputs and it was proposed that they may be sensory neurons.
More recent work[20] showed that fast epsp's can be recorded from AH
cells, and that repetitive stimulation of the nerve fibers evokes
a slow (about 1 min) epsp in AH cells[19] and also in S cells[21]. During
the slow epsp the excitability of AH is greatly augmented[22] and it
was concluded that these neurons are not primary sensory cells but
may be motor neurons or may drive motor neurons [10].

Additional cell categories were defined according to the pattern
of their spontaneous activity. The mechanism that drives this activity
may be either synaptic or intrinsic to the cell (pacemaker). One kind
of spontaneous activity seen in culture consisted of bursts of subthreshold potentials which occasionally evoked an action potential
(Fig. 4). The potentials occurred in groups containing variable numbers
of potentials (usually 2-6) which appeared at irregular intervals.
Similar behavior was observed by Wood[9] and the cells were designated
"erratic bursters". Evidence from extracellular recordings indicates
that this activity is generated by synaptic mechanisms[23] and this
also appears to be the case in culture, as shown by the following
experiments. Current injections in erratic bursters in culture did
not alter the basic activity pattern, but either inhibited the firing
of action potentials (hyperpolarizing currents, Fig. 4A), or facilitated spike discharge (depolarizing currents, Fig. 4B). Application of
the nicotinic blocker hexamethonium greatly suppressed the bursting
activity, which indicates that nicotinic cholinergic synapses are

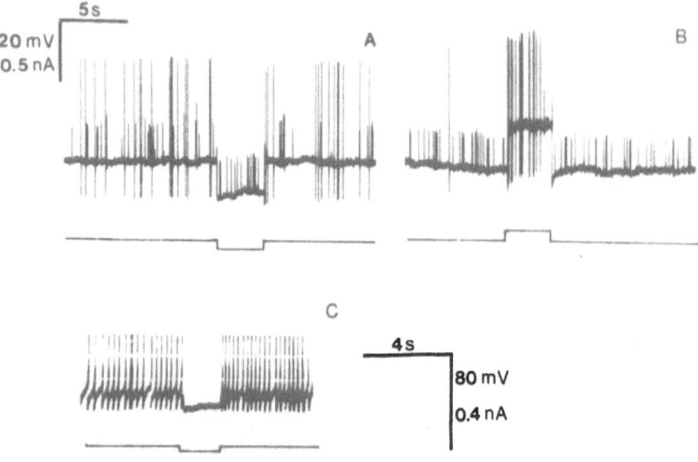

Fig. 4. Patterns of spontaneous activity. A, erratic burster; subthreshold potentials appeared in bursts and occasionally
evoked an action potential. A hyperpolarizing current inhibited the action potentials but had no effect on the low-
amplitude potentials. B, a depolarizing current greatly
increased the spike frequency. C, a pacemaker neuron; the
spontaneous activity was completely abolished by a weak
hyperpolarizing current.

involved in this process. The existence of pacemaker cells has been
proposed on the basis of physiological considerations[9],[10] but in situ
they have been observed only with extracellular electrodes. Such
cells were identified in the cultured myenteric plexus, but seem to
be quite rare (3 in 170). Pacemaker cells fired spikes at a fairly
steady rate for over 2 hours. In the example shown in Fig. 4C the
cell fired at 4 Hz. The spontaneous activity in this cell was very
sensitive to changes in the membrane potential. Weak hyperpolarizing
currents eliminated this activity; note the difference between the
pacemaker cell and the one depicted in Fig. 4A,B. The mechanism which
generates the rhythmic activity is apparently intrinsic but there is
no information about its nature.

It is generally accepted that sensory cells are present in the
ENS, but only little is known on this subject. Using extracellular
electrodes, Wood[24] recorded responses from 3 types of mechanosensitive
units which differ in the pattern of the discharge in response to
mechanical stimuli. Similar cells were not observed by intracellular
recordings, and no attempt has yet been made to identify them in
culture.

Electronmicroscopic work has demonstrated that enteric neurons in culture possess structures which are typical for chemical synapses[16,17]. The occurrence of spontaneous epsp-like potentials also indicated the presence of synaptic inputs. A more direct evidence for active synapses was the recording of evoked synaptic potentials. The electrical stimuli were delivered with fine metal electrodes which were placed on a fiber bundle or on an adjacent aggregate. Brief (0.1-0.5 ms) stimuli evoked in many cases fast epsp's which resembled the spontaneous subthreshold potentials (Figs. 5,6). These potentials were reduced in size, or even completely suppressed by the cholinergic nicotinic antagonists curare and hexamethonium (Fig. 5). The drug effects were reversible in 10-30 min. These results are in accord with previous work in situ which showed that the fast epsp's are nicotinic[6,7].

The cultured neurons are multiply innervated as was shown by two methods: 1. As the stimulus intensity was increased additional

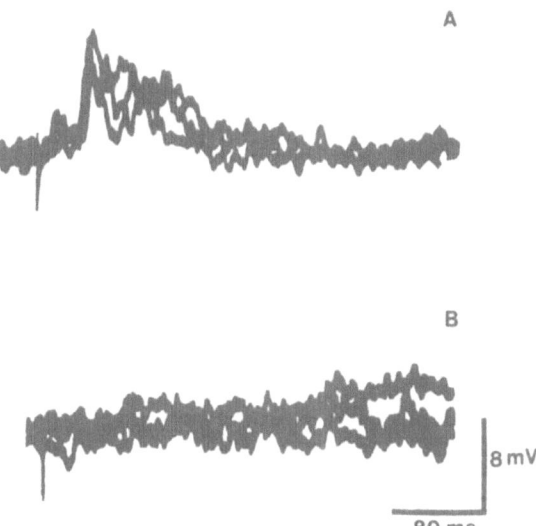

Fig. 5.   Evoked synaptic potentials. The electrical stimulus was delivered at the downwards deflection and 3 responses were superimposed. The width of the responses in A suggests more than a single synaptic input. The response was eliminated after the injection of curare (B). The drug was delivered from a micropipette (containing a 1.3 10^{-4}M curare solution) by a 1.5 s long pressure pulse.

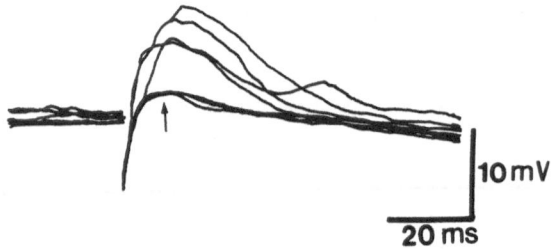

10 mV

20 ms

Fig. 6. The effect of stimulus intensity on the evoked synaptic
        potentials. With low intensity stimulation a synaptic poten-
        tial of low amplitude was evoked (arrow). When the stimulus
        intensity was raised there was an abrupt increase in the
        response amplitude indicating the presence of additional
        synaptic inputs.

epsp's appeared, due to the activation of fibers with higher thresh-
olds (Fig. 6). 2. The stimulating electrode could sometimes be moved
during the recording to other fiber bundles and this allowed the
observation of additional inputs. Up to 6 inputs in a single neuron
were found using these methods, but this is probably an underestimate,
as in no case could all the fiber bundles be stimulated. Multiple
cholinergic synaptic inputs in the ENS have been demonstrated also
in situ[6]. Repetitive electrical stimulation of the fiber bundles
was found to elicit slow synaptic potentials in situ[21,22]. Such potentials were not observed in culture.

The temporal pattern of the stimuli strongly affects the synaptic
potentials. At a stimulating frequencies over 1 Hz there was a progressive reduction of the epsp amplitude (Fig. 7). Such a "run-down"
effect has been observed in situ[7,19] and was shown to be presynaptic
in origin.

PHARMACOLOGY OF CULTURED MYENTERIC NEURONS

The ENS is sensitive to a great variety of neuroactive compounds
and has become a useful tool for studying drug effects. For example,
the actions of substance P (SP) at the cell membrane level were first
studied in detail in myenteric neurons[25]. Information on the site of
action and mechanisms of actions of opiates and enkephalins was obtained from work on this preparation[26,27]. Cultured enteric neurons

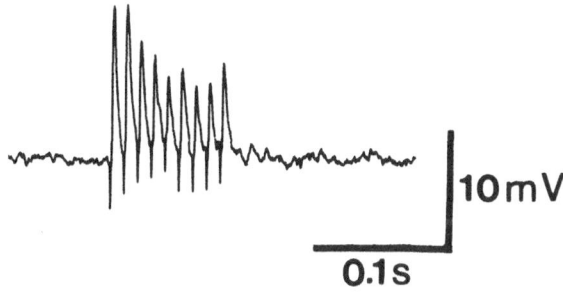

Fig. 7.   Repetitive stimulation. During stimulation of the nerve
           fiber at high frequency there was a progressive decline in
           the epsp amplitude. Stimulus frequency 50 Hz.

are very suitable for such pharmacological studies since no diffusion
barrier exists for drug applications; the cells are clearly visible;
and muscle movement is eliminated.

Ionophoretic application of acetylcholine (ACh) showed that
many neurons in culture are sensitive to this transmitter. The response to a brief pulse of ACh was a fast, epsp-like potential which
could evoke a spike[16]. The reversal potential of the ACh responses
was measured by injecting depolarizing currents, and its value was
about -10 mV[16]. This value is typical for nicotinic synapses[29], and
this indicates that the conductance change caused by ACh involves
the same ionic species as other autonomic nicotinic synapses.

While it is agreed that the mediator of the fast epsp in enteric
neurons is ACh, the identity of transmitter mediating the slow epsp
is controversial. Wood and Mayer[22] presented evidence that this transmitter is serotonin. North and his co-workers[25,29] proposed that it
is SP, and showed that the response to serotonin may also be hyperpolarizing[30]. The actions of these two compounds were tested on myenteric neurons in culture. The drugs were injected by pressure
pulses (10-400 ms long) from micropipettes which were about 10 µm
from the cell surface. A large proportion of the neurons was sensitive
to SP or to serotonin, and many cells responded to both. Most of the
neurons were depolarized by SP and by serotonin, but in most cases
each drug elicited a distinctive response. In about 70% of the cases
the SP-induced depolarization was very prolonged (1-2 min) and had
a latency of 3-5 s (Fig. 8A). Responses to serotonin were much faster:

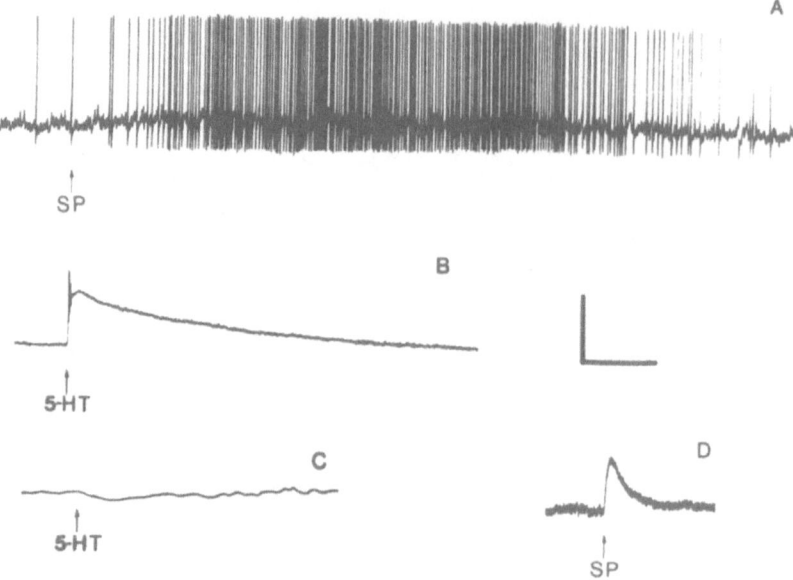

Fig. 8. Comparison of the actions of substance P (SP) and serotonin
(5-HT). The drugs were injected by brief pressure pulses
from pipettes containing SP (3 10^{-5}M) or 5-HT (4 10^{-4}M);
the results are from 4 different cells. A, prolonged response to SP. B, depolarizing response to 5-HT. C, hyperpolarizing response to 5-HT. D, a fast response to SP. Time
calibration: 5 s for A, 2.5 s for B, 0.25 s for C, 2 s for
D; vertical calibration: 20 mV for A and C, 40 mV for B,
10 mV for D.

the duration was 0.5-10 s and the latency 20-50 ms (Fig. 8B,C). The
depolarization caused by SP was usually accompanied by an increased
rate of action potentials (Fig. 8A), whereas during the depolarization evoked by serotonin there was only a short burst of spikes
(Fig. 8B). In about 20% of the cells sensitive to serotonin the response was hyperpolarizing, with a time course similar to that of
the depolarizing response (Fig. 8C). These results indicate that
SP is a more likely candidate as the mediator of the slow epsp.

Previous reports on the actions of SP on myenteric[25] and central[31] neurons have demonstrated the slow responses to this peptide.
Surprisingly, SP evoked in 30% of the cultured enteric neurons a
fast response, which lasted up to only 5 s and with latencies of
30-50 ms (Fig. 8D). This could represent a novel type of SP response

and may be the physiological correlate of the two sub-types of SP receptors found by binding assay[32].

CONCLUSIONS

Tissue culture has become recognized as a reproducible and convenient model of a variety of nervous systems[33]. The introduction of the tissue culture preparation of enteric neurons has opened many interesting possibilities. The recent work on this preparation has demonstrated its suitability as a model for the ENS[15,16], and this is further supported by the results described above. The electrophysiological experiments show that myenteric neurons in culture retain many of the physiological and pharmacological characteristics observed in situ.

The employment of new methods, notably intracellular electrophysiology and immunocytochemistry, has greatly contributed to the understanding of the ENS. Studying this system in culture will enable further work which previously has been difficult or impossible. It appears that this preparation will be particularly useful for investigating synaptic interactions and pharmacology, as shown in the present work. With additional work this system will become more standardized and may be employed for testing the actions of new drugs at the cellular level. Other topics that may be explored using the cultures are the effects of various toxic agents, the development of the ENS and the interactions between the nerves and the intestinal muscle.

ACKNOWLEDGMENTS

This work was supported by grants from the Wellcome Trust and the Leonard Wolfson Foundation for Scientific Research.

REFERENCES

1. G. Gabella, Fine structure of the myenteric plexus in the guinea-pig ileum, J. Anat. 111:69 (1972).
2. G. Gabella, Innervation of the gastrointestinal tract, Int. Rev. Cytol. 59:129 (1979).
3. J.B. Furness and M. Costa, Types of nerves in the enteric nervous system, Neuroscience 5:1 (1980).
4. M.D. Gershon, The enteric nervous system, Ann. Rev. Neurosci. 4:227 (1981).
5. M. Schultzberg, T. Hokfelt, G. Nilsson, L. Terenius, J.H. Rehfeld, M. Brown, R. Elde, M. Goldstein and S. Said, Distribution of

peptide- and catecholamine- containing neurons in the gastrointestinal tract of rat and guinea-pig: immunohistochemical
studies with antisera to substance P, vasoactive intestinal
polypeptide, enkephalins, somatostatin, gastrin/cholecysto-
kinin, neurotensin and dopamine beta-hydroxylase, Neuroscience
5:689 (1980).

6.   G.D.S. Hirst, M.E. Holman and I. Spence, Two types of neurones
     in the myenteric plexus of duodenum in the guinea-pig, J.
     Physiol. (Lond.) 236:303 (1974).

7.   S. Nishi and R.A. North, Intracellular recording from the my-
     enteric plexus of the guinea-pig ileum, J. Physiol. (Lond.)
     231:471 (1973).

8.   R.A. North, Electrophysiology of the enteric nervous system,
     Neuroscience 7:315 (1982).

9.   J.D. Wood, Electrophysiology of the enteric nervous system,
     in: "Physiology of the Gastrointestinal Tract", L.R. Johnson,
     ed., Raven Press, New York (1981).

10. J.D. Wood, Intrinsic neural control of intestinal motility,
     Ann. Rev. Physiol. 43:33 (1981).

11. K.R. Jessen, J.D. McConnell, R.D. Purves, G. Burnstock and J.
     Chamley-Campbell, Tissue culture of mammalian enteric neurons,
     Brain Research 152:573 (1978).

12. K.R. Jessen, M.J. Saffrey and G. Burnstock, The enteric nervous
     system in tissue culture. I. Cell types and their interactions
     in explants of the myenteric and submucous plexuses from
     guinea pig, rabbit and rat, Brain Research 262:17 (1983).

13. K.R. Jessen, R. Mirsky, M.E. Dennison and G. Burnstock, GABA
     may be a transmitter in the vertebrate peripheral nervous
     system, Nature (Lond.) 281:71 (1979).

14. K.R. Jessen, M.J. Saffrey, S. Van Noorden, S.R. Bloom, J.M.
     Polak and G. Burnstock, Immunohistochemical studies of the
     enteric nervous system in tissue culture and in situ: local-
     ization of vasoactive intestinal polypeptide (VIP), substance
     P and enkephalin immunoreactive nerves in the guinea pig gut,
     Neuroscience 5:1717 (1980).

15. K.R. Jessen, M.J. Saffrey, P. Baluk, M. Hanani and G. Burnstock,
     The enteric nervous system in tissue culture. III. Studies
     on neuronal survival and the retention of biochemical and
     morphological differentiation, Brain Research 262:49 (1983).

16. M. Hanani, P. Baluk and G. Burnstock, Myenteric neurons express
     electrophysiological and morphological diversity in tissue
     culture, J. Auton. Nerv. Syst. 5:155 (1982).

17. P. Baluk, K.R. Jessen, M.J. Saffrey and G. Burnstock, The en-
     teric nervous system in tissue culture. II. Ultrastructural
     studies on cell types and their interrelationships, Brain
     Research 262:37 (1983).

18. J.P. Hodgkiss and G.M. Lees, Morphological studies of electro-
     physiologically identified myenteric plexus neurons of the

guinea-pig ileum, Neuroscience 8:593 (1983).

19. J.D. Wood and C.J. Mayer, Intracellular study of electrical activity of Auerbach's plexus in guinea-pig small intestine, Pfluegers Arch. 374:265 (1979).

20. P. Grafe, J.D. Wood and C.J. Mayer, Fast excitatory postsynaptic potentials in AH (type 2) neurons of guinea-pig myenteric plexus, Brain Research 103:349 (1979).

21. S.M. Johnson, Y. Katayama and R.A. North, Slow synaptic potentials in neurones of myenteric plexus, J. Physiol. (Lond.) 301:505 (1980).

22. J.D. Wood and C.J. Mayer, Intracellular study of tonic-type enteric neurons in guinea pig small intestine, J. Neurophysiol. 42:569 (1979).

23. J.D. Wood, Effects of elevated magnesium on discharge of myenteric neurons in cat small intestine, Am. J. Physiol. 229: 657 (1975).

24. J.D. Wood, Sensory mechanisms in enteric ganglia, in: "Motility of the Digestive Tract", M. Wienbeck, ed., Raven Press, New York (1982).

25. Y. Katayama, R.A. North and J.T. Williams, The actions of substance P on neurones of the myenteric plexus of the guinea-pig small intestine, Proc. R. Soc. Lond. B 206:191 (1979).

26. K. Morita and R.A. North, Opiates and enkephalins reduce the excitability of neuronal processes, Neuroscience 6:1943 (1981).

27. K. Morita and R.A. North, Opiate activation of potassium conductance in myenteric neurons: inhibition by calcium ion, Brain Research 242:145 (1982).

28. M.J. Dennis, A.J. Harris and S.W. Kuffler, Synaptic transmission and its duplication by focally applied acetylcholine in parasympathetic neurons in the heart of the frog, Proc. R. Soc. Lond. B 177:509 (1971).

29. S.M. Johnson, Y. Katayama, K. Morita and R.A. North, Mediators of slow synaptic in the myenteric plexus of the guinea-pig ileum, J. Physiol. (Lond.) 32:125 (1981).

30. S.M. Johnson, Y. Katayama and R.A. North, Multiple actions of 5-HT on myenteric neurons of the guinea-pig ileum, J. Physiol. (Lond.) 304:459 (1980).

31. R.A. Nicoll, B.E. Alger and C.E. Jahr, Peptides as putative excitatory neurotransmitters: carnosine, enkephalin, substance P and TRH, Proc. R. Soc. Lond. B 210:133 (1980).

32. L.L. Iversen, Substance P, Brit. Med. Bull. 38:277 (1982).

33. P.G. Nelson and M. Lieberman, eds., "Excitable Cells in Tissue Culture", Plenum, New York (1981).

GASTROINTESTINAL NERVES, HORMONES AND AUTACOIDS IN RELATION TO

HUMAN GASTROINTESTINAL MOTILITY

Alan Bennett

Department of Surgery
King's College School of Medicine and Dentistry
The Rayne Institute
123 Coldharbour Lane
London SE5 9NU   UK

Excellent reviews of the topics in this chapter have been written by various authors in the volumes edited by Bertaccini (1982).   The work here is confined mainly to the human gastrointestinal tract, and discusses both older and recent research.

Types of intramural nerves which affect muscle activity

The motor nerves within the gut wall can be divided pharmacologically into at least 4 types, although in the guinea-pig there are up to 9 morphologically distinguishable types of neurone (Gabella, 1972; Cook & Burnstock, 1976).   The identities of only 2 transmitters are conclusively established, acetylcholine in the cholinergic nerves and noradrenaline in the adrenergic nerves. (In addition, catecholamines can reach the gut via the bloodstream). Acetylcholine and noradrenaline have satisfied the criteria, mainly in animal studies, that their release can be detected following nerve stimulation, and that their addition mimics the effect of nerve stimulation.   In addition, acetylcholine and noradrenaline are stored in neurones which contain their precursors, synthesizing and inactivating pathways.   Drugs that modify nerve responses similarly modify the effects of added acetylcholine or noradrenaline (Furness & Costa, 1982).

The transmitters for the other 2 pathways (nerves which are neither cholinergic nor adrenergic but which produce inhibition or excitation respectively), have not been conclusively identified. Table 1 lists various non-peptide substances and their distributions in the gut, and Table 2 shows peptides that can affect gastro-

TABLE 1.   GUT NON-PEPTIDES THAT CAN AFFECT GASTROINTESTINAL MUSCLE

Substance	Neuronal	Extra-neuronal
Acetylcholine	+	
Noradrenaline/adrenaline	+	
5-Hydroxytryptamine	+	+
Adenosine triphosphate	+	+
γ-Amino butyric acid	?	
Histamine		+
Dopamine		+
Eicosanoids		+

TABLE 2.   GUT PEPTIDES THAT CAN AFFECT GASTROINTESTINAL MUSCLE

Substance	Neuronal	Extra-neuronal
Vasoactive intestinal polypeptide	+	
Cholecystokinin fragments	+	
Pancreatic polypeptide	+	
Angiotensin	+	
Physalaemin	+	
Neurotensin	?	+
Substance P	+	+
Enkephalins	+	+
Somatostatin	+	+
Bombesin	+	+
Cholecystokinin		+
Secretin		+
Gastrin		+
Motilin		+
Gastric inhibitory peptide		+
Enterogastrone		+

intestinal muscle.   Debate exists about whether the inhibitory nerves utilise adenosine triphosphate or vasoactive intestinal polypeptide as a transmitter, a subject covered in depth by Furness & Costa (1982).   Perhaps there are nerves that use one of these transmitters, nerves that use the other transmitter, and some that use both (or, of course, neither).   Different transmitters may co-exist in the same nerve (Burnstock, 1978; Chan-Palay et al. 1978).

5-Hydroxytryptamine (5-HT)

5-HT has potent actions on the human gastrointestinal tract, with marked regional differences.   It inhibits muscle from gastric antrum and colon, both in vitro and in vivo, but it stimulates the small intestine.   The site of action for both the inhibitory and the excitatory effects in these human tissues appears to be directly on the muscle.   The responses are blocked by methysergide, a drug used to treat the diarrhoea due to 5-HT produced by carcinoid tumours.   Since methysergide blocks muscle 5-HT receptors but not those on nerves, a presynaptic role for 5-HT in nerve transmission in human gut is unlikely, in contrast to some other species.   It is not known if 5-HT has a physiological role in human gut motility. 5-HT is discussed more fully by Bennett & Whitney (1966) and Bennett (1970).

Histamine

The actions of histamine on human gastrointestinal muscle are even more varied than those of 5-HT (see Bennett & Whitney, 1966, and Bennett, 1970), and histamine does not seem to play important roles in normal or disordered human gut motility.   However, histamine H_2 receptors may help regulate gastric emptying since in monkeys the selective H_2 agonist dimaprit increased gastric emptying whereas cimetidine caused a decrease (Dubois et al., 1977, 1978); H_1 receptors may play a similar role in the rat (Scarpignato et al, 1981).   The possible physiological role of histamine in gastrointestinal motility has been discussed by Bertaccini et al. (1980).

Dopamine

There is no evidence for gut dopamine-containing neurones, and little evidence for a role of dopamine in gut motility, but dopamine interacts with receptors in the gastrointestinal tract.   Although metoclopramide is a dopamine antagonist, it stimulates upper gastrointestinal motility by a non-dopaminergic mechanism, as discussed by Sanger (1984) elsewhere in this book.

Prostaglandins, leukotrienes and related substances

Prostanoids (prostaglandins and other cyclo-oxygenase products) seem to be involved in various aspects of gut activity, as described in the review by Bennett & Sanger (1984) elsewhere in this book and by Bennett & Sanger (1982) and Robert & Ruart (1982). Little is known about the possible roles of leukotrienes and other lipoxygenase products in gastrointestinal motility, but their ability to stimu-late colonic secretion may play a role in diarrhoea (Musch et al 1982).

Peptides

Numerous polypeptides occur within the gastrointestinal tract or can reach it through the blood stream. Table 2 lists peptides found in the gut. Tables 3-6 list the diverse actions of many peptides on the motility of the human lower oesophageal sphincter, stomach, small intestine and colon. They sometimes show different responses according to the region and the muscle layer, and different responses in vivo and in vitro. The interpretations of the findings are difficult and complex, and there are also many other factors to consider. With hormones that normally reach the gut via the blood-stream, infusion of exogenous pure hormone into the blood may mimic the physiological or pathological events in vivo. However, when a substance is normally released within a tissue, how appropriate is administration via the blood supply? Perhaps diffusion into iso-lated muscle strips more closely mimics release within tissues (Bennett, 1968). As in all gut motility studies it is not feasible to extrapolate from muscle activity to movement of contents, since propulsion results from a pressure gradient which can be produced by contraction and/or relaxation. Other factors are the amounts, source and purity of peptides used, interactions between peptides and other substances, and species differences. Furthermore, some peptides can release others, eg gastrin, cholecystokinin (CCK), secretin, gastric inhibitory peptide (GIP), somatostatin and cal-citonin release insulin; secretin, bombesin, and insulin release pancreatic polypeptide (Adrian et al. 1978, De Magistris et al. 1979; Floyd et al. 1977). Bombesin also stimulates the release of human enteroglucagon, motilin, neurotensin, vasoactive intes-tinal polypeptide (VIP) and glucagon, and somatostatin inhibits the release of insulin, glucagon, gastrin, enteroglucagon, CCK and secretin (see Bertaccini, 1982, Table 1, p3).

Of the hormones discussed, CCK, gastrin and secretin are those for which there is most evidence for a physiological role in modu-lating gastrointestinal motility. Other peptides generally affect gut muscle only at substantially higher blood concentrations than occur with the naturally released substances. The use of the term "physiological concentration" is justified with regard to blood levels, but may not be appropriate for the local concentrations achieved by substances released within muscles; local concentra-tions are not known, but if they are comparable to concentrations

TABLE 3.   EFFECTS OF PARACRINE OR ENDOCRINE PEPTIDES ON HUMAN
            LOWER OESOPHAGEAL SPHINCTER MOTILITY IN VIVO

Peptide

Angiotensin	↑ Haulica et al., 1980
Bombesin	↑ F. Marletta, cited by Bertaccini 1982
Calcitonin	O, but inhibits gastrin ↑ , Waldeck et al. 1973, Debat et al. 1976
CCK and cerulein	↓ Resin et al. 1973, Sturdevant & Kun 1974, Fisher et al. 1975, Scheurer & Halter 1976, Pandolfo et al. 1977
Gastrin	↑ Cohen et al. 1971, Lipshutz et al. 1973, Waldeck et al. 1973, Christiansen & Borgeskov 1974, Jaffer et al. 1974, Siewert et al. 1974, Walker et al. 1975, Corazziari et al. 1978, Henderson et al. 1976, Jensen et al. 1978, Lane et al. 1979, Orlando & Bozymski 1979 ↑ or ↓ Scheurer & Halter 1976
Glucagon	↓ Jennewein et al. 1973, Waldeck et al 1973, Christiansen & Borgeskov 1974, Jaffer et al. 1974, Hogan et al. 1975, Christiansen et al. 1977
Insulin	↓ during hypoglycaemia Castell 1971
Motilin	↑ Lux et al. 1976, Rösch et al. 1976
Neurotensin	↓ Thor et al. 1980a
Secretin	O Cohen & Lipshutz 1971, Lipshutz 1976, Itoh et al. 1978 ↓ Christiansen & Borgeskov 1974, Scheurer & Halter 1976
Vasopressin	↑ Boesby & Pedersen 1974

↑ contraction,   O no effect,   ↓ relaxation

This topic has been reviewed by Christensen (1975), Goyal &
Rattan (1978), and Fisher & Cohen (1980).   In vitro, gastrin
or pentagastrin can contract strips of human lower oesophageal
sphincter (Bennett et al. 1967, Bennett 1968, Burleigh 1979).

TABLE 4. EFFECTS OF PARACRINE OR ENDOCRINE PEPTIDES ON HUMAN GASTRIC MOTILITY

Peptide	In vivo	In vitro
Angiotensin		↑ LC Bertaccini et al.1974b ↑ LC Bertaccini et al.1974a,b
Bombesin Bradykinin	↑ antrum, body/fundus Bertaccini et al.1974b	↑ LC Bertaccini et al.1974b Bertaccini 1982
CCK and cerulein	O Fisher & Cohen 1973 ↑ pylorus ↓ antrum: Bortolotti et al.1970, Grossi et al.1970, Munk et al.1978 ↓ stomach Bortolotti et al.1975 ↑ antrum Szekely et al.1975 ↓ or ↑ antrum Kwong et al.1972 ↓ gastric emptying: Johnson et al.1966, Dinoso et al.1969, Chey et al.1970, Stertz et al.1974	↑ LC Cameron et al.1970, Bertaccini et al.1974b, Vizi et al.1973
Gastrin/pentagastrin	↑ : Misiewicz et al.1967, Szekely et al.1969, Kwong et al.1972, Monges & Salducci 1972 ↓ pylorus: Fisher et al.1973, Fisher & Boden 1976 ↑ pylorus ↓ antrum White & Keighley 1978 ↑ pylorus and antrum Munk et al.1978 ↓ gastric emptying: Hunt & Ramsbottom 1967, Meves et al.1975, Hamilton et al.1976, MacGregor et al.1978 ↑ gastric emptying in peptic ulcer patients, Gamblin et al.1977, Dubois & Castell 1978 ↑ gastric emptying in normal subjects at pH7 Fiddian-Green & Quinn 1978, Pittinger et al.1978	↑ or O LC Bennett et al.1967 ↑ or ↓ Cameron et al.1970 ↑ LC Vizi et al.1973
Glucagon	↓ Stunkard et al.1955, Necheles et al.1966, Bortolotti et al.1975	O LC Cameron et al.1970

Peptide	In vivo	In vitro
Glucagon	↓ emptying Hradsky et al.1973, Meves et al.1975, Chernish et al.1978, Miller et al.1974a,1978a	
Insulin	↑ or ↓ see review by Bachrach 1953 for early references ↓ Shapiro & Woodward 1959	
Motilin	↓ emptying Ruppin et al.1975 ↑ emptying Bloom et al.1978, Christofides et al.1979a,b	↑ LC Strunz et al.1975
Neurotensin	↓ Blackburn et al.1980	
Secretin	↓ Kwong et al.1972, Bortolotti et al.1975 ↓ emptying: Dinoso et al.1969, Chey et al.1970, Vagne & Andre 1971, Meves et al.1975	↓ LC Cameron et al.1970
Substance P		O LC Bertaccini et al.1974b
TRH	↑↓ Dolva et al.1978, Dolva & Stadaas 1979	
VIP		↓ Strunz et al.1978

↑ contraction, O no effect, ↓ relaxation, L longitudinal muscle, C circular muscle.

93

TABLE 5. EFFECTS OF PARACRINE OR ENDOCRINE PEPTIDES ON THE MOTILITY OF HUMAN SMALL INTESTINE

Peptide	In vivo	In vitro
Angiotensin		↑ LC Bertaccini et al. 1971, 1974b
Bombesin	↓ Bertaccini et al. 1974b, Corazziari et al. 1974	↑ LC Bertaccini et al. 1974a,b, 1979
Bradykinin		↑ L, ↓ or OC Fishlock 1966 ↑ L Duodenum, Bertaccini et al. 1979
CCK & cerulein	↑ Post-duodenum: Monod 1964, Morin et al. 1966, Dahlgren 1967, Parker & Beneventano 1970, Ramorino et al. 1970, Bertaccini & Agosti 1971, Bertaccini et al. 1971, Hedner & Rorsman 1972, Bertaccini 1973, Gutierrez et al. 1974a, Levant et al. 1974, Dollinger et al. 1975, Novak 1975, Öigaard et al 1975, Corazziari et al. 1976, Rapela et al. 1976, Fleckstein & Öigaard 1977, Lorber 1980, Robbins et al. 1980, Sargent et al. 1980	↑ LC post-duodenum, Bertaccini et al. 1971, 1974b
	↑ Duodenum: Guttierrez et al. 1974a	
	O Duodenum: Fleckstein & Öigaard 1977	
	↓ Duodenum: Aldercreutz et al. 1960, Torsoli et al. 1961, Bertaccini & Agosti 1971, Bertaccini et al. 1971, Labò et al. 1972, Öigaard et al. 1975, Osnes 1975, Labò & Bortolotti 1976	↓ ? Duodenum, Bertaccini et al. 1971 ↓ L Duodenum, Bertaccini et al. 1979
Gastrin/ pentagastrin	↑ Smith & Hogg 1966, Waterfall et al. 1972 Inconclusive, Logan & Connell 1976	O LC Bennett et al. 1967

94

Peptide	In vivo	In vitro
Glucagon	↓ Doteval & Koch 1963, Chernish et al.,1972, Hicks & Turnberg 1974, Whalen 1974, Corazziari 1976, Labò & Bortolotti 1976 ↑↓ Miller et al.,1978b	
Insulin	↑ Quigley & Solomon 1929/1930 ↓ Shapiro & Woodward 1959	
Motilin	↑ Ruppin et al.,1976, Lux et al.1978, Ruppin et al.,1979, Vantrappen et al.,1979	↑ C Strunz et al.,1975
Neurotensin	Produces fed myoelectric pattern, Thor et al., 1980b	
Secretin	↓ Chey et al.,1967, Waterfall et al.1972, Gutierrez et al.,1974a,b, Dollinger et al.,1975, Osnes 1975, Corazziari 1976, Labò & Bortolotti 1976	
Substance P	↑ Liljedahl et al.,1958, Pernow 1960, 1963	↑ L Duodenum,Bertaccini et al.1979, Pernow 1960, 1963
Vasopressin	↑ Brazeau 1975	

↑ Contraction, O no effect, ↓ relaxation, L longitudinal muscle, C circular muscle, ? muscle layer not stated

95

TABLE 6. EFFECTS OF PARACRINE OR ENDOCRINE PEPTIDES ON HUMAN COLONIC MOTILITY

Peptide	In vivo	In vitro
Angiotensin		↑ LC Fishlock & Gunn 1970, Bertaccini et al.1971, 1974b
Bombesin	↓ or O Bertaccini et al.1974b	↑ LC Bertaccini et al. 1974b
Bradykinin	↓ Murrell & Deller 1967	↓ ↑ L, ↓ C Fishlock 1966
CCK and cerulein	↑ Ramorino et al.1970, Bertaccini et al.1971, Dinoso et al.1973	↑ L Egberts & Johnson 1977, ↑ LC Bertaccini et al 1971, 1974b
Enkephalins		O Weiss et al.1976 Weak ↑ LC and inhibit ↑ to nerve stimulation Sanger et al. 1982
Gastrin/penta-gastrin	↑ Smith & Hogg 1966 ↑ or ↓ Logan & Connell 1966 weak ↓ Misiewicz et al.1967	LC O or weak ↑ Bennett et al.1967
Glucagon	↓ Taylor et al.1975	↑ L Egberts & Johnson 1977
Insulin	↓ Shapiro & Woodward 1959, Killenberg & Cornwell 1964	
Motilin	↑ Rennie et al.1980	↑ L, O C Strunz et al. 1975
Neurotensin		↑ LC Sanger et al. 1982
Secretin	↓ Dinoso et al. 1973	
Substance P		↑ LC Bertaccini et al.1974b ↑ C Bennett 1975
VIP		↑ LC Sanger et al. 1982
Vasopressin	↑ Gothlin 1972, Brazeau 1975	

↑ contraction, O no effect, ↓ relaxation, L longitudinal muscle, C circular muscle.

of acetylcholine released from stimulated nerves they may be in the mM range. The extent to which injections of single substances are relevant to physiology is not clear. Apart from the fact that interacting mixtures of hormones are released in vivo, some released hormones (eg gastrin), may be present in several forms which contribute to the total biological activity.

The list of peptides in Table 3-6 is incomplete because in some cases there has been no work done in man or with human isolated gastrointestinal muscles (eg calcitonin, coherin, gastric inhibitory peptide, pancreatic polypeptide, thyrotropin releasing hormone (TRH), and VIP). The latter substance would appear to be a strong candidate as the (a ?) transmitter at non-adrenergic-non-cholinergic inhibitory nerves (see Furness & Costa, 1982). However, relatively little work has been done with this peptide on human alimentary muscle.

Adenosine triphosphate (ATP)

The possibility that ATP acts as a transmitter at non-adrenergic-non-cholinergic inhibitory nerve endings in the gut is one of considerable debate. ATP often relaxes some parts of the human gut in vitro, but there may be no effect or even contraction (Stockley & Bennett, 1977).

Relationships between gastrointestinal intrinsic innervation and motility

The studies described above show that there may be marked regional differences in the responses of gut muscles, as well as differences between the longitudinal and circular muscles from the same region. Experiments on hundreds of human gastrointestinal muscles from human surgical specimens also demonstrate variations in neurogenic responses to nicotine or electrical stimulation (Bennett & Whitney, 1966; Bennett & Stockley, 1975). The findings are discussed fully in those papers, but in brief there are usually opposite effects on stimulation of the cholinergic or adrenergic nerves. The cholinergic excitatory drive to the gastrointestinal tract is predominant in the highly motile small intestine, overshadowing the adrenergic inhibitory nerves, whereas adrenergic inhibition predominates in the less-motile colon and distal ileum. With strips of stomach, responses to stimulation of the intrinsic nerves are more difficult to elicit than with intestinal strips, consistent with the fact that gastric motor activity relies heavily on the extrinsic vagal innervation, unlike the intestine. The electrical stimulation experiments also indicate some differences in the innervation of the longitudinal and circular muscles, with the circular muscles from various regions often showing greater inhibitory responses than in longitudinal strips (Bennett & Stockley,

1975). Regional differences in gastrointestinal innervation, together with other regional dissimilarities (eg intrinsic muscle activity and eelctrical slow waves), account for the marked variations in gastrointestinal motility which enable each region to perform its special functions.

There is no doubt about the physiological importance of the cholinergic nerves for motility in vivo, but the role of the adrenergic nerves is less clear. For example, to what extent are adrenergic responses in vitro are due to the abnormal overflow of noradrenaline, eg from vasomotor nerves? With regard to pathology, however, increased adrenergic activity may be important in paralytic ileus (Neely & Catchpole, 1971).

REFERENCES

Adlercreutz, E., Pettersson, T., Adlercreutz, H., Gribbe, P. & Wegelius, C. (1960). Effect of cholecystokinin on duodenal tonus and motility. Acta Med Scand 167: 339-342.

Adrian, T.E., Bloom, S.R., Besterman, H.S. & Bryant, M.G. (1978). PP-physiology and pathology. In: Bloom, S.R. (ed) Gut Hormones. Churchill Livingstone, Edinburgh pp254-260.

Bachrach, W.H. (1953). Action of insulin hypoglycemia on motor and secretory functions of the digestive tract. Physiol Rev 33: 566-592.

Bennett, A. (1968). The biological effects of gastrin. J.Roy. Coll. Physns., Lond. 2: 269-273.

Bennett, A. (1968). The relationship between in vitro studies of gastrointestinal muscle and motility of the gastrointestinal tract in vivo. Am J Dig Dis 13, 410-414.

Bennett, A. (1970). Control of gastrointestinal motility by substances occurring in the gut wall. Rendic. R. Gastroenterol. 2: 133-142.

Bennett, A (1975). Pharmacology of colonic muscle. Gut 16: 307-311.

Bennett, A., Misiewicz, J.J. & Waller, S.L. (1967). Analysis of the motor effects of gastrin and pentagastrin on the human alimentary tract in vitro. Gut 8: 470-474.

Bennett, A. & Sanger, G.J. (1982). Prostaglandins. In: Mediators and Drugs in Gastrointestinal Motility II. Handb. Exp. Pharm. 59/II, ed G. Bertaccini, Springer Verlag, Berlin, pp 219-248.

Bennett, A. & Stockley, H.L. (1975). The innervation of the human alimentary tract and its relation to function. Gut 16: 443-453.

Bennett, A. & Whitney, B. (1966). A pharmacological study of the motility of the human gastrointestinal truact. Gut 7: 307-316.

Bertaccini, G. (1973). Action of caerulein on the motility of the biliary system and the gastrointestinal tract in man. Med. Chir Dig 2: 133-138.

98

Bertaccini, G. (1982). In: Mediators and Drugs in Gastrointestinal Motility II Handbook of Experimental Pharmacology 59/II, ed G. Bertaccini, Springer-Verlag, Berlin.

Bertaccini, G., Agosti, A. (1971). Action of caerulein on intestinal motility in man. Gastroenterology 60: 55-63.

Bertaccini, G. Agosti, A. & Impicciatore, M. (1971). Caerulein and gastrointestinal motility in man. Rend. Gastroenterol. 3: 23-27.

Bertaccini, G., Impicciatore, M., Molina, E. & Zappia, L. (1974a). Action of some natural and synthetic peptides on the motility of human gastrointestinal tract in vitro. In: Daniel,E.E. (ed) Fourth Int.Symp.Gastrointest. Motility. Mitchell, Vancouver, pp287-292.

Bertaccini, G., Impicciatore, M., Molina, E. & Zappia, L. (1974b). Action of bombesin on human gastrointestinal motility. Rend. Gastroenterol. 6: 45-51.

Bertaccini, G., Scarpignato, C. & Coruzzi, G. (1980). Histamine receptors and gastrointestinal motility. In: Torsoli, A. Lucchelli, P.E & Brimblecombe, R.W. (eds). European symposium of further experience with H_2-receptor antagonists in peptic ulcer disease and progress in histamine research. Excerpta Medica., Amsterdam, pp251-261.

Bertaccini, G. Zappia, L. & Molina, E. (1979). "In vitro" duodenal muscle in the pharmacological study of natural compounds. Scand. J. Gastroenterol. (Suppl 54) 14: 87-93.

Blackburn, A.M., Bloom, S.R., Long, R.G., Fletcher, D.R., Christofides, N.D., Fitzpatrick, M.L. & Baron, J.H. (1980). Effect of neurotensin on gastric function in man. Lancet 1: 987-989.

Bloom, S.R., Christofides, N.D., Modlin, I. & Fitzpatrick, M.L. (1978). Effect of motilin on gastric emptying of solid meals in man. Gastroenterology 74: A1010.

Boesby, S. & Pedersen, S.A. (1974). The effect of vasopressin on resting gastroesophageal sphincter pressure in man. Scand. J. Gastroenterol, 9: 587-590.

Bortolotti, M., Miglioli, M., Lanfranchi, G.A. & Barbara, L. (1970). L'azione della caeruleine sull' attivita elettrica e meccanica dello stomaco nell'uomo. Gastroenterologia 22: 147-179.

Bortolotti, M., Sanavio, C., Sansone, G. & Labò, G. (1975). Modifications in human gastric motility induced by secretin and by glucagon. Rend Gastroenterol. 7: 240.

Bortolotti, M., Sansone, G. & Sanavio, C. (1975). Effects of some gut hormones on gastric myoelectric and mechanical activity in man. Rend Gastroenterol. 7: 135.

Brazeau, P. (1975). Agents affecting the renal conservation of water. In: Goodman, L.S. & Gilman, A. (eds) The Pharmacological basis of therapeutics. Macmillan, New York, pp848-859.

Burleigh, D.E. (1979). The effects of drugs and electrical field stimulation on the human lower oesophageal sphincter. Arch. Int. Pharmacodyn Ther. 240: 169-176.

Burnstock, G. (1978).   Do some sympathetic neurones release both
    noradrenaline and acetylcholine?   Progr Neurobiol 11: 205-222.
Cameron, A.J., Phillips, S.F. & Summerskill, W.H.J. (1967).
    Effect of cholecystokinin on motility of human stomach and
    gallbladder muscle "in vitro'.   Clin Res 15: 416-420.
Cameron, A.J., Phillips, S.F. & Summerskill, W.H.J. (1970).   Com-
    parison of effects of gastrin, cholecystokinin-pancreozymin,
    secretin, and glucagon on human stomach muscle in vitro.
    Gastroenterology 59: 539-545.
Castell, D.O. (1971).   Changes in lower esophageal sphincter pres-
    sure during insulin-induced hypoglycemia.   Gastroenterology
    61: 10-15.
Chan-Palay, V., Jonsson, G. & Palay, S.L. (1978).   Serotonin and
    substance P co-exist in neurons of the rat's central nervous
    system.   Proc. Nat. Acad. Sci. USA 75: 1582-1586.
Chernish, S.M., Miller, R.E., Rosenak, B.D. & Schulz, N.E. (1972).
    Hypotonic duodenography with the use of glucagon.   Gastro-
    enterology 63: 392-398.
Chernish, S.M., Brunelle, R.R., Rosenak, B.D. & Ahmadzai, S. (1978).
    Comparison of the effects of glucagon and atropine sulfate on
    gastric emptying.   Am. J. Gastroenterol. 70: 581-586.
Chey, W.Y., Lorber, S.H., Kusakcioglu, O. & Hendricks, J. (1967).
    Effect of secretin and pancreozymin-cholecystokinin on motor
    function of stomach and duodenum.   Fed. Proc. 26: 383, A710.
Chey, W.Y., Hitanant, S., Hendricks, J. & Lorber, S.H. (1970).
    Effect of secretin and cholecystokinin on gastric emptying and
    gastric secretion in man.   Gastroenterology 58: 820-827.
Christensen, J. (1975).   Pharmacology of the esophageal motor fun-
    tion.   Annu. Rev. Pharmacol. Toxicol. 15: 243-258.
Christiansen, J. & Borgeskov, S. (1974).   The effect of glucagon
    and the combined effect of glucagon and secretin on lower
    esophageal sphincter pressure in man.   Scand. J. Gastro-
    enterol. 9: 615-618.
Christiansen, J., Lauritzen, K., Moesgaard, J. & Holst, J.J. (1977).
    Effect of endogenous and exogenous glucagon on pentagastrin-
    stimulated lower esophageal sphincter pressure in man.   Scand.
    J. Gastroenterol. 12: 33-36.
Christofides, N.D., Long, R.G., Fitzpatrick, M.L. & Bloom, S.R.
    (1979a).   Motilin increases the rate of gastric emptying of
    glucose.   Gut 20: A924.
Christofides, N.D., Modlin, I.M., Fitzpatrick, M.L. & Bloom, S.R.
    (1979b).   Effect of motilin on the rate of gastric emptying
    and gut hormone release during breakfast.   Gastroenterology
    76: 903-907.
Cohen, S. & Lipshutz, W.H. (1971).   Hormonal regulation of human
    lower esophageal sphincter competence: interaction of gastrin
    and secretin.   J. Clin. Invest. 50: 449-454.
Cohen, S., Lipshutz, W. & Hughes, W. (1971).   Role of gastrin
    supersensitivity in the pathogenesis of lower esophageal
    sphincter hypertension in achalasia.   J.Clin.Invest.50:1241-1247.

Cook, R.D. & Burnstock, G. (1976). The ultrastructure of Auerbach's plexus in the guinea-pig. I. Neuronal elements. J. Neurocytol. 5: 171-194.

Corazziari, E. (1976). Mechanical activity of the second portion of human duodenum. Rend. Gastroenterol. 8: 64.

Corazziari, E., Pozzessere, C., Dani, S., Anzini, F. & Torsoli, A. (1978). Lower oesophageal sphincter response to intravenous infusions of pentagastrin in normal subjects, antrectomized and achalasic patients. Gut 19: 1121-1124.

Corazziari, E., Tonelli, F., Pozzessere, C., Dani, S., Anzini, F. & Torsoli, A. (1976). The effects of graded dosed of caerulein on human jejunal motor activity. Rend. Gastroenterol. 8: 190-193.

Corazziari, E., Torsoli, A., Delle Fave, G.F., Melchiorri, P., Habib, I. & Fortunee (1974). Effects of bombesin on the mechanical activity of the human duodenum and jejunum. Rend. Gastroenterol. 6: 55-59.

Dahlgren, S. (1967). The effect of cholecystokinin on duodenal motility. Acta. Chir. Scand. 133: 403-405.

Debas, H.T., Farooq, O. & Grossman, M.I. (1975). Inhibition of gastric emptying is a physiological action of cholecystokinin. Gastroenterology 68: 1211-1217.

Debat, J., Couturier, D., Roze, C. & Debray, C. (1976). Effects of thyrocalcitonin on pentagastrin induced contraction of the lower esophageal sphincter in normal and in patients with achalasia. Gastroenterology 70: 876.

De Magistris, L., Delle Fave, G., Khon, A. & Schwartz, T.W. (1979). Stimulation of pancreatic polypeptide and gastrin secretion by bombesin in man. Ital. J. Gastroenterol. 11: 139A.

Dent, J., Dodds, W.J., Hogan, W.J. & Arndorfer, R.C. (1978). CCK-OP: a useful agent for evaluating lower esophageal sphincter (LES) denervation in human. Gastroenterology 74: A1025.

Dinoso, V., Chey, W.Y., Hendricks, J. & Lorber, S.H. (1969). Intestinal mucosal hormones and motor function of the stomach in man. J. Appl. Physiol. 26: 326-329.

Dinoso, V.P., Meshkinpour, H. Lorber, S.H. Gutierrez, J.G. & Chey, W.Y. (1973). Motor responses of the sigmoid colon and rectum to exogenous cholecystokinin and secretin. Gastroenterology 65: 438-444.

Dollinger, H.C., Berz, R., Raptis, S., Üexkull, T. Von, & Goebell, H. (1975). Effects of secretin and cholecystokinin on motor activity of human jejunum. Digestion 12: 9-16.

Dolva, L.O., Stadaas, J.O. (1979). Action of thyrotropin-releasing hormone on gastrointestinal functions in man. III. Inhibition of gastric motility in response to distension. Scand. J. gastroenterol. 14: 419-423.

Dolva, L.O., Hanssen, K.F., Stadaas, J. & Berstad, A. (1978). Thyrotropin releasing hormone inhibits the pentagastrin stimulated gastric secretion and gastric motility in man. Scand. J. Gastroenterol (Suppl 49) 13: 49.

Doteval, G. & Koch, N.G. (1963). The effect of glucagon on intestinal motility in man. Gastroenterology 45: 364-367.

Dubois, A. & Castell, D.O. (1978). Abnormal gastric emptying response to pentagastrin in duodenal ulcer. Scand. J. Gastroenterol. (Suppl 49) 13: 50.

Dubois, A., Hamilton, B. & Castell, D.O. (1977). Histamine H_2 receptor involved in gastric emptying. Gastroenterology 72: A1051.

Dubois, A., Nompleggi, D., Myers, L. & Castell, D.O. (1978). Histamine H_2 receptor stimulation increases gastric emptying. Gastroenterology 74: A1028.

Egberts, E-H. & Johnson, A.G. (1977). The effect of cholecystokinin on human taenia coli. Digestion 15: 217-222.

Fiddian-Green, R.G. & Quinn, T.S. (1978). Physiological actions of luminal gastrin in human gastric juice. Gut 19: A435.

Fisher, R.S. & Boden, G. (1976). Gastrin inhibition of the pyloric sphincter. Am. J. Dig. Dis. 21: 468-472.

Fisher, R.S. & Cohen, S. (1973). Pyloric sphincter dysfunction in patients with gastric ulcer. N. Engl. J Med. 288: 273-276.

Fisher, R.S. & Cohen, S. (1980). Effects of gut hormones on gastrointestinal sphincters. In: Jerzy Glass G. (ed) Gastrointestinal hormones. Raven, New York, pp 613-638.

Fisher, R.S. Lipshutz, W. & Cohen, S. (1973). The hormonal regulation of pyloric sphincter function. J. Clin. Invest. 52: 1289-1296.

Fisher, R.S. Lipshutz, W. & Cohen S. (1973). The hormonal regusmall and large intestine. Nature, 212: 1533-1535.

Fishlock, D.J. & Gunn, A. (1970). The action of angiotensin on the human colon "in vitro". Br. J. Pharmacol. 39: 34-39.

Fleckenstein, P. & Öigaard, A. (1977). Effects of cholecystokinin on the motility of the distal duodenum and the proximal jejunum in man. Scand. J. Gastroenterol. 12: 375-378.

Floyd, J.C., Fajans, S.S. Pek, S. & Chance, R.E. (1977). A newly recognised pancreatic polypeptide; plasma levels in health and disease. Rec. Prog. Horm. Res. 33: 519-570.

Furness, J.B. & Costa, M. (1982). Identification of gastrointestinal neurotransmitters. In: Mediators and Drugs in Gastrointestinal Motility I. Handb. Exp. Pharmacol. ed G Bertaccini, Springer-Verlag, Berlin, pp383-462.

Gabella, G. (1972). Fine structure of the myenteric plexus in the guinea-pig ileum. J. Anat. 111: 69-97.

Gamblin, G.T., Dubois, A. & Castell, D.O. (1977). Contrasting effect of pentagastrin on gastric emptying in normals and patients with gastric ulcer. Clin.Res. 25: A17.

Göthlin, J. (1972). Vasopressin in the elimination of intestinal gas. Acta.Radiol. Diagn. 12: 100-112.

Goyal, R.K. & Rattan, S. (1978). Neurohumoral, hormonal, and drug receptors for the lower esophageal sphincter. Gastroenterology 74: 598-619.

Grossi, F., Del Duca, T., Spada, S. & Grassi, M. (1970). Influenze della caeruleina sulla motilita gastrointestinale nell'uomo. Clin. Ter. 54: 321-327.

Gutiérrez, J.G., Chey, W.Y. & Dinoso, V.P. (1974a). Actions of cholecystokinin and secretin on the motor activity of the small intestine in man. Gastroenterology 67: 35-41.

Gutiérrez, J.G., Chey, W.Y., Shah, A. & Holzwasser, G. (1974b). Use of secretin in hypotonic duodenography. Radiology, 113: 563-566.

Hamilton, S.G., Sheiner, H.J. & Quinlan, M.F. (1976). Continuous monitoring of the effect of pentagastrin on gastric emptying of solid food in man. Gut, 17: 273-279.

Hara, Y. (1980). Actions of tetragastrin on smooth muscles of human stomach. Eur. J. Physiol. 386: 127-134.

Haulica, I., Stanciu, C.W., Frasin, M., Cijevschi, C., Balan, G. & Pancu, D. (1980). Effects of angiotensin on the human lower esophageal sphincter. Abstr. XI Int. Congr. Gastroenterol. Thieme, Stuttgart, p28.

Hedner, P. & Rorsman, G. (1972). Acceleration of the barium meal through the small intestine by the C-terminal octapeptide of cholecystokinin. Am. J. Roentgenol, 116: 245-248.

Henderson, J.M., Lidgard, G., Osborne, D.H., Carter, D.C. & Heading, R.C. (1978). Lower oesophageal sphincter response to gastrin Pharmacological or physiological? Gut 19: 99-102.

Hicks, T. & Turnberg, L.A. (1974). Influence of glucagon on the human jejunum. Gastroenterology, 67: 1114-1118.

Hogan, W.J., Dodds, W.J., Hoke, S.E., Reid, D.P., Kalkhoff, R.K. & Arndorfer, R.C. (1975). Effect of glucagon on esophageal motor function. Gastroenterology 69: 60-65.

Hradsky, M., Stockbrügger, R. & Oestberg, H. (1973). The effect of glucagon on gastric motility, the pylorus and reflux of bile into the stomach during gastroscopic examination. Scand. J. Gastroenterol. (Suppl 20) 8: 26.

Hunt, J.N. & Ramsbottom, N. (1967). Effect of gastrin II on gastric emptying and secretion during a test meal. Br. Med. J. 4: 386-387.

Jaffer, S.S., Makhlouf, G.M., Schorr, B.A. & Zfass, A.M. (1974). Nature and kinetics of inhibition of lower esophageal sphincter pressure by glucagon. Gastroenterology 67: 42-46.

Jennewein, H.M., Waldeck, F., Siewert, R., Weiser, F. & Thimm, R. (1973). The interaction of glucagon and pentagastrin on the lower oesophageal sphincter in man and dog. Gut 14: 861-864.

Jensen, D.M., McCallum, R.W. & Walsh, J.H. (1978). Failure of atropine to inhibit gastrin-17 stimulation of the lower esophageal sphincter in man. Gastroenterology 75: 825-827.

Johnson, L.P., Brown, J.C. & Magee, D.F. (1966). Effect of secretin and cholecystokinin-pancreozymin extracts on gastric motility in man. Gut 7: 52-57.

Killenberg, P.G. & Cornwell, G.G. (1964). Effect of insulin hypoglycemia on the human sigmoid colon. Am. J. Dig. Dis. 9:221-228.

Kwong, N.K., Brown, B.H., Whittaker, G.E. & Duthie, H.L. (1972). Effect of gastrin I, secretin and cholecystokinin-pancreozymin on the electrical activity, motor activity, and acid output of the stomach in man. Scand. J. Gastroenterol. 7: 161-170.

Labò, G. & Bortolotti, M. (1976). Effect of gut hormones on myoelectric and manometric activity of the duodenum in man. Rend. Gastroenterol. 8: 64.

Labò, G., Barbara, L., Lanfranchi, G.A., Bortolotti, M. & Miglioli, M. (1972). Modification of the electrical activity of the human intestine after serotonin and caerulein. Dig. Dis. Sci. 17: 363-373.

Lane, W.H., Ippoliti, A.F. & McCallum, R.W. (1979). Effect of gastrin heptadecapeptide (G17) on oesophageal contractions in patients with diffuse oesophageal spasm. Gut, 20: 756-759.

Levant, J.A., Kun, L., Jachna, J., Sturdevant, R.A.L. & Isenberg, J.I. (1974). The effects of graded doses of C-terminal octapeptide of cholecystokinin on small intestinal transit time in man. Am. J. Dig. Dis. 19: 207-209.

Liljedahl, S.O., Mattsson, O. & Pernow, B. (1958). The effect of substance P on intestinal motility in man. Scand. J. Clin. Lab. Invest. 10: 16-25.

Lipshutz, W.H. (1976). Physiology of the gastro-oesophageal junction and hiatus hernia. In: Bouchier, I.D. (ed) Recent Advances in Gastroenterology, vol 3, Churchill Livingstone, Edinburgh, London, pp1-26.

Lipshutz, W., Gaskins, R.D., Lukash, W.M. & Sode, J. (1973). Pathogenesis of lower esophageal sphincter incompetence. N. Engl. J. Med. 289: 182-184.

Logan, C.J.H. & Connell, A.M. (1966). The effect of a synthetic gastrin-like pentapeptide (I.C.I. 50, 123) on intestinal motility in man. Lancet I: 996-999.

Lorber, S.H. (1980). Small bowel transit time. Am. J. Roentgenol. 135: 648-649.

Lux, G., Rösch, W., Domschke, S., Domschke, W., Wünsch, E., Jaeger, E. & Demling, L. (1976). Intravenous 13-Nle-motilin increases the human lower esophageal sphincter pressure. Scand. J. Gastroenterol (Suppl 39) 11: 75-79.

Lux, G. Strunz, U., Domschke, S., Femppel, J., Rösch, W. & Domschke, W. (1978). 13-Nle-motilin and interdigestive motor and electrical activity of human small intestine. Gastroenterology, 74: A1058.

MacGregor, I.L., Wiley, Z.D. & Martin, P.M. (1978). Effect of pentagastrin infusion on gastric emptying rate of solid food in man. Am. J. Dig. Dis. 23: 72-75.

Manville, I.A. & Chuinard, E.G. (1934). Studies on gastric hunger mechanisms. Am. J. Dig. Dis. 1: 688-693.

Meves, M., Beger, H.G. & Hüthwohl, B. (1975). The effect of some gastrointestinal hormones on gastric evacuation in man. In: Vantrappen, G (ed) Fifth International Symposium on Gastrointestinal Motility. Typoff, Herentals, pp 327-332.

104

Miller, R.E., Chernish, S.M., Skucas, J., Rosenak, B.D. & Rodda, B.E. (1974). Hypotonic roentgenography with glucagon. Am.J. Roentgenol. Radium. Ther. Nuc. Med. 121:264-274.

Miller, R.E., Chernish, S.M., Brunelle, R.L. & Rosenak, B.D. (1978a). Dose response to intramuscular glucagon during hypotonic radiography. Radiology 127:49-53.

Miller, R.E., Chernish, S.M., Brunelle, R.L. & Rosenak, B.D. (1978b). Double-blind radiographic study of dose-response to intravenous glucagon for hypotonic duodenography. Radiology, 127: 55-59.

Misiewicz, J.J., Holdstock, D.J. & Waller, S.L. (1967). Motor responses of the human alimentary tract to near-maximal infusions of pentagastrin. Gut 8: 463-469.

Monges, H. & Salducci, J. (1972). Variations of the gastric electrical activity in man produced by administration of pentagastrin and by introduction of water or liquid nutritive substance into the stomach. Am. J. Dig. Dis. 17: 333-338.

Monod, E. (1964). Action entéro-kinétique de la cécékine. Arch. Mal. Appar. Dig. 53: 607-608.

Morin, G., Besançon, F., Grall, A., Jouve, R., Garat, J.P. & Debray, C. (1966). La cholécystokinine appliquée au radiodiagnostique de l'intestine grêle: nouvelle technique de radiocinématographie complète en quelques minutes, avec 62 observations. Entret Bichat Radiol. 247-250.

Munk, J.F., Hoare, M. & Johnson, A.G. (1978). Hormonal influence of pyloric diameter and antral motility in man: Gut 19: A435.

Murrell, T.G.C. & Deller, D.J. (1967). Intestinal motility in man: the effect of bradykinin on the motility of the distal colon. Dig. Dis. Sci. 12: 568-576.

Musch, M.W., Miller, R.J., Field, M. & Siegel, M.I. (1982). Stimulation of colonic secretion by lipoxygenase metabolites of arachidonic acid. Science 217: 1255-1256.

Necheles, H., Sporn, J. & Walker, L. (1966). Effect of glucagon on gastrointestinal motility. Am. J. Gastroenterol. 45: 34-39.

Neely, J. & Catchpole, B.N. (1971). Ileus: the restoration of alimentary tract motility by pharmacological means. Br.J. Surg. 58: 21-28.

Novak, D. (1975). Beschleunigung der Dünndarmpassage mit Caerulein. Dtsch. Med. Wochenschr. 100: 2488-2491.

Öigaard, A., Dorph, S., Christensen, K.C. & Christiansen, L. (1975). The effect of cholecystokinin on electrical spike potentials and intraluminal pressure variations in the human small intestine. Scand. J. Gastroenterol. 10: 257-262.

Osnes, M. (1975). The effect of secretin and cholecystokinin on the duodenal motility in man. Scand. J. Gastroenterol (Suppl 35) 10: 22-26.

Orlando, R.C. & Bozymski, E.M. (1979). The effects of pentagastrin in achalasia and diffuse esophageal spasm. Gastroenterology 77: 472-477.

Pandolfo, N., Bortolotti, M., Nebiacolombo, G., Sansone, G. & Mattioli, F. (1977). Action of caerulein on lower oesophageal sphincter pressure. In: Speranza V, Basso N, Lezoche E. (eds) Symp. Gastrointestinal Horm. and Pathol. of the Dig. System. Rome, June 13-15. Arti. Grafiche. Tris, Rome.

Parker, J.G. & Beneventano, T.C. (1970). Acceleration of small bowel contrast study by cholecystokinin. Gastroenterology 58: 679-684.

Pernow, B. (1960). Effect of substance P on smooth muscle. In: Polypeptides Which Affect Smooth Muscles and Blood Vessels. Ed M. Schachter, Pergamon Press, Oxford pp 171-178.

Pernow, B. (1963). Pharmacology of substance P. Ann. NY. Acad. Sci. 104: 393-402.

Pittinger, G. Kothary, P. & Fiddian-Green, R.G. (1978). The effect of luminal gastrin on the rate of gastric emptying. Clin. Res. 26: A665.

Quigley, J.P. (1928/1929). Action of insulin on the gastric motility of man. Proc. Soc. Exp. Biol. Med. 26: 769-770.

Ramorino, M.L., Ammaturo, M.V. & Anzini, F. (1970). Effects of caerulein on small and large bowel motility in man. Rend. Gastroenterol. 2: 172-175.

Rapela, R.O., Gutstein, D., Naveiro, J.J. & Morel, J. (1976). Acción de la ceruleina sobre la motilidad intestinal. Rev. Argent. Chir. 30: 14-16.

Rennie, J.A., Christofides, N.D., Ellis, M.R., Michener, P., Johnson, A.G. & Bloom, S.R. (1980). Effect of motilin on human colonic activity. Clin. Sci. 58: 12.

Robbins, A.H., Wetzner, S.M. & Landy, M.D. (1980). Ceruletide-assisted examination of the small bowel. Am. J. Roentgenol. 134: 343-347.

Robert, A. & Ruart, M.J. (1982). Effects of prostaglandins on the digestive system. In: Prostaglandins. Ed J.B. Lee, Elsevier, New York, pp 113-176.

Rosch, W., Lux, G., Domschke, S., Domschke, W., Wünsch, E., Jaeger, E. & Demling, L. (1976). Effect of 13-NLE-motilin on lower esophageal sphincter pressure in man. Gastroenterology 70: A931.

Ruppin, H., Domschke, S., Domschke, W., Wünsch, E., Jaeger, E. & Demling, L. (1975). Effects of 13 -Nile-motlin in man - inhibition of gastric evacuation and stimulation of pepsin secretion. Scand. J. Gastroenterol. 10: 199-202.

Ruppin, H., Sturm, G., Westhoff, D., Domschke, S., Domschke, W., Wünsch, E. & Demling, L. (1976). Effect of 13-Nle-motilin on small intestinal transit time in healthy subjects. Scand. J. Gastroenterol. (Suppl 39) 11: 85-88.

Ruppin, H., Soergel, K.H., Dodds, J.W., Wood, C.M. & Domschke, W. (1979). Effects of the inter-digestive motor complex (IMC) and 13-norleucine motilin (NLEM) on fasting intestinal flow rate and velocity in man. Gastroenterology, 76: 1231.

Sanger, G.J., Jackson, A. & Bennett, A. (1982), unpublished.

Sargent, E.N., Halls, J.M., Colletti, P. & Wieler, M. (1980). Efficacy and tolerance of ceruletide in radiography of the small intestine. Radiology, 136: 57-60.

Scarpignato, C., Loruzzi, G. & Bertaccini, G. (1981). The effect of histamine and related compounds on gastric emptying of the rat. Pharmacology, 23: 185-191.

Schapiro, H. & Woodward, E.R. (1959). The action of insulin hypoglycemia on the motility of the human gastrointestinal tract. Am. J. Dig. Dis. 4: 787-791.

Scheurer, U. & Halter, F. (1976). Lower esophageal sphincter reflux in reflux esophagitis. Scand. J. Gastroenterol. 11: 629-634.

Siewert, R., Weiser, F., Jennewein, H.M. & Waldeck, F. (1974). Clinical and manometric investigations of the lower esophageal sphincter and its reactivity to pentagastrin in patients with hiatus hernia. LES-pentagastrin-test. Digestion, 10: 287-297.

Smith, A.N. & Hogg, D. (1966). Effect of gastrin II on the motility of the gastrointestinal tract. Lancet 1: 403-404.

Sterz, P., Guth, P. & Sturdevant, R. (1974). Gastric emptying in man: delay by octapeptide of cholecystokinin and L-tryptophan. Clin. Res. 22: A174.

Stockley, H.L. & Bennett, A. (1977). Relaxations mediated by adrenergic and non-adrenergic nerves in human isolated taenia coli. J. Pharm. Pharmac. 29: 533-537.

Strunz, U., Domschke, W., Mitznegg, P. et al (1975). Analysis of the motor effects of 13-norleucine motilin on the rabbit, guinea-pig, rat, and human alimentary tract in vitro. Gastroenterology, 68: 1485-1491.

Strunz, U., Domschke, W., Domschke, S., Mitznegg, P., Wünsch, E., Jaeger, E. & Demling, L. (1976). Gastroduodenal motor response to natural motilin and synthetic position 13-substituted motilin analogues: a comparative in vitro study. Scand. J. Gastroenterol. (Suppl 39) 11: 199-203.

Strunz, U., Mitznegg, P., Domschke, S., Domschke, W., Wünsch, E. & Demling, L. (1978). VIP antagonizes motilin-induced antral contractions in vitro. In: Duthie, H.L. (ed) Gastrointestinal motility in health and disease. MTP Press, Lancaster, pp 125-131.

Stunkard, S.J., Van Itallie, T.B. & Reis, B.B. (1955). The mechanism of satiety. Effect of glucagon on gastric hunger contraction in man. Proc. Soc. Exp. Biol. Med. 89: 258-261.

Sturdevant, R.A.L. & Kun, T. (1974). Interaction of pentagastrin and the octapeptide of cholecystokinin on the human lower oesophageal spincter. Gut 15: 700-702.

Szekely, A., Major, T. & Romvari, H. (1975). Röntgenkymographische Untersuchung der die Magenperistaltik steigernden Wirkung von intravenös gegebenem Caerulein. Fortschr Roentgenstr 122: 167-169.

Szekely, A., Major, T. & Romvari, H. (1969). Über die Wirkung von Pentagastrin auf die Magenmotilität. Fortsch. Geb. Roentgenstr. Ver. Roentgenprax. 111: 841-846.

Taylor, I., Duthie, H.L. Cumberland, D.C. & Smallwood, R. (1975). Glucagon and the colon. Gut 16: 973-978.

Thor, K., Rosell, S., Rokaeus, A., Nyquist, O., Levenhaupt, A., Kager, L. & Folkers, K. (1980a). Plasma concentrations of neurotensin-like immunoreactivity (NTLI) and lower esophageal sphincter (LES) pressure in man following infusion of (Gln^4)-neurotensin. Abstr. XIth Int. Congr. Gastroenterol. Thieme, Stuttgart, p 28.

Thor, K., Rokaeus, A., Kager, L., Folkers, K. & Rosell, S. (1980b). (Gln^4)-neurotensin inhibits the interdigestive migrating motor complex in man. In: Bloom S.R., Polak, J.M. (eds) Regulatory peptides, suppl 1. Elsevier/North-Holland Biomedical. Amsterdam, Oxford, New York, p S114.

Torsoli, A., Ramorino, M.L. Colagrande, C. & Demaio, G. (1961). Experiments with cholecystokinin. Acta. Radiol. (Stockh) 55: 193-206.

Vagne, M. & André, C. (1971). The effect of secretin on gastric emptying in man. Gastroenterology, 60: 421-424.

Vantrappen, G., Janssens, J., Peeters, T.L., Bloom, S.R., Christofides, N.D. & Hellemans, J. (1979). Motilin and the interdigestive migrating motor complex in man. Dig. Dis. Sci. 24: 497-500.

Vizi, S.E., Bertaccini, G., Impicciatore, M. & Knoll, J. (1973). Evidence that acetylcholine released by gastrin and related polypeptides contributes to their effect on gastrointestinal motility. Gastroenterology, 64: 268-277.

Waldeck, F., Sievert, R., Jennewein, H.M. & Weiser, F. (1973). Das Druckprofil im unteren Ösophagussphinkter beim Menschen und seine Beeinflussung durch Gastrin, Calcitonin und Glucagon. Dtsch. Med Wochenschr. 98: 1059-1063.

Walker, C.O., Frank, S.A., Manton, J. & Fordtran, J.S. (1975). Effect of continuous infusion of pentagastrin on lower esophageal sphincter pressure and gastric acid secretion in normal subjects. J. Clin. Invest. 56: 218-225.

Waterfall, W.E., Brown, B.H., Duthie, H.L. & Whittaker, G.E. (1972). The effects of humoral agents on the myoelectrical activity of the terminal ileum. Gut, 13: 528-534.

Weiss, S.M., Hughes, S.R., Paskin, D.L. & Lipshutz, W.H. (1976). Effects of drugs and hormones on human colon muscle. Clin. Res. 24: A293.

Whalen, G.A. (1974). Glucagon and the small gut. Gastroenterology 67: 1284-1286.

White, C.M. & Keighley, M.R.B. (1978). An explanation of the paradoxical effect of pentagastrin on gastric motility. Gut, 19: A434-A435.

Yamagishi, T. & Debas, H.T. (1978). Cholecystokinin inhibits gastric emptying by acting on both proximal stomach and pylorus. Am. J. Physiol. 234: E375-E378.

DISTRIBUTION OF GUT PEPTIDES AND THEIR ACTIONS

Susan M. Wood

Department of Medicine

Hammersmith Hospital, Du Cane Road, London, W12

INTRODUCTION

Secretin was the first peptide to be identified within the gastrointestinal tract, and provided the prototype for the classical hormones, in that it is released by acid from endocrine cells in the duodenum and passes via the circulation to its effector organ, the exocrine pancreas[1]. The discovery of gastrin was soon to follow[2], but it was some twenty years later before further active components were identified from gut extracts. The major limitation of these studies, which showed that intravenous gut extracts could mimic the biological actions normally induced by enteric stimuli, such as acid or food, was the inability at that time to isolate the active substances from the crude extracts. It was not until the 1960s that the techniques of purification and structural analysis pioneered by Gregory and Mutt, allowed investigation of the active substances extracted from the gut, to advance[3,4]. Many of the classical hormones and a continuing stream of new peptides have now been purified and sequenced by these methods[5,6].

The development of the technique of radioimmunoassay[7] was the next major step forward for it provided a method of measuring the gut peptides which are often present at very low concentrations in plasma and tissue. The highly specific antisera produced for radioimmunoassay were soon applied to another technique, that of immunocytochemistry. Together these two techniques have provided powerful tools in the investigation of the distribution, and actions of gut peptides. With these techniques it has been shown that many of the peptides initially thought to be present only in the gut, are also abundant in the brain[8]. Furthermore as well as being present in endocrine cells, some peptides have also been found in nerves[9,10], while a few occur exclusively in one or other of these cell types (Table 1). Gut peptides therefore can no longer be regarded purely as classical circulating hormones, as many would seem to be able to assume a neurotransmitter, neuromodulator or paracrine function as well. The versatility of these peptides has far reaching implications to intercellular regulatory mechanisms, and has revolutionised our concepts of neural and hormonal regulation.

MOLECULAR HETEROGENEITY OF GUT PEPTIDES

The gut peptides have been found to exist in a number of molecular forms. In some cases these are fragments of the precursor molecule occurring as an essential byproduct of the peptide synthetic process. It is not yet known whether a single large precursor peptide may give rise to several existing gut peptides, as has been previously described for corticotrophins and endorphins[11]. The new technology of gene isolation and sequencing will provide a more feasable way of studying this[12] to show whether the many known groups of homologous peptides are the products of one giant peptide. In many instances a number of different active forms of the same peptide exist in tissue and plasma, as in the case of gastrin, cholecystokinin and somatostatin[12,13]. The tissue distribution of these various forms often differ, as does their cellular localisation. The functional significance of molecular heterogeneity of peptides remains unclear but could provide a mechanism for their differential selectivity of action.

THE GUT ENDOCRINE CELLS

The endocrine cells of the gut apart from those in the oxyntic area of the stomach are mainly of the open type[14] in that their apical surfaces consist of microvilli which extend into the gut lumen and so are in close proximity to their nutrient stimulants. Unlike most endocrine organs the gut consists of a widely dispersed network of endocrine cells, with ultrastructural appearances characteristic of their peptide products, each cellular type tending to have a defined distribution[15]. For instance, endocrine cells containing cholecystokinin (CCK), secretin, motilin, gastric inhibitory poly-peptide (GIP) and neurotensin are found only in upper small intestine, and gastrin cells in the antrum and upper duodenum. Cells containing insulin, glucagon and pancreatic polypeptide (PP) are almost entirely confined to the pancreas, in contrast enteroglucagon and somatostatin staining cells are more widely distributed in stomach, small intestine, colon and pancreas. Doubt still remains as to the localisation to endocrine cells of certain peptides, including bombesin, VIP and enkephalin like peptides[14,15,16].

Of the peptides found principally in endocrine cells, those shown to be released into the circulation by specific enteric signals at concentrations that are sufficient to produce characteristic biological actions, reproducable by similar concentrations of exogenous peptide, can be regarded as hormones. Gastrin, secretin, glucagon and insulin amply satisfy these requirements, the evidence is almost as good for GIP, PP and motilin, and probably for CCK although in the latter case radio-immunoassay remains unreliable[16,17]. Although somatostatin, neurotensin and enteroglucagon have been shown to be released into the circulation, the concentrations achieved have not been demonstrated to produce the known effects of these peptides, thus they as yet do not fulfil the criteria for a hormone.

Table 1. Gastroenteropancreatic Peptides and their Distribution in Neurons, Endocrine Cells and Plasma

Peptide	Neurons	Endocrine Cells	Plasma
Cholecystokinin	+	+	+
Gastrin	+	+	+
Secretin	+	+	+
Gastric Inhibitory Peptide (GIP)*	−	+	+
Vasoactive Intestinal Polypeptide	+	−	+/−
Peptide Histidine Isoleucine (PHI)	+	−	+/−
Glucagon	−	+	+
Enteroglucagon	−	+	+
Insulin	+	+	+
Somatostatin	+	+	+
Pancreatic Polypeptide	−	+	+
Peptide Tyrosine Tyrosine (PYY)	?	+	?
Bombesin/Gastrin releasing peptide	+	−	−
Neurotensin	+	+	+
Motilin	+	+	+
Enkephalin	+	+	?
Substance P	+	+	+/−

+ = present   − = absent
? = unknown   +/− = low concentrations
* also known as glucose dependent insulinotropic peptide

The identification of peptides within nerves has relied on immunocytochemical methods for their detection. Cross reactivity with other peptides is often a problem, necessitating the use of additional techniques such as chromatographic separation and immuno-assay with a variety of antisera to confirm the presence of a particular peptide[18,19].

The extrinsic autonomic nerve supply to the gut comes from the vagus nerve, the sacral spinal outflow and from prevertebral sympathetic ganglia. Although substance P, enkephalin and VIP have been identified in the vagus, and somatostatin in many of the principal adrenergic ganglion cells of the coeliac and mesenteric ganglia, the majority of the peptidergic nerves appear to be intrinsic in origin[19]. Together with cholinergic and adrenergic fibres these form plexi within the various layers of the gut wall involved in the primary regulation of gut function, which remains intact despite extrinsic denervation[20]. Numerous neuropeptides have now been identified in the peptidergic nerves of the gut, these include VIP, PHI, substance P, enkephalin, somatostatin, gastrin/CCK in both nerve cell bodies and fibres, and neurotensin and bombesin-like peptides in nerve terminals[18,19,21]. This list cannot pretend to be comprehensive in view of the very rapid rate at which new peptides are being identified.

It is of interest that some peptides have been shown to be present in the same peripheral autonomic nerves as the more classical neurotransmitters. For instance somatostatin has been found in the adrenergic ganglion cells of the inferior and superior mesenteric ganglion complex, suggesting that it co-exists with noradrenaline. There is also evidence from ultrastructural studies and acetyl-cholinesterase staining, that in some situations acetylcholine and VIP co-exist[19].

The identification of a peptide within a nerve is only the first step in demonstrating that it may act as a neurotransmitter. In addition, it has become the practice to satisfy a number of other criteria, including evidence for synthesis, and subsequent storage of the putative neurotransmitter within granules in the nerve ending; its release by electrical stimulation of nerves; and the demonstration that its exogenous application can mimic the biological effects of neurotransmission. A method of degradation or uptake of the neuro-transmitter into cells has been regarded as important for the cholinergic and adrenergic neurotransmitters but is probably of less relevance to the peptides[22]. The evidence for a neurotransmitter function for the gut neuropeptides has in most cases not gone beyond the first stage of their immunocytochemical localisation within nerves. Further progress in this field is greatly hindered by lack of the specific antagonists, which were so instrumental in the characterisation of cholinergic and adrenergic effects. It is likely that confirmation of specific functions of the neuro-peptides will have to await the development of these peptidergic antagonists.

Despite this handicap there is considerable evidence to suggest that VIP is a neurotransmitter in the gut. Electrical stimulation of the pelvic nerves in the cat is accompanied by a rise of VIP in the venous effluent plasma[23]; the resultant vasodilatation of the colonic and intestinal vasculature can be mimicked by exogenous VIP. There is good evidence from studies also in the cat, investigating the effects of stimulation of the chorda tympani, that VIP is released from postganglionic parasympathetic nerves and results in the atropine resistant vasodilatation observed in the submaxillary gland.Intra-arterial infusion of VIP to mimic the concentration released after chorda stimulation results in an equivalent vaso-dilatation, while intra-arterial acetylcholine does not release VIP and is a less potent submaxillary vasodilator[24]. Recent studies in the same organ and species show that VIP enhances muscarinic ligand binding, suggesting that if VIP and acetylcholine are co-released their interaction at the receptor may modify the ultimate response[25]. A fascinating series of experiments has shown that variation in the frequency and delivery of experimental electrical stimulation can result in different tissue responses as a result of preferential release of a particular neurotransmitter. Thus it has been shown that a higher stimulus frequency is required to release VIP compared to acetylcholine from postganglionic parasympathetic nerve terminals in the cat[24]. Recordings of the frequency of impulses passing along nerve terminals has shown that this varies in vivo[24], and is not just an experimental manipulation. Thus such a mechanism of varying neurotransmitter release may occur physiologically.

Although the evidence remains incomplete it seems highly likely that the neuropeptides are the neurotransmitters of a third division of the autonomic nervous system, with regulatory functions comparable to the cholinergic and adrenergic divisions.

PARACRINE MECHANISMS

It has been suggested that one of the mechanisms whereby peptides produce their effects is by direct release from endocrine type cells onto neighbouring cells, rather than by passing via the circulation, or by release from nerve terminals. Somatostatin is probably the only peptide for which there is some evidence for such a mechanism, and this rests on morphological studies that have demonstrated long cytoplasmic processes projecting from antral somatostatin cells onto gastrin producing cells[26]. The study of gastrin release from the isolated perfused stomach, and insulin from isolated islet preparations show that changes in either of these are accompanied by the expected parallel change in somatostatin and vice versa[27], supporting a possible paracrine interaction between these cell types in the stomach and islet. There is however now considerable evidence suggesting that somatostatin is a circulating hormone and is probably also released by nerves[27].

CONCLUSIONS

The biologically active peptides described above are now known to be widely dispersed throughout the gut in both endocrine cells and nerves. There is much evidence to suggest that these peptides play an important regulatory role as circulating hormones, neuro-transmitters or neuromodulators, and possibly as paracrine and trophic agents. However many questions remain unanswered which will require the combined efforts of many scientific disciplines before a unified concept of peptide function can be reached.

REFERENCES

1. W.M. Bayliss and E.H. Starling, On the causation of the so called peripheral reflex secretion of the pancreas, Proc. Roy. Soc. (London) 69: 352 (1902).
2. J.S. Edkins, On the chemical mechanism of gastric secretion, Proc. Roy. Soc. (London) 76: 376 (1905).
3. R.A. Gregory, and H.J. Tracy, The constitution and properties of two gastrins extracted from hog antral mucosa, Gut 5: 103 (1964)
4. V. Mutt, J.E. Jorpes, and S. Magnussen, Structure of porcine secretin. The amino acid sequence, Eur. J. Biochem. 15: 513 (1970).
5. S.I. Said, and V. Mutt, Polypeptide with broad biological activity: Isolation from small intestine, Science 1969: 1217 (1970).
6. T.J. McDonald, H. Jornvall, G. Nilsson, M. Vagne, M. Ghatei, S.R. Bloom, and V. Mutt, Characterisation of a gastrin releasing peptide from porcine non antral gastric tissue, Biochem. and Biophys Res. Commun. 90: 227 (1979).
7. R.S. Yalow, and S.A. Berson, Assay of plasma insulin by immuno-logical methods, Nature 184: 1648 (1959).
8. G.J. Dockray, Immunochemical evidence of cholecystokinin like peptides in brain, Nature 264: 568 (1976).
9. K.R. Jessen, J.M. Polak, S. Van Noorden, S.R. Bloom, and G. Burnstock, Peptide containing neurones connect the two ganglionated plexuses of the enteric nervous system, Nature 283: 391 (1980).

10. M. Costa, Y. Patel, J.B. Furness, and A. Arimura, Evidence that some intrinsic neurons of the intestine contain somatostatin, Neurosci. Lett. 6: 215 (1977).
11. R.E. Mains, B.A. Eipper, and N. Ling, Common precursor to corticotrophins and endorphins, Proc. Natl. Acad. Sci. 74: 3014 (1977).
12. V. Mutt, Gastrointestinal hormones: A field of increasing complexity, Scand. J. Gastroenterol. Supp 77: 133 (1982).
13. J.H. Walsh, Circulating gastrin, Ann. Rev. Physiol. 37: 81 (1975).
14. T. Fujita, and S. Kobayashi, The cells and hormones of the gastroenteropancreatic endocrine system, in: Gastro-entero-pancreatic endocrine. A cell biological approach, T. Fujita, ed., Igaku Shoin, Tokyo (1973).
15. E. Solcia, J.M. Polak, L.I. Larsson, A.M.J. Buchan and C. Capella, Update on Lausanne classification of endocrine cells, in: Gut Hormones. Bloom S.R. and Polak J.M. ed., Churchill Livingstone, London (1981).
16. J.H. Walsh, Nature of gut peptides and their possible function, in: Cellular basis of chemical messengers in the digestive tract. J. Lechago, M.I. Grossman, Walsh J.M. ed., Academic Press, New York (1980).
17. M.I. Grossman, Physiological effects of gastrointestinal hormones, Fed. Proc. 36: 1930 (1977).
18. J.B. Furness, M. Costa, R. Franco, and J.J. Llewellyn-Smith, Neuronal peptides in the intestine: distribution and possible function in: Advances in biochemical psychopharmacology, neural peptides and neuronal communications. E. Costa, M. Trabucchi eds., Raven Press, New York (1980).
19. A.E. Bishop, G.L. Ferri, L. Probert, S.R. Bloom and J.M. Polak, Peptidergic nerves, Scand. J. Gastroenterol. 17 Supp 71: 43 (1982).
20. M.D. Gershon, and S.M. Erde, The nervous system of the gut, Gastroenterology 80: 1571 (1981).
21. J.B. Furness, and M. Costa, Types of nerves in the enteric nervous system, Neuroscience 5: 1 (1980).
22. J.B. Furness, M. Costa, R. Murphy, A.M. Beardsley, J.R. Oliver, I.J. Llewellyn-Smith, R.L. Eskay, A.A. Shulkes, T.W. Moody, and K.K. Meyer, Detection and characterisation of neurotransmitters, particularly peptides, in the gastrointestinal tract, Scand.J. Gastroenterol. 17, Supp 71: 61 (1981).
23. J. Fahrenkrug, U. Haglund, M. Jodal, O. Lundgren, L. Olbe, and O.B. Schaffalitzky de Muckadell, Nervous release of vasoactive intestinal polypeptide in the gastrointestinal tract of cats: Possible physiological implications, J. Physiol. 284: 291 (1978).
24. A.V. Edwards, and S.R. Bloom, Recent physiological studies of the alimentary autonomic innervation, Scand. J. Gastroenterol. 17, Supp 71: 78 (1981).

25. J.M. Lundberg, B. Hedlund, and T. Burtfai, Vasoactive
    intestinal polypeptide enhances muscarinic ligand binding
    in cat submandibular salivary gland, Nature 295: 147 (1982).
26. L.I. Larsson, N. Goltermann, L. de Magistra, J.F. Rehfeld,
    and T.W. Schwartz, Somatostatin cell processes as pathways
    for paracrine secretion, Science 205: 1393 (1979).
27. V. Schusdziarra, Somatostatin – a regulatory modulator connecting
    nutrient entry and metabolism, Horm. Metab. Res. 12: 563 (1980).

HISTAMINE AND THE DIGESTIVE FUNCTIONS

Giulio Bertaccini and Gabriella Coruzzi

Institute of Pharmacology
University of Parma
43100 Parma, Italy

Histamine occurs along the whole gastrointestinal tract of different animal species with remarkable quantitative variations according to the species and the different areas of the gut. The amine is mainly contained in the mast cells but also in the so called ECL (enterochromaffin-like) cells. Its content varies, in the human gut mucosa, between about 7 micrograms per g of the large intestine and approximately 17 micrograms per g in the gastric corpus (Lorenz et al., 1973).

Even if a physiological role of histamine in the gastrointestinal tract is not completely established the amine is likely to be involved in two main functions that is gastric secretion and bowel motility.

The involvement of histamine in the gastric acid secretory response was first reported in 1920 by Popielski but afterwards a number of contrasting findings on the physiological role of histamine appeared in the literature (for review see Johnson, 1971).

An exceptionally important step in the history of histamine was the discovery by Black and co-workers (1972) of the so called H2 receptors which, together with the H1 receptors described by Ash and Schild (1966), mediated the action of histamine in the various tissues. The distribution of the two types of receptors is extremely variable: in some regions (like the gastric mucosa) the H2 receptors are largely predominant; in others (like the gut muscle) the opposite is true, in still others (like the central nervous system) both kinds of receptors occur in high amount whereas in some tissues (like the rat uterus) only H2 receptors seem to be present (for review see Bertaccini and Coruzzi, 1983).

There is a noticeable parallelism between histamine H1 and H2 and adrenergic alpha and beta receptors. In the smooth muscle, for instance, H1 receptors mediate excitation and H2 receptors usually mediate relaxation but exceptions are also possible (Bertaccini, 1982). Also the post-receptors events present some resemblance with those of the adrenergic system. Usually excitation of the H2 receptors causes an increase in cAMP intracellular levels whereas that of H1 receptors leads to increased levels of cGMP probably connected with increased cellular levels of calcium ions. It has been suggested that, at least in some tissues the H1 receptor is coupled to the phosphatidyl-inositol cycle which is thought to act as a calcium gating mechanism in the cell membrane (Johnson, 1982).

In the present article only some aspects concerning histamine and digestive functions will be considered since they have been the object of numerous monographs, textbooks and review articles. Particular emphasis will be given to some controversial points or to very recent data concerning a) gastric secretion, b) pancreatic exocrine secretion and c) gastrointestinal motility.

a) Gastric Secretion.

As far as gastric secretion is concerned, in spite of the fact that the role of histamine and of H2 receptors seems to be a major one in the physiological regulation of acid secretion (for review see Code, 1982), remarkable controversies exist because of the extreme variability of data obtained in the different experimental conditions: "in vivo" versus "in vitro" experiments, isolated whole stomach or gastric fundus or finally preparations of oxyntic cells and different ways of evaluating gastric secretion (aminopyrine accumulation, oxygen consumption, carbonic anhydrase activity), the availability of new drugs capable of stimulating or inhibiting gastric secretion, have been factors which have multiplied discrepancies and have permitted different interpretations on the role of histamine and its receptors to be made.

The early experiments pointed out the importance of H2 receptors ruling out that of H1 receptors. Subsequent studies, however, suggested that also H1 receptors could be involved in gastric secretion. According to some investigators H1 stimulation caused inhibition of acid secretion, whereas in other experimental conditions the opposite was true. Apparently all the experiments were performed correctly by the use of selective stimulants and/or inhibitors, therefore only differences in the techniques may explain the different the different conclusions (Vinik et al., 1983).

Another controversial point is that of basal acid secretion in isolated preparations. In most cases excepting in kittens, frogs and mice, H2 antagonists do not modify basal secretion thus suggesting a minor if any role of histamine in isolated preparations. In our personal experience concerning isolated fundus of the rat, we confirmed the lack of inhibitory effect of most H2 antagonists but we observed a remarkable effect of the new H2 antagonist oxmetidine which was mimicked only by administration of KSCN and omeprazole (Fig. 1).

As for the post-receptor events again the early experiments were different from the more recent ones. Cyclic AMP considered the second messenger after excitation of H2 receptors, was found to be affected also by excitation of H1 receptors, though quantitative differencies (2 to 20 times) were found by different Authors (for review see Teppermann et al., 1979).

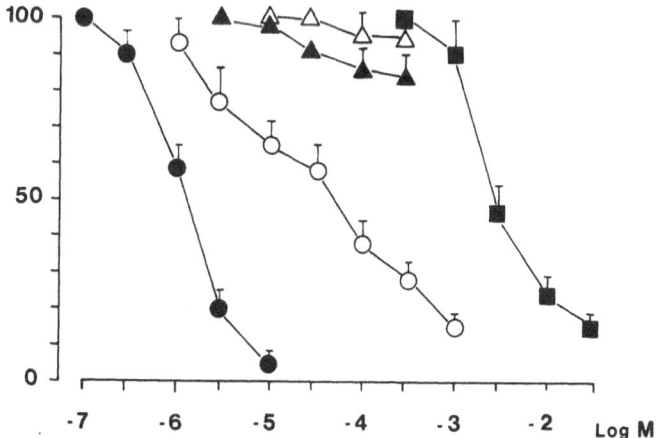

Fig. 1. Acid secretion from isolated rat fundus. Basal levels taken as 100; percent reduction following omeprazole (●); oxmetidine (O); ranitidine (▲); cimetidine (Δ) and KSCN (■). Each value represents the mean of the values obtained from 4 to 7 experiments; vertical bars are standard errors.

Recent studies showed that guinea pig gastric cells apparently possess two different binding sites for histamine which may be both part of the H2 receptor or only one is the H2 receptor and in any case only one site mediates cAMP generation (Batzri et al., 1982). In this connection we have to remember that, whereas so far a good correlation between cAMP content and gastric secretion was constantly found, recent experiments performed in man by Francavilla et al., 1983) showed that impromidine could elicit a high increase in the volume of gastric juice without a significant increase in cAMP levels.

Another controversial point concerns the interference between histamine and calcium ions. Apart from the guinea pig in which apparently calcium-entry blockers inhibit the effect of histamine (Kirkegaard et al., 1982; Sewing and Hannemann, 1983), in other species histamine seems to be calcium-independent as shown by the use of calcium-free solutions or calcium-antagonists. Surprisingly enough in some experiments histamine appeared to be actually potentiated by decreasing the calcium concentration of the nutrient fluid (Main and Pearce, 1978; Bunce et al., 1979).

The availability of rather "selective" agonists and antagonists provided some interesting tools for examining the different histamine receptors: on the other hand results obtained with such compounds were often misleading because of quite a lot of unsuspected side-effects, especially present in the group of the agonists, which may remarkably influence the drug-receptor interaction. A peculiar example of such a situation is the inhibitory (instead of a stimulatory) effect of dimaprit and impromidine on histamine-induced gastric secretion in the bullfrog (for review see Bertaccini and Coruzzi, 1983bis). An even more paradoxical situation is that pointed out by Arrang and coworkers (1983) who found that impromidine together with burimamide represent the best inhibitors of a subgroup of histamine receptors in the rat brain which they called "H3".

All the above considerations seem to point out that, in spite of several assumptions on the major role of histamine in the physiological regulation of acid secretion, there are still many problems to be clarified and it is difficult to accept that so many phenomena can be altered only by changing the experimental conditions.

b) Pancreatic Exocrine Secretion.

There are really a few papers concerning histamine and pancreatic secretion, most of the investigators being interested in the effect of the H2-antagonists rather than in that of histamine. Apparently histamine stimulates pancreatic exocrine secretion in

the rabbit (Liebow and Franklin, 1980) and in the dog in which the
effect was mimicked by H2-agonists like 4-methylhistamine and inhibited by H2-antagonists like metiamide and cimetidine. In our personal experience we confirmed these data (Dobrilla et al., 1980) and
recently we extended the study to dimaprit and impromidine, among
the agonists, and to cimetidine, ranitidine and oxmetidine, among
the antagonists; therefore the role of H2 receptors seems to be well
established. Moreover we found a noticeable interference between histamine receptors and the action of the hormone cholecystokinin ina-
smuch as the H2-blockers, starting from threshold doses of 2 to 5
mg/kg, inhibited dose-dependently the volume and protein content of
pancreatic juice stimulated by ceruletide. One exception was represented by ranitidine which actually potentiated, instead of inhibiting, the effect of ceruletide (from 0.5 to 2 mg/kg) (Fig. 2).

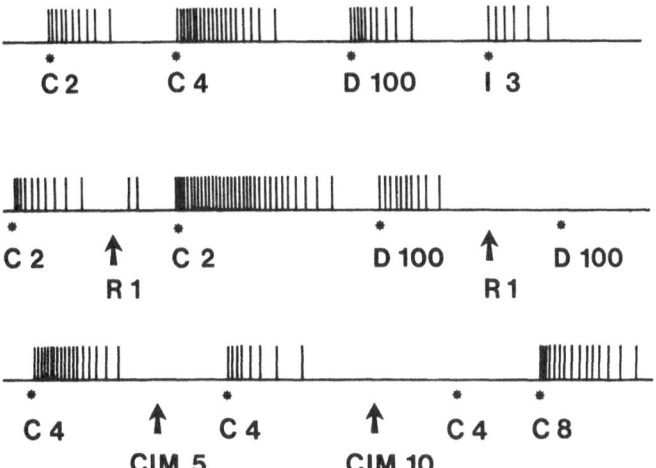

Fig. 2.   Pancreatic secretion of the anaesthetized dog. In the re-
          cord of the drop-counter each stroke represents one drop of
          secretion collected from the Wirsung duct. C = ceruletide
          (in ng/kg); D = dimaprit and I = impromidine (in μg/kg);
          R = ranitidine and CIM = cimetidine (in mg/kg).

This is not surprising when considering that ranitidine was found to possess a remarkable cholinergic-like effect in different preparations of different species (Bertaccini and Coruzzi, 1982; Bertaccini et al., 1983) and this may explain the potentiation of the ceruletide effect. Indeed both the effect of ceruletide and the potentiation induced by ranitidine were prevented by administration of small doses of atropine (0.02 mg/kg i.v.).

    c) Gastrointestinal Motility.

    Although gastrointestinal motility was not investigated as extensively as gastric secretion, there are some review articles in which the problem of histamine receptors involved in gut motility is debated rather thoroughly (Bertaccini et al., 1980; Parsons, 1982; Bertaccini, 1982).

    The guinea pig ileum is one of the most widely employed tool for the study of stimulatory substances and most of the early studies concerning histamine were performed on this preparation. This may be considered the starting point for the study of histamine on gut motility; in fact subsequent studies demonstrated that the amine is capable of stimulating all the different areas of the gastrointestinal tract from the oesophagus to the rectum in the different animal species.

    The stimulatory effect of histamine is mainly connected with the excitation of H1 receptors, H2 receptors being much less numerous and almost always causing relaxation of the intestinal muscle. A few exceptions are possible and apparently they were found in the human lower esophageal sphincter, in the dog antrum and in the guinea pig taenia coli where H2- receptor stimulation caused contraction of the smooth muscle.

    The mechanism of action of histamine is thought to be associated with depolarization and increase in the action potential discharge on the muscle membrane. As a consequence of the interaction with H1 receptors histamine increases the permeability to Na^+ and K^+ and may also enhances that to Ca^{++}ions (Uchida, 1980; Bolton and Clark, 1981).

    Relaxation following H2 receptor stimulation was reported in different areas of the gut, however it must be mentioned that several experiments were performed with an incorrect technique, that is to say by the use of a single agonist or antagonist of histamine receptors with the consequent erroneous extrapolation to the function of H2 receptors.

    Some very peculiar phenomena were observed by using in separated experiments the four classes of compounds necessary for the identification of receptors, i.e. H1 agonists and antagonists from one side and H2 agonists and antagonists from the other. With this correct methodological procedure gut muscle showed in some cases not to be a simple structure in which histamine act as a stimulatory agent through H1 receptors and as an inhibitory agent through H2 receptors: several experiments showed that the activity of histamine could be mimicked by selective H2 agonists but not blocked by the corresponding antagonists and that at the same time other effects of histamine could be inhibited by the H2 antagonists but not mimicked by the corresponding agonists; finally there are still other effects of histamine which are not blocked by a mixture of H1 plus H2 antagonists. These peculiar situations which are not infrequent in the gut muscle, seem to point out the occurrence of subtypes of histamine H2 receptors which have different characteristics in comparison with the classical ones. Of course it is also possible that these observations reflect artifacts due to the technique used or only the lack of a truly selectivity in the action of the compounds employed (for review see Bertaccini et al., 1980).

Another point of enormous importance and so far not sufficiently investigated is that of presynaptic histamine receptors which, in many respects, resemble the presynaptic adrenergic receptors. Both types of histamine receptors were found in either adrenergic or cholinergic fibers in different tissues where apparently they may act as modulators of the neurotransmitter release. Early experiments performed on the opossum LES suggested that activation of H1 receptors on intramural inhibitory neurons causes inhibition of the sphincter probably following release of relaxant unidentified substances (Rattan and Goyal, 1978). On the other hand in the rat intestine Sakai (1979) demonstrated that histamine caused a dose-dependent contraction abolished by tetrodotoxin, hexamethonium and morphine but not by atropine or methysergide; this suggests that the primary action of histamine is on the myenteric nervous plexus involving cholinergic interneurones which in turn lead to stimulation of non-cholinergic non-tryptaminergic terminal fibers. Also in the rabbit colon histamine seems to potentiate endogenous acetylcholine (released by electrical stimulation) through activation of presynaptic H1 receptors (Marshall and Roberts, 1983).

In the guinea pig ileum there is not a common agreement concerning histamine presynaptic receptors: according to the different investigators they may be of the H1, of the H2 type and actually of a H2-subtype, but in any case their stimulation causes an increase in the transmitter release which may be represented by acetylcholine or by other stimulatory substances (SP? 5-HT?) (Barker and Ebersole, 1982; Zavecz and Yellin, 1982; Kilbinger, personal communication).

As already said the study of presynaptic histamine receptors is at its very beginning and it is certainly destined to improve in the near future, throwing new light on the mechanism of action of histamine. We may add to these considerations our knowledge on the series of endogenous substances which may release or may be released by histamine. Thus the amine may represent one of the most important steps in the complex chain of events which involves autacoids, hormones, neurotransmitters etc. (see Fig. 3).

On the light of all the above considerations it seems cautious to avoid any possible oversimplification when considering the action of histamine on the digestive functions only for its interaction with the "classical" H1 and H2 receptors.

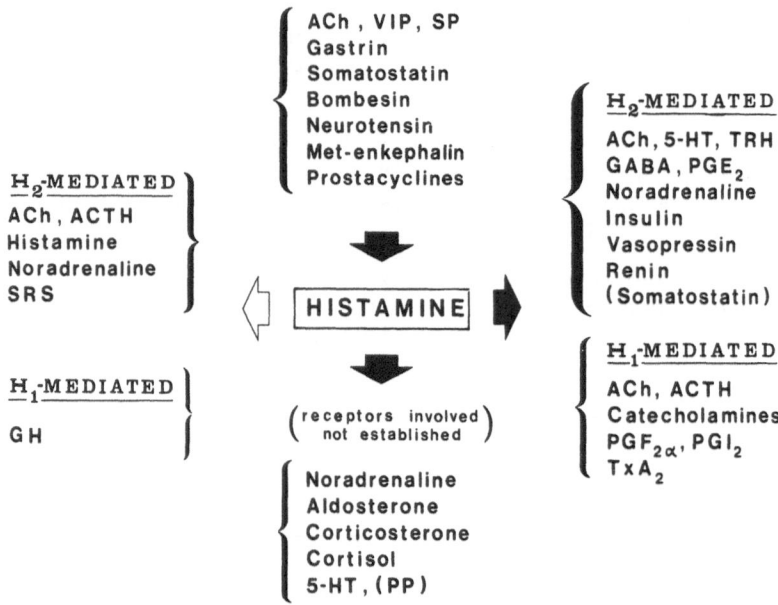

Fig. 3. Interaction between histamine and other endogenous active substances. Black arrow = stimulation of release; white arrow = inhibition of release.

ACKNOWLEDGEMENT

Original work of the authors was supported by a grant from the Smith Kline & French, S.p.A. Milan

REFERENCES

Arrang, J.M., Garbarg, M. and Schwartz, J.C., 1983, Auto-inhibition of brain histamine release mediated by a novel class (H3) of histamine receptor, Nature, 302: 832.

Ash, A.S.F. and Schild, H.O., 1966, Receptors mediating some actions of histamine, Br. J. Pharmacol., 27: 427.

Barker, L.A. and Ebersole, B.J., 1982, Histamine H2-receptors on guinea pig ileum myenteric plexus neurons mediate the release of contractile agents, J. Pharm. Exp. Ther., 221:69.

Batzri, S., Harmon, J.W. and Thompson, W.F., 1982, Interaction of histamine with gastric mucosal cells. Effect of histamine agonists on binding and biological response, Mol. Pharmacol., 22:33.

Bertaccini, G., 1982, Amines: Histamine, in: "Mediators and drugs in gastrointestinal motility" II, G. Bertaccini ed., Springer-Verlag, Berlin.

Bertaccini, G. and Coruzzi, G., 1982, Cholinergic-like effects of the new histamine H2-receptor antagonist ranitidine, Agents and Actions, 12: 168.

Bertaccini, G. and Coruzzi, G., 1983 in press, Extragastric H2-receptors, in: "Receptors and the upper G.I. tract", B.I. Hirschowitz and J.G. Spenney eds., Adis Press, New York.

Bertaccini, G. and Coruzzi, G., 1983 bis, Histamine H2-receptors: a homogeneous population?, Ital. J. Gastroenterol., 15: 51.

Bertaccini, G., Coruzzi, G. and Vizi, E.S., 1983, Further observations on the motor activity of some new histamine H2-receptor antagonists on the digestive system. Int. J. Tiss. Reac., 5:257.

Bertaccini, G., Scarpignato, C. and Coruzzi, G., 1980, Histamine receptors and gastrointestinal motility: an overview, in: "H2 antagonists", A. Torsoli, P.E. Lucchelli and R.W. Brimblecombe, eds., Excerpta Medica, Amsterdam.

Black, J.W., Duncan, W.A.M., Durant, C.J., Ganellin, C.R. and Parsons, E.M., 1972, Definition and antagonism of histamine H2-receptors, Nature, 236: E42.

Bolton, T.B. and Clark, J.P., 1981, Effects of histamine, high potassium and carbachol on ^{42}K efflux from longitudinal muscle of guinea pig intestine, J. Physiol., 320: 347.

Bunce, K.T., Honey, A.C. and Parsons, M.E., 1979, Investigation on the role of extracellular calcium in the control of acid secretion in the isolated whole stomach of the rat, Br. J. Pharmacol., 67: 123.

Code, C.F., 1982, Histamine receptors and gastric secretion, in: "Pharmacology of histamine receptors", C.R. Ganellin and M.E. Parsons, eds., Wright. PSG, Bristol.

Dobrilla, G., Bonoldi, M.C., Chilovi, F. and Bertaccini, G., 1980, Effects of cimetidine on pancreatic function and disease, in: "H2-Antagonists", A. Torsoli, P.E. Lucchelli and R.W. Brimblecombe, eds., Excerpta Medica, Amsterdam.

Francavilla, A., Polimeno, L.? Amoruso, A. and Ierardi, E., 1983, Effetto dell'impromidina, agonista degli H2-recettori, sulla produzione di succo gastrico nell'uomo, SIMAD 3, Bari (Italy), June 27 - July 1, ab. 15.

Johnson, C.L., 1982, Histamine receptors and cyclic nucleotides, in: "Pharmacology of histamine receptors", C.R. Ganellin and M.E. Parsons, eds., Wright-PSG, Bristol.

Johnson, L.R., 1971, Control of gastric secretion: No room for histamine?, Gastroenterology, 61: 106.

Kirkegaard, P., Christiansen, J., Petersen, B. and Skov Olsen, P., 1982, Calcium and stimulus-secretion coupling in gastric fundic mucosa, Scand. J. Gastroenterol., 17: 533.

Liebow, C. and Franklin, J.E., 1980, Characterization of histamine stimulation of pancreatic protein secretion, Fed. Proc., 39:377.

Lorenz, W., Matejka, E., Schmal, A., Seidel, W., Reiman, H.J. and Mann, G., 1973, A phylogenetic study on the occurrence and distribution of histamine in the gastrointestinal tract and other tissues of man and various animals, Comp. gen. Pharmac., 4:229.

Main, I.H.M. and Pearce, J.B., 1978, Effects of calcium on acid secretion from the rat isolated gastric mucosa during stimulation with histamine, pentagastrin, metacholine and dibutyryl cyclic adenosine-3',5'-monophosphate, Br. J. Pharmacol., 64: 359.

Marshall, I. and Roberts, P.M., 1983, Histamine potentiates responses of rabbit isolated distal colon to pelvic nerve stimulation, Br. J. Pharmacol. 78: 145P.

Parsons, M.E., 1982, Histamine receptors in alimentary and genitourinary smooth muscle, in: "Pharmacology of histamine receptors", C.R. Ganellin and M.E. Parsons, eds., Wright-PSG, Bristol.

Popielski, L., 1920, Imidazolylathylamin und die Organextrakte. Eester Teil: beta-Imidazolylathylamin als machtiger Erreger der Magendrusen, Pflugers Arch. ges. Physiol., 178: 214.

Rattan, S. and Goyal, R.K., 1978, Effects of histamine on the lower esophageal sphincter in vivo: evidence for action at three different sites, J. Pharm. Exp. Ther., 204: 334.

Sakai, K., 1979, A pharmacological analysis of the contractile action of histamine upon the ileal region of the isolated blood-perfused small intestine of the rat, Br. J. Pharmacol., 67: 587.

Sewing, K.F. and Hannemann, H., 1983, Calcium channel antagonists
    verapamil and gallopamil are powerful inhibitors of acid secre-
    tion in isolated and enriched guinea pig parietal cells. Pharma-
    cology, 27: 9.
Tepperman, B.L., Jacobson, E.D. and Rosenfeld, G.C., 1979, Histamine
    H2-receptors in the gastric mucosa: role in acid secretion.
    Life Sciences, 24: 2301.
Uchida, M., 1980, Histamine-induced decrease of membrane-bound cal-
    cium ions in the membrane fraction of the rabbit taenia coli,
    Eur. J. Pharmacol., 64: 357.
Vinik, A.I., Heldsinger, A.A. and Skoglund, M.L., 1983, Evidence for
    histamine H1 and H2 receptors in guinea pig oxyntic cells. J.
    Pharm. Exp. Ther., 227: 115.
Zavecz, J.H. and Yellin, T.O., 1982, Histamine receptors in the myen-
    teric plexus-longitudinal muscle of the guinea pig ileum: H1-
    and H2-receptor-mediated potentiation of the contractile respon-
    se ro electrical stimulation, J. Pharm. Exp. Ther., 223: 177.

RELATIONSHIPS OF PROSTAGLANDINS TO GASTROINTESTINAL MOTILITY AND

SECRETION

Alan Bennett and Gareth J. Sanger

Department of Surgery, King's College School of Medicine
and Dentistry, The Rayne Institute, London, UK and
Department of Pharmacology, Beecham Pharmaceuticals
Harlow, Essex

INTRODUCTION

The relationships of prostaglandins and gastroenterology have
been subjects of considerable study over the last 15 years.   Most
of the early work concerned prostaglandins of the E and F series,
because it was not until 1976 that thromboxanes and prostacyclin
were identified;   less is known about the leukotrienes which were
identified 3 years later (Samuelsson et al, 1979).

General reviews of the early work on prostaglandins and the
gut include Bennett & Fleshler, 1970; Bennett, 1972, 1973, 1976a,
b, 1977; Wilson, 1972; Main, 1972; Waller, 1973; Karim &
Ganesan, 1974; Robert, 1974, and more recent reviews include those
by Bennett & Sanger (1982) and Robert & Ruart (1982).   There are
also reviews concerning prostaglandins and specific gut functions.
The subject is now so large that it would be outside the scope of
the present chapter to include all aspects.   Further details will
be found in the above reviews, particularly those published in 1982.

Formation of prostaglandins by gastrointestinal tissues

Many studies show that PGE and PGF compounds can be extracted
from a wide variety of gastrointestinal tissues (see Bennett,
1976a,b). Since prostaglandins are not stored, but are formed when
their precursor substances (mostly arachidonate in Western man)
are released, it is important to be cautious in referring to the
tissue content of prostaglandins.   Measurements obtained when
tissue enzyme activity is inhibited, so stopping the new formation
of prostaglandins, probably represent the basal turnover of prostaglandins in the tissue.   When enzyme activity is not inhibited and

the extraction procedure involves damage to the tissue and subsequent release of prostaglandin precursors, the prostaglandin yield depends on the synthetic capacity of the tissue. This aspect hampers the interpretation of prostaglandin involvement in physiological responses, since in many studies tissue damage during preparation may cause inappropriate release of prostaglandins. The condition of such tissues might therefore be more akin to pathological rather than to physiological states. Furthermore, gastrointestinal tissues consist of many cell types, including blood vessels and blood constituents, and it is not yet possible to determine the contribution of each gastrointestinal cell type to the prostaglandin yield. Some cells preferentially produce one type of prostanoid - eg blood platelets produce thromboxanes and blood vessel endothelium produces PGI_2.

The human gastrointestinal tract has been studied for its ability to produce prostaglandins in different sections cut through the gut wall from mucosa to serosa (Bennett et al, 1968c, 1977b). These findings relied on bioassay using rat gastric fundus which is most sensitive to PGE compounds. They indicate that mucosa from human stomach and terminal ileum produces more prostaglandin-like material (presumably mainly PGE_2 and $PGF_{2\alpha}$) than the muscle, whereas the reverse seems to be true in the colon.

More recently, studies using gas chromatography-mass spectrometry, indicate that human gastrointestinal mucosa and muscle can produce PGD_2, PGE_2, $PGF_{2\alpha}$, 6-keto-$PGF_{1\alpha}$ (formed from PGI_2), TXB_2 (formed from TXA_2) and the lipoxygenase product 12-HETE (Bennett et al., 1981, 1983). Prostaglandins and related substances have also been found in extracts of gut tissue from various animals (see Bennett & Sanger, 1982), and again there may be regional differences in synthesis.

Using radio-immunoassay, Peskar et al.,(1980) found that the incubates of microsomes or small pieces of human gastric mucosa formed more PGE_2 than 6-keto-$PGF_{1\alpha}$, as did gastric juice aspirated after giving pentagastrin sc. In contrast, when we homogenized human gastric tissues in Krebs solution, mass spectrometric measurements showed more 6-keto-$PGF_{1\alpha}$ than PGE_2, $PGF_{2\alpha}$ and TXB_2 (Stamford et al., 1983). This suggested that the 6-keto-$PGF_{1\alpha}$:PGE_2 ratio may be greater in homogenates than with incubated pieces. We examined this possibility using radio-immunoassay of prostaglandins from human gastric mucosa, and found that the 6-keto-$PGF_{1\alpha}$: PGE_2 ratio was greater in 4/6 homogenates (P O Collins & A Bennett, unpublished).

Several other investigators have measured prostaglandins in human gastric juice, but the interpretation of the results is difficult. Are these prostaglandins secreted, are they released from cells sloughed off from the gastric mucosa, how much comes from

swallowed saliva or refluxed duodenal contents, and what is the
extent of degradation in the acid medium?

The ability of human gastric mucosa to inactivate prostaglandins has been studied by Peskar et al. (1976). They found three
prostaglandin-metabolising enzymes, namely prostaglandin-15-hydroxy-
dehydrogenase, delta 13-reductase and 9-keto-reductase in the high-
speed supernatant of homogenized mucosa from human gastric fundus.
Peskar (1978) found the same types of enzyme in mucosa of human
oesophagus, stomach, duodenum, colon and rectum.

Possible physiological roles

Prostaglandins may have physiological roles relating to gastrointestinal secretions, muscle activity, and blood flow.

Gastric secretion

Much of the early work concerns the inhibition gastric acid
secretion in various species by PGE and PGA compounds. Numerous
studies show that the volume of secretion and the acid concentration
in response to secretagogues such as histamine, pentagastrin and
food are reduced, usually with little effect on pepsin (see Robert
& Ruart, 1982). However, PGE_2 did not inhibit the stimulation of
acid. secretion in rats by dibutyryl-cAMP (Main & Whittle, 1974).
More recent work shows inhibition of acid secretion by PGI_2 (Gerkens
et al, 1978). These effects are produced by prostaglandins administered parenterally or orally in laboratory animals but in human
subjects natural prostaglandins inhibit acid secretion only when
given parenterally (Horton et al, 1968; Bhana et al, 1973; Karim
et al, 1973), and stable prostaglandin analogues such as 15(R)- and
15(S)- methyl-PGE_2, 16,16-dimethyl-PGE_2, and 11,16,16-trimethyl PGE_2
are needed to exert an antisecretory effect orally (Robert & Ruart,
1982). Degradation of the natural prostaglandin compounds is unlikely to explain entirely their lack of activity, because prostaglandins by mouth can cause diarrhoea (see later).

The fall in acid secretion is not mediated by a reduction of
gastric mucosal blood flow, as shown by clearance studies (Main &
Whittle, 1973), by the finding that acid secretion is inhibited in
isolated tissues which do not have a blood supply (Way & Durbin,
1969), and by the increase in blood flow that often occurs with
PGI_2. The role of cAMP in gastric acid secretion has been the
subject of controversy, partly because of the different cell types
in the gastric mucosa. Studies on relatively pure parietal cells
from dog fundic mucosa indicate that PGE_2 inhibits the response to
histamine by blocking the stimulation of cAMP (Soll, 1978). Antisecretory prostaglandins will also be discussed later in the context
of mucosal protection ("cytoprotection").

In animals such as the rat and dog, there is evidence that endogenous prostaglandins play a regulatory inhibitory role in gastric
acid secretion; there is no evidence for a similar role in man.
Indomethacin given for a month did not alter basal or histamine-
stimulated acid output (Winship & Bernhard, 1970) and indomethacin
did not increase acid output during submaximal stimulation with
pentagastrin (Bennett et al. 1973).   Although we cannot exclude
the possibility that indomethacin stimulated a back-diffusion of
acid which masked an increase in acid output, these data argue
against a regulatory role of gastric mucosal prostanoids in human
gastric acid secretion.

Intestinal secretion

Prostaglandins induce diarrhoea in man and laboratory animals
by reducing the absorption of water and electrolytes, increasing
secretion, and probably also by a primary effect on muscle activity.
Relationships of these effects to diarrhoea of various causes are
discussed later.   The various routes of administration by which
prostaglandins can cause diarrhoea in man include oral, intraduodenal and parenteral (Misiewicz et al. 1969; Matuchansky &
Bernier, 1973; Milton-Thompson et al. 1975).

The anti-ulcer effect of some prostaglandin analogues is limited
by their gastrointestinal side effects, and an important aim has been
to synthesize compounds without intestinal activity.   Quantification
of the diarrhoeagenic potential, at least as far as fluid transport
is concerned, can be achieved using an "enteropooling" assay to
measure intraluminal fluid accumulation in rat small intestine
(Robert et al. 1976).   Motility changes are probably also necessary
to convert this into diarrhoea, and Robert & Ruart (1982) concluded
that 16,16-dimethyl PGE_2 directly stimulates rat colon in vivo since
tying the ileocaecal junction did not alter the accelerated transit
(Ruart et al. 1978).   However, it is not clear to what extent this
involves colonic secretion, absorption and/or motility.   Whereas
many prostaglandins stimulate intestinal fluid secretion, in rats
PGD_2 and PGI_2 actually inhibit "enteropooling" (Robert et al. 1979).
In man PGI_2 iv can cause colicky pain which might be indicative
of distension or muscle contraction (O'Grady et al. 1979).

Gastric anti-ulcer effect and mucosal protection

Because prostaglandins and their analogues can inhibit gastric
acid secretion, they would be expected to exert anti-ulcer activity.
The ability of these substances to inhibit gastric ulceration
(mainly in rats) by pyloric ligation, stress, bile salts, nonsteroidal anti-inflammatory drugs, reserpine, 5-hydroxytryptamine, and
corticosteroids is widely documented; prostaglandins also inhibit
duodenal ulceration caused by cysteamine, propionitrile, and histamine alone and with carbachol or pentagastrin (see Robert & Ruart,

132

1982).   In patients too, there is an anti-ulcer effect, but the
results are not entirely clear-cut.   Although some studies showed
a faster rate of gastric ulcer healing, as judged endoscopically in
patients given 15(R)-15-methyl-PGE$_2$, its methyl ester or PGE$_2$ (Fung
et al, 1974a,b; Fung & Karim, 1976), in another study 15(R)- or
15(S)-methyl-PGE$_2$ methyl ester or 16,16-dimethyl PGE$_2$ appeared to
enhance the healing of duodenal but not gastric ulcers (Rybicka &
Gibinski, 1978).   Patients given PGE$_2$ had less faecal blood loss
following aspirin ingestion (Cohen, 1978).

Prostaglandins can protect the gastric mucosa against damage
by various agents, including acid, alkali, heat, hypertonic NaCl,
ethanol, bile acids, nonsteroidal anti-inflammatory drugs and corticosteroids.   This protection can occur with doses of prostaglandins
that do not affect acid output.   It seems likely that in damage
caused by anti-inflammatory drugs the administered prostaglandins
perform a role normally carried out by the endogenous prostaglandins
whose synthesis has been inhibited.   Robert & Ruart (1982) and
Miller (1983) have written excellent reviews of the subject.

Gastric mucosal processes that may involve endogenous prostaglandins,or may be affected by exogenous prostaglandins that protect the gastric mucosa, include maintenance of the gastric mucosal
barrier, inhibition of acid secretion (see above), increase of mucosal blood flow (Kauffman & Whittle, 1982), stimulation of mucus and
bicarbonate secretion (Bolton et al, 1978; Allen & Garner, 1980),
and stimulation of the sodium pump (Choudhury & Jacobson, 1978).
Fuller details and other references are given by Miller (1983),
together with other effects of prostaglandins on the gastric mucosa
including stimulation of chloride transport, surface-active phospho-
lipids, and macromolecular synthesis (DNA, RNA and protein), stabi-
lization of lysosomes, effects on sulphydryl compounds and mucosal
folds, and changes in cAMP.

The protection of the gastric mucosa by prostaglandins is often
called "cytoprotection" (Robert, 1979), but in some ways this is
misleading.   "Cyto" refers to cells, and there is no evidence that
prostaglandins protect at the cellular level.   Indeed, "cytoprotection" can occur despite extensive mucosal damage as shown by
microscopy (Lacy & Itoh, 1982).   "Mucosal protection" is therefore
a better term with no implication of unsubstantiated mechanisms.
It may well be that several processes combine to produce the protection, and their contribution may vary with the damaging agent.
Furthermore, there may be simple explanations for apparently mira-
culous results.   For example, the protection against damage "even
by boiling water" might be due merely to cooling and heat removal.
The local temperature must reach a critical point for gross mucosal
damage to occur.   "Boiling" water would be partly cooled by the time
it reaches the stomach and would presumably be more greatly cooled

in the stomach of prostaglandin-treated rats than in untreated controls because of the greater amount of mucus present after treatment with prostaglandins. The heat would have to diffuse through a greater thickness of mucus before reaching the mucosa, and would be dissipated more quickly by a prostaglandin-mediated increase in mucosal blood flow. The hypothesis could be checked in various ways, such as with a heat-sensitive probe in the mucosa. Similar hypotheses could be made for other damaging agents, and could include other aspects such as stimulation of bicarbonate secretion in the protection against damage by acid.

Claims have been made that other types of anti-ulcer drugs are also "cytoprotective". For example, cimetidine or probanthine inhibited rat gastric lesions produced by acidified aspirin (Guth et al, 1979). This was confirmed by Robert et al (1979b) but they found that when the HCl was increased to 0.35M, 16,16-dimethyl PGE$_2$ was protective but cimetidine or probanthine had much less effect. Perhaps this relates to stimulation of bicarbonate secretion, mucus secretion and increased mucosal blood flow with the prostaglandin analogue.

Protection of intestinal mucosa

Nonsteroidal anti-inflammatory drugs can cause necrosis in the small intestine leading to ulceration, perforation and fatal peritonitis. These events can be prevented by giving various prostaglandins (Robert, 1975; Fitzpatrick & Wyndalda, 1976), as can the damage produced by prednisolone which inhibits prostaglandin precursor release (Lancaster & Robert, 1978). Inhibition of prostaglandin synthesis may be important for breaching the defence mechanisms of the intestinal mucosa, so allowing bacteria to invade and produce the lesions (Whittle, 1981).

It has been suggested that sulphasalazine, which reduces relapse in ulcerative colitis, may act by decreasing protaglandin breakdown and so protects the colonic mucosa (Hoult & Moore, 1978). This mechanism is unlikely to be important, since 5-aminosalicylic acid seems to be the active moiety of sulphasalazine (Khan et al. 1977).

GASTROINTESTINAL MUSCLE

In vitro

As with secretion the early studies involved PGE and PGF compounds, and many of these are discussed in the review by Bennett & Fleshler (1970). Details on other compounds can be found in the reviews by Bennett & Sanger (1982) and Robert & Ruart (1982). As a general rule, PGE compounds contract gastrointestinal longitudinal muscle but relax the circular muscle, whereas PGF compounds contract both layers, but there are exceptions. Most other prostaglandins cause contraction, as with PGD_2 in longitudinal muscle strips from rat or human stomach, rabbit jejunum and guinea-pig intestine (Horton & Jones, 1974; Hamberg et al., 1975; Bennett & Sanger, 1980; Bennett et al., 1981); PGD_2 also contracts circular muscle of guinea-pig colon (Bennett & Sanger, 1978). PGH_2 and its expoxymethano analogues, PGG_2, PGI_2 and its degradation products, and thromboxanes contract the longitduinal muscle of rat stomach and colon, gerbil colon, guinea-pig ileum and chick rectum (Hamberg et al., 1975; Bunting et al., 1976; Boot et al., 1977; Chijimatsu et al., 1977; Gorman et al., 1977; Bennett et al. 1980). In most tissues from laboratory animals PGE_2 seems to be the most potent prostanoid, unlike human tissues in which endoperoxide analogues (thromboxane mimetics; Coleman et al., 1980) are the most potent. This indicates differences in the prostaglandin receptor populations (see later).

PGI_2 also relaxes some tissues, such as human stomach and colon (Bennett et al., 1981, 1983). Contractions of guinea-pig circular colon muscle to PGI_2, PGD_2 and the U-46619 epoxymethano analogue of PGH_2 were converted by the prostaglandin antagonist SC-19220 (Sanner 1969) to inhibitory effects (Sanger & Bennett, 1980). The inhibitory effect of PGI_2 on human tissues is somewhat selective: in the longitudinal muscle of human stomach PGI_2 reduced contractions to PGE_2 or $PGF_{2\alpha}$, but not to U-46619 or acetylcholine, whereas with gastric circular muscle PGI_2 reduced the contraction to U-46619 but not to acetylcholine (Bennett & Sanger, 1980).

The effects of prostanoids (prostaglandins and other cyclo-oxygenase products) on gastrointestinal muscle can obviously depend greatly on the species, the gut region and the types of products formed. One way of investigating possible roles in motility is to use drugs which block prostaglandin formation, but there are many points that may affect the interpretation of the findings. Inhibition of cyclo-oxygenase would reduce the formation of all prostanoids, some of which may have markedly different actions on the tissues. The net response to a synthesis inhibitor would reflect the balance between different effects of endogenous prostaglandins. An inhibitor might not penetrate to all sites in the tissue, it might not be effective on all tissue cyclo-oxygenases, and it may affect other enzymes and tissue functions (Flower, 1974). Furthermore, block of cyclo-oxygenase may divert substrate metabolism into lipoxygenase products (Higgs et al., 1980) some of which have potent musculotropic substances. We also have to consider that the experimental techniques may damage the tissues and cause inappropriate prostaglandin release, so that the effects of prostaglandin synthesis inhibitors may correspond to their effects in diseased rather than in normal tissues.

It nevertheless seems likely that endogenous prostanoids can affect gut muscle tone and reactivity. The tone of gastrointestinal longitudinal muscle from several species is reduced by drugs that inhibit prostaglandin action (Bennett & Posner, 1971) or synthesis (eg in human small intestine, Bennett & Stockley, 1977). In contrast, indomethacin often increases the tone and spontaneous activity of the circular muscle (eg Bennett & Stockley, 1977). The opposite response of the two muscle layers may reflect the different effects of PGE_2, as discussed earlier. With in vivo studies, which mainly avoid the release of prostaglandins by tissue damage, indomethacin increased the tone of the lower oesophageal sphincter (Dilawari et al. 1975). This agrees with the in vitro studies on other circular muscles, and with experiments in anaesthetized guinea-pigs in which the synthesis inhibitor 5,8,11,14,-eiosatetravnoic acid (TYA) applied serosally reduced intra-ileal pressure changes (Willis et al. 1974).

Sites of prostaglandin action

This subject is dealt with in detail by Bennett & Sanger (1982). In all cases prostaglandins seem able to affect the activity of isolated gut muscle at least partly by a direct action on the muscle cells, as demonstrated by prostaglandin-induced responses in the presence of neurone-blocking drugs or antagonists of transmitters. In some isolated tissues the prostaglandin receptors seem to be only on the muscle cells (eg many human gastrointestinal muscles), but in some longitudinal muscles part of the action is on intramural nerves. Thus contractions to PGE and PGF compounds in longitudinal muscle from guinea-pig ileum or colon, dog stomach or colon, and occasionally human ileum and colon are reduced by toxins which block autonomic nerve activity, or by drugs that block muscarinic receptors (see Bennett & Fleshler, 1970; Bennett & Sanger, 1982). Some tissues therefore seem to contain cholinergic nerves with excitatory prostaglandin receptors.

In guinea-pig ileum, some reports indicate that PGE compounds can increase acetylcholine output. The reduction of PGE- or PGF-induced contractions of guinea-pig ileum by enkephalins (Jaques, 1977; Spruegel et al. 1977) may be due to block of prostaglandin-induced acetylcholine release. With regard to other nerve types, PGE compounds in rabbit and guinea-pig intestine can inhibit noradrenaline release and action (see Bennett & Sanger, 1982). Non-adrenergic non-cholinergic inhibitory responses in guinea-pig taenia caecum or opossum lower oesophageal sphincter were not affected by PGE_1, PGE_2, $PGF_{2\alpha}$ or indomethacin (Kadlec et al. 1974; Burnstock et al. 1975; Sakato & Shimo, 1976; Daniel et al. 1979). However, the contractions following the cessation of nerve stimulation could be reduced by prostaglandin synthesis inhibitors (Kadlec et al. 1974; Burnstock et al. 1975; Sakato, 1975; Bennett & Stockley, 1977).

Other actions of PGE compounds include stimulation of 5-hydroxytryptamine release from guinea-pig ileum (Kadlec et al. 1975) but not from rat stomach and jejunum (Thompson & Angulo, 1968). In rat stomach fundus, PGE_1-induced contraction was accompanied by a decrease in cAMP content and an increase in cGMP (Shearin & Pancoe, 1976).

The investigation of prostaglandin receptors has been made difficult by the lack of selective antagonists for most prostanoids, although there are now good thromboxane antagonists (Coleman et al., 1981; Jones et al., 1982). It seems likely that there are separate receptor types for various prostanoids, and a useful classification has been suggested by Kennedy et al.,(1982). In addition, there has long been evidence for at least 2 types of PGE receptor, since SC-19220 blocks the excitatory response of guinea-pig colon to PGE_2, but not the relaxation of the circular muscle (Bennett & Posner, 1971). The topic of prostaglandin receptors in the gut is complex, because of differences between species, muscle layers, and regions, and the many different prostanoids. This subject is dealt with in detail by Bennett & Sanger (1982). A prostaglandin antagonist selective for specific receptor types might have various gastrointestinal uses, perhaps including muscle spasm, inflammation, peptic ulceration (blockade of thromboxane-induced mucosal ischaemia and platelet aggregation (Bennett, 1983)), some types of diarrhoea and food intolerance, etc, as will become clearer in the subsequent section on prostanoids in disordered gastrointestinal motility.

Possible roles of prostanoids in motility

The fact that many prostanoids which can be formed in the gut have potent musculotropic activities is consistent with a role in either normal or deranged motility. However, these facts alone are far from enough evidence; other substances which are potent in vitro, such as histamine and 5-hydroxytryptamine, can be formed throughout the human gastrointestinal tract, but there is no evidence for a role in gut motor activity. Another consideration is the type of activity that a substance might induce, and this cannot be deduced from the muscle strip work described earlier. Muscle contraction does not necessarily induce propulsion, and may in fact cause stasis (eg with morphine-induced spasm of colonic circular muscle) or retropulsion. Movement of contents along the alimentary tract requires a pressure gradient, and this can be caused by muscle relaxation in front of a bolus and/or by contraction behind it. The importance of the relaxation is likely to vary with the gut region, probably being more important with solid contents in the large bowel than with liquid contents in the small intestine.

Most studies have been made with segments of guinea-pig intestine in vitro. PGE_1 or PGE_2 applied serosally, but not mucosally, enhanced the peristaltic contractions of the ileal longitudinal muscle; the circular muscle activity was depressed by higher concentrations of PGE but enhanced by low concentrations (Bennett et al.

1968a; Radmanovic 1972; Sanger & Watt, 1978). Methodological differences may also affect the results (see Bennett & Sanger, 1982). PGF compounds stimulated activity in both muscle layers (Radmanovic, 1972; Eley et al. 1977). In guinea-pig isolated colon, the PGE compounds applied serosally increased both longitduinal and circular muscle activity during peristalsis elicited by raising the intra-luninal pressure (Eley et al. 1977) but they did not alter fluid propulsion, whereas Ishizawa & Miyazaki (1973a) found that they increased the propulsion of a small plastic ball. The PGF compounds also stimulated guinea-pig colon segments (Ishizawa & Miyazaki, 1973a,b, 1975; Eley et al. 1977). The possible role of endogenous prostaglandins is indicated by the reduction of peristaltic activity in guinea-pig isolated ileum and colon with indomethacin or aspirin (Bennett et al. 1976; Fontaine et al. 1977). Since the reduction was modest, and the effect of aspirin was sometimes temporary despite its continued presence, it seems that prostaglandins are not essential for peristalsis in guinea-pig intestine but may play a contributory role. This accords with clinical evidence that prostaglandin synthesis inhibitors generally have little effect on bowel function.

In vivo studies

Various in vivo studies indicate the involvement of prostaglandins in some aspects of gut motility, but again there are wide species variations. In humans the inhibitory effect of PGE_1 or PGE_2 on the pentagastrin-stimulated lower oesophageal sphincter, and the stimulatory effect of indomethacin, suggest an inhibitory role for endogenous prostaglandin E_2 or possibly other inhibitory prostanoids eg PGI_2 (Goyal et al. 1974; Sorensen et al. 1974; Dilawari et al, 1975; Mukhopadhyay et al. 1975; Kruidinier et al. 1978). However, in the opossum a role of endogenous prostanoids in the motility of this region is less likely since indomethacin had little or no effect (Daniel et al. 1979). Nevertheless, PGE_2 inhibited the opossum lower oesophageal sphincter (Goyal et al. 1973) and PGE_2 or PGI_2 were inhibitory in cats (Sinar et al. 1979), but PGE_2 caused an increase in the dog (Maher et al. 1978).

With regard to the human stomach, PGE_1 iv depressed antral motility (Classen et al. 1973, as did 16,16-dimethyl PGE_2 given orally (Nylander & Andersson, 1975). However, Newman et al.(1975) found that PGE_2 infused iv did not affect the frequency of antral contractions, whereas $PGF_{2\alpha}$ caused an increase. Oral 16,16-dimethyl PGE_2 increased the gastric emptying of barium in human subjects (Johansson & Ekeland, 1977; Nylander & Mattson, 1978) and PGE_1 given orally to human subjects produced biliary reflux, consistent with pyloric (circular muscle) relaxation (Horton et al. 1968). As with other parts of the gastrointestinal tract, it is hazardous to equate motility and transit changes.

In rats gastric motility in vivo was stimulated by PGE_1 ip (Shearin & Pancoe, 1976), but gastric emptying was inhibited by sc 16,16-dimethyl PGE_2 (Robert et al. 1976) or $PGF_{2\alpha}$ (Nilsson & Ohrn, 1974). In monkeys, parenteral PGI_2 inhibited gastric emptying (Shea-Donohue, 1980), whereas the 15(S)-methyl derivatives of PGE_2 or $PGF_{2\alpha}$ caused an increase (Nompleggi et al. 1979, 1980), PGE_1 iv in rabbits stimulated gastric motility (Smejkal, 1969). Again, a normal role of endogenous prostanoids is in doubt since indomethacin had little or no effect on gastric emptying in rats (Ruart et al. 1979) or monkeys (Nompleggi et al. 1979, 1980).

Intestinal studies in vivo also show a range of effects which are difficult to interpret. $PGF_{2\alpha}$ iv inhibited human small intestinal motility and increased intestinal secretion, but transit did not change (Cummings et al. 1973; Milton-Thompson et al. 1973). Oral PGE_1 speeded intestinal transit, and 15-methyl- or 16,16-dimethyl-PGE_2 given intraduodenally, increased the rate at which barium reached the colon, although duodenal motility was less (Nylander & Andersson, 1975; Nylander & Mattson, 1975). A contributory factor may be the faster emptying of the gastric meal. More rapid gastric emptying also occurred with oral 16,16-dimethyl-PGE_2, but jejunal transit was less (Ekelund et al. 1977; Johansson & Ekelund, 1977). Many factors have to be evaluated in interpreting these results. For example, how is propulsion affected by the experimental procedures and by prostaglandin-induced changes in gastric acid and intestinal secretion, and by gastric and intestinal motility?

Findings in laboratory animals are also complex. $PGF_{2\alpha}$ sc in rats inhibited the intestinal transit of an oral charcoal meal, but gastric emptying was also inhibited (Nilsson & Ohrn, 1974). PGE_2 sc increased intestinal transit (Robert & Ruart, 1982), and parenteral PGE_1 or analogues of PGE_2 increased the intraluminal pressure in rat small intestine (Bennett et al. 1968b; Main & Whittle, 1974). In dogs parenteral PGE_1 decreased the intraluminal pressure (Shehadeh et al. 1969; Ohashi et al. 1973); $PGF_{2\alpha}$ increased the intraluminal pressure (Ohashi et al. 1973), stimulated contractions of both muscle layers, and increased tone in the circular muscle but decreased it in the longitudinal muscle (Dajani et al. 1979). PGE_2 increased the myoelectric activity in fasted but not fed conscious dogs (Mukhopadhyay et al. 1974), and PGE_2 or its 15-methyl derivative blocked the interdigestive myoelectric complexes and induced the type of activity seen in fed animals (Konturek, 1978).

Although prostaglandins can alter gut motility, and evidence cited later suggests that they may be involved in pathology, an important role in normal function seems unlikely in view of the lack of dramatic effect of non-steroidal or steroidal anti-inflammatory drugs on bowel function. Indomethacin did not affect small intestinal transit in rats (Summers et al. 1970; Ruart et al. 1979) or monkeys (Nompleggi et al. 1978).

With regard to the colon in vivo, iv PGE_2 but not $PGF_{2\alpha}$ inhibited sigmoid motility in human subjects (Hunt et al, 1975).   Oral PGE_1 accelerated colonic transit as measured by telemetry (Misiewicz et al, 1969).   The extent to which the occurrence of watery stools with oral PGE_1 (Horton et al. 1968), or iv $PGF_{2\alpha}$ is a primary effect on colonic transit is not known, since an effect on water and electrolyte transport appears to be important.   A high infused dose of PGI_2 caused colicky pain in 1 of 5 subjects (O'Grady et al. 1979). In anaesthetized dogs iv $PGF_{2\alpha}$ did not affect colonic motility, although the small intestine was stimulated (Shehadeh et al. 1969; Dajani et al. 1979).

PROSTAGLANDINS AS FACTORS IN GASTROINTESTINAL DISEASES

The discussions above cast considerable doubt that prostaglandins are involved in many physiological processes within the gut. The main exceptions are likely to be those involved with mucosal protection, and may therefore include secretion of mucus and bicarbonate, contribution to the maintenance of mucosal blood flow and the gastric mucosal sodium pump.   In contrast, there is substantial evidence for roles of prostaglandins in various gastrointestinal disorders.   Some of these are discussed briefly below.

Gastric ulcers

Although prostaglandin production by the gastric mucosa seems to exert a protective role, evidence is beginning to emerge that thromboxane generation may cause gastric ulcers.   When arachidonic acid is injected into the blood supplying dog gastric mucosa, using a delay coil to allow thromboxane generation, mucosal ischaemia occurred.   With taurocholic and hydrochloric acids bathing the gastric mucosa, the ischaemia developed into severe necrosis (Whittle et al, 1981).   This damage was prevented by a thromboxane synthesis inhibitor.   In rats, a thromboxane synthesis inhibitor lessened the gastric mucosal damage caused by taurocholic acid but not that by ethanol.

Inflammatory bowel disease

It would be expected that since prostaglandins are involved in acute inflammation they may play an important part in conditions such as ulcerative colitis.   Much of the early evidence argued in favour of this view (see Bennett, 1976a,b), but more recent work is contrary.   Treatment with prostaglandin synthesis inhibitors has no effect or worsens the disease (Campieri et al. 1978, 1980; Gilat et al. 1979; Rampton & Sladen, 1981).   Perhaps this is due to diversion of arachidonate metabolism into lipoxygenase products.   It

appears that the important moiety of sulphasalazine, used to maintain remission of ulcerative colitis and Crohn's disease of the
large bowel, is 5-amino-salicylic acid (Khan et al. 1977). This
substance is a weak inhibitor of cyclo-oxygenase, but it can also
inhibit various lipoxygenases (Stenson & Lobos, 1982; Sircar, 1983).
This fact, together with the potent anti-inflammatory effect of
corticosteroids which inhibit precursor release and reduce the formation of both lipoxygenase and cyclo-oxygenase products, indicates
that lipoxygenase products (eg leukotrienes) may be important in
bowel inflammation. Another possibility is that actions of 5-amino-
salicylic acid and sulphapyridine include interference with super-
oxide production and myeloperoxidase-mediated cytotxicity (Molin
& Stendahl, 1979).

Gastro-oesophageal reflux

The inhibitory effect of PGE_2 on the lower oesophageal sphincter,
discussed earlier, suggests an involvement in oesophageal reflux.
PGI_2 might also be involved, since although its effect on the human
lower oesophageal sphincter has not been studied, PGI_2 relaxes human
stomach muscle. Perhaps the relief of "upset stomach" by Alka
Seltzer, a highly buffered form of acetysalicylate, involves a reduction of prostaglandin-aided oesophageal reflux.

Gastrointestinal disturbances

Several emetic, purgative or irritant compounds (such as capsaicin) can stimulate prostaglandin synthesis, and this action might
account for their unpleasant side effects (Collier et al. 1975, 1976).
Hypertonic solutions increase prostaglandin synthesis in rat stomach,
and there may be a link between prostaglandins and the hyperosmolar
dumping syndrome which can occur after partial gastrectomy (Assouline
et al. 1977; Knapp et al. 1978).

Diarrhoea

The involvement of prostaglandins in diarrhoea has been reviewed
recently by Rask-Madsen and Bukhave (1979) and Korman et al. (1981).
In man they probably act by increasing fluid accumulation in the
small intestine, which in turn increases propulsive activity, possibly aided by direct prostaglandin actions on the muscles. The increased amount of fluid entering the colon overloads its absorptive
capacity. Effects of prostaglandins on colonic absorption and motility could also be important. The implication of prostaglandins
as factors in diarrhoea or gastrointestinal disturbances includes
their raised levels which may be found in the blood or in faeces.
Distension of rat stomach or guinea-pig ileum releases prostaglandin-
like material (Bennett et al. 1967; Takai et al. 1974; Yagasaki et
al. 1974) and perhaps prostanoids are released within the gut partly

by hyperactivity. However, peripheral blood PGE levels, determined by radioimmunoassay, are raised only in some types of diarrhoea (Jaffe & Condon, 1976). It may be that other prostanoids contribute to the diarrhoea, and/or that PGE released by gut hyperactivity does not reach the peripheral venous blood because it is rapidly metabolised in the pulmonary circulation (Ferreira & Vane, 1967). Since prostanoids occur within the gut wall, may contribute to gut activity, and can be released by distension, treatment with inhibitors of prostaglandin synthesis might help alleviate all types of diarrhoea, (see below) regardless of whether the diarrhoeagenic stimulus releases prostaglandins.

Small bowel pseudo-obstruction, which results in diarrhoea, may be accompanied by raised prostaglandin levels in blood and gastric juice (Chouseterman et al. 1977; Luderer et al. 1977; Book et al. 1979) and when the condition resolved spontaneously or after giving prostaglandin synthesis inhibitors the levels normalized.

Bacterial endotoxins can release prostaglandins. In mice, diarrhoea caused by iv Salmonella enteritidis endotoxin was prevented by indomethacin (Harper & Skarnes, 1972), and E.coli endotoxin iv in rabbits increased prostaglandin output from the ex vivo intestine (Herman & Vane, 1975). Cholera diarrhoea in various species might involve prostaglandins (see Bennett, 1976a,b; Bennett & Sanger, 1982 for earlier studies). More recently it has been found that cholera toxin caused a highly organised myoelectric "migrating action potential complex" in loops of rabbit distal ileum, and this could be blocked by indomethacin (Mathias et al. 1977). Fluid accumulation in rat small intestine with cholera toxin injected in the upper jejunum of anaesthetised rats was reduced by indomethacin (Robert et al. 1979c). Reports claiming that there is no relationship between cholera toxin and prostaglandins contain dubious aspects. In some there were methodological problems or incorrect analysis of data. The use of pure toxin might also have been inappropriate (Bennett, 1976c) since the vibrios release crude material, and purification might reduce the diarrhoeagenic activity, as may be surmised from the data of Bedwani & Okpako (1975).

This once-active area of research has now been almost abandoned, even though relatively simple experiments would help determine clearly the role of prostaglandins in cholera (Bennett, 1976c). Careful experimental design is needed, and it may be important to use in vivo conditions since cholera toxin seems to have a systemic component contributing to diarrhoea in rabbits (Vaughan-Williams & Dohadwalla, 1969). Prostaglandins are unlikely to be the only factor involved in the response to cholera toxin (which stimulates adenylate cyclase directly), but they may well make some contribution to the accumulation of intraluminal fluid and stimulation of propulsion.

142

Diarrhoea resistant to conventional forms of treatment may follow irradiation for cancer of the cervix. However, the relief of the diarrhoea by aspirin suggests prostaglandin release by incidental radiation damage to the gut (Mennie & Dalley, 1973; Mennie et al, 1975). Irradiation in mice increased small intestinal motility and the release of prostaglandin-like material (Borowska et al. 1979). Both of which were reduced by indomethacin. Raised amounts of prostaglandin-like material extracted from several mouse tissues after whole-body irradiation may have been due, at least partly, to reduced prostaglandin-15-hydroxy-dehydrogenase activity (Eisen & Walker, 1976, 1978).

Many tumours can synthesise increased amounts of prostaglandin-like material (see Bennett, 1979), and to some extent this is true of human colonic cancers (Jaffe, 1974; Bennett et al. 1977b), but the significance of this is not understood. Diarrhoea is common with many endocrine tumours (for reviews see Bennett, 1976a,b, 1978, 1979; Jaffe & Condon, 1976; Rask-Madsen & Bukhave, 1979; Korman et al. 1981). The extent to which prostaglandins released into the bloodstream contribute to the diarrhoea is not known, particularly since many are substantially inactivated on passage through the pulmonary circulation and the amounts reaching the gut may be small. Nevertheless, although inactivation of PGE and PGF compounds is high in dogs and rabbits (Ferreira & Vane, 1967) only about 70% of a dose of PGE_1 was inactivated in one passage though human lungs (Golub et al. 1975). Various nonendocrine tumours are associated with raised blood levels of 6-keto-$PGF_{1\alpha}$ (Demers et al. 1979; Khan et al. 1981), and although PGI_2 is not destroyed in the pulmonary circulation diarrhoea is not usually a feature of these diseases.

Other substances produced by endocrine tumours (eg calcitonin, vasoactive intestinal peptide (VIP) and human pancreatic polypeptide) might contribute to diarrhoea by stimulating gut prostaglandin synthesis (see Rask-Madsen & Bukhave, 1979), but the evidence is not conclusive. In rats, VIP-induced intestinal fluid secretion was inhibited by indomethacin 5mg/kg, but a selective effect of indomethacin on prostanoid synthesis was questioned (Albuquerque et al. 1979).

Diarrhoea commonly occurs in the irritable colon syndrome. Rask-Madsen & Bukhave (1978) found increased amounts of PGE_2 in jejunal secretions of two fasting patients with this condition. Indomethacin treatment resulted in more-solid, smaller stools which were passed less frequently; relapse occurred after treatment was stopped.

In patients given foods to which they showed gastrointestinal intolerance, blood and stool concentrations of prostaglandins were usually raised (Buisseret et al., 1978). Pretreatment with prosta-glandin synthesis inhibitors usually prevented the symptoms. Lieb (1978) found that aspirin prevented gastrointestinal disturbances associated with his lactose intolerance after eating dairy products, and that aspirin prevented abdominal cramps and diarrhoea evoked in a woman by black coffee (Lieb, 1980).

Increased gastrointestinal motility (Fochem, 1955) and defaeca-tion (McCance & Pickles, 1960) can occur in menstruation, and breast-fed babies can suffer diarrhoea during menstruation of the lactating mother (Naish, 1952). Nausea, vomiting and diarrhoea are common in patients with dysmenorrhoea (Kauppila & Ylikorkala, 1977). Men-struation and, in particular, dysmenorrhoea are associated with in-creased endometrial prostaglandin synthesis (see Collins & Willman, 1978). In dysmenorrhoea, prostaglandin synthesis inhibitors re-lieve both uterine pain and gastrointestinal disturbances (Kapadia & Elder, 1978; Lundström, 1978). Perhaps prostaglandins reach the gut from the uterus, or increased gut prostaglandin synthesis occurs (see Sanger & Bennett, 1979).

Idiopathic postural hypotension is characterised by parasym-pathetic and sympathetic denervation. One conventionally treated patient had recurrent profuse diarrhoea which improved with aspirin (Smythies & Russell, 1974).

Treatment of diarrhoea with nutmeg

As discussed by Bennett (1978) nutmeg is commonly used in some countries to treat human diarrhoea. Case reports of the response to nutmeg include medullary carcinoma of the thyroid (Fawell & Thompson, 1973; Barrowman et al., 1975) and Crohn's disease (Shafran et al. 1977). Excellent prevention or treatment of scouring in calves and bowel oedema in piglets has been obtained (Stamford et al., 1978, 1980). Nutmeg may act by inhibiting prostaglandin syn-thesis (Bennett et al., 1974; Shafran et al., 1977).

BENEFICIAL EFFECTS OF PROSTANOIDS IN GASTROINTESTINAL MOTILITY DISORDERS

This aspect is the converse of the association of prostaglandins with diarrhoea. Thus in postoperative ileus, Fukunishi et al.,(1977) restored depressed gut mechanical and electrical activity with $PGF_{2\alpha}$ without appreciable side effects when infused into patients iv ($0.5\mu g$ kg^{-1} min^{-1} for 2h, 3 times daily for 3 days after surgery). Postoperative ileus also responded to $PGF_{2\alpha}$ in rabbits (Fiedler, 1979), and to 16,16-dimethyl PGE_2 in rats and guinea-pigs (Ruwart et al., 1980).

Some laxatives may act, at least in part, by stimulating prostaglandin synthesis (Beubler & Juan, 1978, 1979; Capasso et al. 1983; Luderer et al. 1980). Kelly et al. (1974) found that PGE, A or B compounds administered intraduodenally to rats caused expulsion of worms, but PGE compounds were not effective in the experiments of Kassai et al. (1979).

REFERENCES

Assouline, G., Leibson, V. & Danon, A. (1977). Stimulation of prostaglandin output from rat stomach by hypertonic solution. Eur. J. Pharmacol. 44: 271-273.

Barrowman, J.A., Bennett, A., Hillenbrand, P., Rolles, L., Pollock, D.J. & Wright, J.T. (1975). Diarrhoea in medullary carcinoma of the thyroid: evidence for the role of prostaglandins and the therapeutic effect of nutmeg. Br Med J 3: 11-12.

Bedwani, J.R. & Okpako, D.T. (1975). Effects of crude and pure cholera toxin on prostaglandin release from the rabbit ileum. Prostaglandins 10: 117-127.

Bennett, A. (1972). Effects of prostaglandins on the gastrointestinal tract. In: Karim, S.S.M. (ed) The prostaglandins: progress in research. Medical and Technical, Oxford, pp205-221.

Bennett, A. (1973). Prostaglandins and the gut. In: Truelove, S.C., Jewell, D.P. (eds) Topics in gastroenterology. Blackwell Scientific, Oxford, pp 281-293.

Bennett, A. (1976a). Prostaglandins and the gut. Annu. Res. Rev., Eden Press, Montreal.

Bennett, A. (1976b). Prostaglandins as factors in diseases of the alimentary tract. Adv. Prostaglandin Thromboxane Res. 2: 547-555.

Bennett, A. (1977). The role of prostaglandins in gastrointestinal tone and motility. In:Berti, F., Samuelsson, B., Velo, G.P. (eds) Prostaglandins and Thromboxanes, Plenum Press, New York, pp 275-285.

Bennett, A. (1978). Prostaglandins. In: Turner, P., Shand, D.G. (eds) Recent advances in clinical pharmacology. Churchill Livingstone, Edinburgh, pp 17-30.

Bennett, A. (1979). Prostaglandins and cancer. In: Karim, S.S. M. (ed) Practical applicantions of prostaglandins and their synthesis inhibitors. MTP Press, Lancaster, pp 149-188.

Bennett, A. (1983). Roles of thromboxanes in gastrointestinal physio pathology. Tissue Reactions, 5: 237-239.

Bennett, A., Del Tacca, M., Stamford, I.F. & Zebro, T. (1977b). Prostaglandins from tumours of human large bowel. Br J. Cancer, 35: 881-884.

Bennett, A., Eley, K.G. & Scholes, G.B. (1968a). Effects of prostaglandins E_1 and E_2 on human, guinea-pig, and rat isolated small intestine. Br.J.Pharmacol, 34: 630-638.

Bennett, A., Eley, K.G. & Scholes, G.B. (1968b). Effect of prostaglandins E_1 and E_2 on intestinal motility in the guinea-pig and rat. Br. J. Pharmacol, 34: 639-647.

145

Bennett, A., Eley, K.G. & Stockley, H.L. (1976). Inhibition of peristalsis in guinea-pig isolated ileum and colon by drugs that block prostaglandin synthesis. Br. J. Pharmacol, 57: 335-340.

Bennett, A. & Fleshler, B. (1970). Prostaglandins and the gastrointestinal tract. Gastroenterology, 59: 790-800.

Bennett, A., Friedmann, C.A. & Vane, J. R. (1967). Release of prostaglandin E_1 from the rat stomach. Nature, 216: 873-876.

Bennett, A., Gradidge, C.F. & Stamford, I F. (1974). Prostaglandins, nutmeg and diarrhoea. N. Engl. J. Med. 290: 110-111.

Bennett, A., Hensby, C.N., Sanger, G.J. & Stamford, I.F. (1981). Metabolites of arachidonic acid formed by human gastrointestinal tissues and their actions on the muscle layers. Br. J. Pharmacol. 74: 435-444.

Bennett, A., Jarosik, C., Sanger, G.J. & Wilson, D.E. (1980). Antagonism of prostanoid-induced contractions of rat gastric fundus muscle by SC-19220, sodium meclofenamate, indomethacin or trimethoquinol. Br. J. Pharmacol, 71: 169-175.

Bennett, A., Murray, J.G. & Wyllie, J.H. (1968c). Occurrence of prostaglandin E_2 in human stomach and a study of its effects on human isolated gastric muscle. Br. J. Pharmacol. Chemother. 32: 339-349.

Bennett, A., Posner, J. (1971). Studies on prostaglandin antagonists. Br. J. Pharmacol. 42: 584-594.

Bennett, A., Sanger, G.J. (1978). The effects of prostaglandin D_2 on the circular muscle of guinea-pig isolated ileum and colon. Br. J. Pharmacol. 63: 357-358P.

Bennett, A. & Sanger, G.J. (1980). Prostacyclin relaxes the longitudinal muscle of human isolated stomach and antagonizes contractions to some prostanoids. J. Physiol. (Lond). 298: 45-46P.

Bennett, A. & Sanger, G.J. (1982). Prostaglandins. In: Mediators and Drugs in Gastrointestinal Motility II. Handb. Exp. Pharm, 59/II, ed G. Bertaccini, Springer-Verlag, Berlin, pp 219-248.

Bennett, A., Sanger, G.J., Stamford, I.F. & Hensby, C.N. (1983). Prostanoids formed by human gastrointestinal tissues and their effects on muscle activity. Adv. in Prostaglandin, Thromb. and Leukotriene Res., 12: 379-381.

Bennett, A., Stamford, I.F. & Unger, W.G. (1973). Prostaglandin E_2 and gastric acid secretion in man. J. Physiol. 229: 349-360.

Bennett, A. & Stockley, H.L. (1977a). The contribution of prostaglandins in the muscle of human isolated small intestine to neurogenic responses. Br. J. Pharmacol. 61: 573-578.

Beubler, E. & Juan, H. (1978). Is the effect of diphenolic laxatives mediated via release of prostaglandin E? Experientia 34: 386-387.

Bhana, D., Karim, S.M.M., Carter, D.C. & Ganesan, P.A. (1973). The effect of orally administered prostaglandins A_1, A_2, and 15-epi-A_2 on human gastric secretion. Prostaglandins, 3: 307-316.

Book, L.S., Johnson, D.G., Jubiz, W. & Roberts, C. (1979). Elevated prostaglandin E in children with chronic idiopathic intestinal pseudo-obstruction syndrome (CIIPS): Effects of prostaglandin synthetase inhibitors on gastrointestinal motility. Clin. Res. 27: 100A.

Boot, J.R., Dawson, W., Cockerill, A.F., Mallen, D.N.B. & Osborne, D.J. (1977). The pharmacology of prostaglandin-like substances released from guinea-pig lungs during anaphylaxis. Prostaglandins 13: 927-932.

Buisseret, P.D., Youlten, L.J.F., Heinzelmann, D.I. & Lessof, M.H. (1978). Prostaglandin-synthesis inhibitors in prophylaxis of food intolerance. Lancet 1: 906-908.

Bunting, S., Moncada, S. & Vane, J.R. (1976). The effects of prostaglandin endoperoxides and thromboxane A_2 on strips of rabbit coeliac artery and other smooth muscle preparations. Br. J. Pharmacol. 57: 462P.

Burnstock, G., Cocks, T., Paddle, B. & Staszewska-Barczak, J. (1975). Evidence that prostaglandin is responsible for the "rebound contraction" following stimulation of non-adrenergic, non-cholinergic ("purinergic") inhibitory nerves. Eur. J. Pharmacol. 31: 360-362.

Campieri, M., Lanfranchi, G.A., Bazzocchi, G., Brignola, C., Benatti, A., Boccia, S. & Labo, G. (1980). Prostaglandins, indomethacin and ulcerative colitis. Gastroenterology, 78: 193.

Campieri, M., Lanfranchi, G.A., Bazzocchi, G., Brignola, C., Corazza, G., Cortini, C., Michelini, M. & Labo, G. (1978). Salicylate other than 5-aminosalicylic acid ineffective in ulcerative colitis. Lancet 2: 993.

Capasso, F., Mascolo, N., Autore, G. & Duraccio, M.R. (1983). Effect of indomethacin on aloin and 1,8 dioxyanthraquinone-induced production of prostaglandins in the isolated rat colon. Prostaglandins, 26: 547-552.

Chijimatsu, Y., Nguyen, T.V. & Said, S.I. (1977). Effects of prostaglandin endoperoxide analogues on contractile elements in lung and gastrointestinal tract. Prostaglandins, 13: 909-916.

Chouseterman, M., Petite, J.P., Housset, E. & Hornych, A. (1977). Prostaglandins and acute intestinal pseudo-obstruction. Lancet 2: 138-139.

Classen, M., Sturzanhofecker, P., Koch, H. & Demling, L. (1973). The effect of prostaglandin E_1 on the secretion and the motility of the human stomach. Acta. Hepatogastroenterol. 20: 159-162.

Cohen, M.M. (1978). Mucosal cytoprotection by prostaglandin E_2. Lancet 2: 1253-1254.

Coleman, R.A., Humphrey, P.P.A., Kennedy, I., Levy, G.P. & Lumley, P. (1980). U-46619, a selective thromboxane A_2-like agonist? Br. J. Pharmacol. 68: 127-128P.

Coleman, R.A., Humphrey, P.P.A., Kennedy, I., Levy, G.P. & Lumley, P. (1981). Further evidence that AH19437 is a specific thromboxane receptor blocking drug.　Br.J. Pharmac. 73: 258P.

Collier, H.O.J., McDonald-Gibson, W.J. & Saeed, S.A. (1975).　Stimulation of prostaglandin biosynthesis by capsaicin, ethanol, and tyramine.　Lancet 1: 702.

Collier, H.O.J., McDonald-Gibson, W.J. & Saeed, S.A. (1976).　Stimulation of prostaglandin biosynthesis by drugs: effects in vitro of some drugs affecting gut function.　Br. J. Pharmacol. 58: 193-199.

Collins, W.P., Willman, E.A. (1978).　Prostaglandins and uterine function.　Top.Horm. Chem. pp 180-215.

Cummings, J.H., Newman, A., Misiewicz, J.J., Milton-Thompson, G.J. & Billings, J.A. (1973).　Effect of intravenous prostaglandin $F_{2\alpha}$ on small intestinal function in man.　Nature (London) 243: 169.

Dajani, E.Z., Bertermann, R.E., Rose, E.A.W., Schweingruber, F.L. & Woods, E.M. (1979).　Canine gastrointestinal motility effects of prostaglandin $F_{2\alpha}$ in vivo.　Arch. Int. Pharmacodyn. 237: 16-24.

Daniel, E.E., Sarna, S., Waterfall, W. & Crankshaw, J. (1979).　Role of endogenous prostaglandins in regulating the tone of opossum lower esophageal sphincter in vivo.　Prostaglandins 17: 641-648.

Demers, L.M. Schweitzer, J., Lipton, A. & Harvey, H. (1979).　Blood 6-keto-$PGF_{1\alpha}$ levels as potential tumour marker.　Cancer Treat. Rep. 63: 1210.

Dilawari, J.D., Newman, A., Poleo, J. & Misiewicz, J.J. (1975).　Response of the human cardiac sphincter to circulating prostaglandins $F_{2\alpha}$ and E_2 and to anti-inflammatory drugs.　Gut 16: 137-143.

Eisen, V. & Walker, D.I. (1976).　Effect of ionizing radiation on prostaglandin-like activity in tissues.　Br.J. Pharmacol, 57: 527-532.

Eisen, V. & Walker, D.I. (1978).　Effect of ionizing radiation on prostaglandin 15-OH-dehydrogenase (PGDH).　Br. J. Pharmacol. 62: 461P.

Ekelund, K., Johansson, C. & Nylander, B. (1977).　Effects of 16, 16-dimethyl prostaglandin E_2 on food stimulated pancreatic secretion and output of bile in man.　Scand. J. Gastroenterol. 12: 457-460.

Eley, K.G., Bennett, A. & Stockley, H.L. (1977).　The effects of prostaglandins E_1, E_2, $F_{1\alpha}$, and $F_{2\alpha}$ on the guinea-pig ileal and colonic peristalsis.　J. Pharm. Pharmacol, 29: 280-296.

Fawell, W.N. & Thompson, G. (1973).　Nutmeg for diarrhoea of medullary carcinoma of the thyroid.　N. Engl. J. Med. 289: 108-109.

Ferreira, S.H. & Vane, J.R. (1967).　Prostaglandins, their disappearance from, and release into the circulation.　Nature, 216: 868-873.

Fiedler, L. (1979).　$PGF_{2\alpha}$ - a new therapy for paralytic ileus?

148

Abstracts 4th International Prostaglandin Conference, Washington, DC, p 33.

Fitzpatrick, F.A. & Wynalda, M.A. (1976).   In vivo suppression of prostaglandin biosynthesis by non-steroidal anti-inflammatory agents.   Prostaglandins 12, 1037-1051.

Flower, R J. (1974).   Drugs which inhibit prostaglandin biosynthesis.   Pharmacol. Rev. 26: 33-67.

Fontaine, J., Van Nueten, J.M. & Reuse, J.J. (1977).   Effects of prostaglandins on the peristaltic reflex of the guinea-pig ileum.   Arch. Int. Pharmacodyn. Ther. 226: 341-343.

Fukunishi, S., Amano, S., Saijo, H., Matsumoto, K., Iriyama, K. & Fujino, T. (1977).   The effect of intravenous prostaglandin $F_{2\alpha}$ on the motility of the gastrointestinal tracts after major abdominal surgery.   Jpn. J. Smooth Muscle Res. 13: 141-152.

Fung, W.P. & Karim, S.M.M. (1976).   Effect of prostaglandin E_2 on the healing of gastric ulcers: A double-blind endoscopic trial.   Aust. NZ J. Med. 6: 121-122.

Fung, W.P., Karim, S.M.M. & Tye, C.Y. (1974a).   Effect of 15(R)-15-methyl prostaglandin E_2 methyl ester on healing of gastric ulcers.   Controlled endoscopic study.   Lancet 2: 10-12.

Gerkens, J.F., Gerber, J.G., Shand, D.G. & Branch, R.A. (1978).   Effect of PGI_2, PGE_2 and 6-keto-$PGF_{1\alpha}$ on canine gastric blood flow and acid secretion.   Prostaglandins 16: 815-823.

Gilat, T., Ratan, J., Rosen, P. & Peled, Y. (1979).   Prostaglandins and ulcerative colitis.   Gastroenterology, 76: 1083.

Golub, M., Zia, P., Matsumo, M. & Horton, R. (1975).   Metabolism of prostaglandins A_1 and E_1 in man.   J. Clin. Invest. 56: 1404-1410.

Gorman, R.R., Sun, F.F., Miller, O.V. & Johnson, R.A. (1977).   Prostaglandin H_1 and prostaglandin H_2 - convenient biochemical synthesis and isolation - further biological and spectroscopic characterization.   Prostaglandins 13: 1043-1054.

Goyal, R.K., Mukhopadhyay, A. & Rattan, S. (1974).   Effect of prostaglandin E_2 on the lower esophageal sphincter in normal subjects and patients with achalasia.   Clin. Res. 22: 358A.

Goyal, R.K., Rattan, S. & Hersh, T. (1973).   Comparison of the effects of prostaglandins E_1, E_2, and A_2, and of hypovolemic hypotension on the lower esophageal sphincter.   Gastroenterology, 65: 608-612.

Guth, P.H., Aures, D. & Paulsen, G. (1979).   Topical aspirin plus HCl gastric lesions in the rat.   Cytoprotective effect of prostaglandin, cimetidine and probanthine.   Gastroenterology, 76: 88-93.

Hamberg, M., Hedqvist, P., Strandberg, K., Svensson, J. & Samuelsson, B. (1975).   Prostaglandin endoperoxides. IV.   Effects on smooth muscle.   Life Sci. 16: 451-462.

Harper, M.J.K. & Skarnes, R.C. (1972).   Inhibition of abortion and fetal death produced by endotoxin or prostaglandin $F_{2\alpha}$.   Prostaglandins, 2: 295-309.

Herman, A.G. & Vane, J.R. (1975). Endotoxin and production of prostaglandins by the isolated rabbit jejunum. Influence of indomethacin. Arch. Int. Pharmacodyn. Ther. 213:328-329.

Higgs, G.A., Eakins, K.E., Mugridge, K.G., Moncada, S. & Vane, J.R. (1980). Effects of non-steroid anti-inflammatory drugs on leucocyte migration in carrageenin-induced inflammation. Eur. J. Pharmac. 6: 81-86.

Horton, E.W. & Jones, R.L. (1974). Biological activity of prostaglandin D_2 on smooth muscle. Br. J. Pharmacol. 52: 110-111P.

Horton, E.W., Main, I.H.M., Thompson, C.J. & Wright, P.M. (1968). Effect of orally administered prostaglandin E_1 on gastric secretion and intestine motility in man. Gut, 9: 655-658.

Hoult, J.R.S. & Moore, P.K. (1978). Sulphasalazine is a potent inhibitor of prostaglandin 15-hydroxydehydrogenase: Possible basis for therapeutic action in ulcerative colitis. Br. J. Pharmacol. 64: 6-8.

Hunt, R.H., Dilawari, J.B. & Misiewicz, J.J. (1975). The effect of intravenous prostaglandin $F_{2\alpha}$ and E_2 on the motility of the sigmoid colon. Gut, 16: 47-49.

Ishizawa, M. & Miyazaki, E. (1973a). Action of prostaglandins on gastrointestinal motility. Sapporo Med. J. 42: 366-373.

Ishizawa, M. & Miyazaki, E. (1973b). Effect of prostaglandins on the movement of guinea-pig isolated intestine. Jpn. J. Smooth Muscle Res. 9: 235-237.

Ishizawa, M. & Miyazaki, E. (1975). Effect of prostaglandin $F_{2\alpha}$ on propulsive activity of the isolated segmental colon of the guinea-pig. Prostaglandins, 10: 759-768.

Jaffe, B.M. (1974). Prostaglandins and cancer: an update. Prostaglandins 6: 453-461.

Jaffe, B.M. & Condon, S. (1976). Prostaglandins E and F in endocrine diarrheagenic syndromes. Ann. Surg. 184: 516-523.

Jaques, R. (1977). Inhibition effect of methionine-enkephalin and leucine-enkephalin on contractions of guinea-pig ileum elicited by PGE_1. Experientia, 33: 374-375.

Johansson, C. & Ekelund, K. (1977). Effects of 16,16-dimethyl prostaglandin E_2 on the integrated response to a meal. In: Duthie, H.L. (ed) Gastrointestinal motility in health and disease. Proc. 6th Int. Symp. Gastrointest. Motility, Edinburgh, MTP Press, Lancaster, pp 195-204.

Jones, R.L. Peesapati, V. & Wilson, N.H. (1982). Antagonism of the thromboxane-sensitive contractile systems of the rabbit aorta, dog saphenous vein and guinea-pig trachea. Br. J. Pharmac. 76: 423-438.

Kadlec, O., Masek, K. & Seferna, I. (1974). A modulating role of prostaglandins in contractions of the guinea-pig ileum. Br. J. Pharmacol. 51: 565-570.

Kadlec, O., Masek, K. & Seferna, I. (1975). The role of prostaglandins in the output of neurotransmitters from the isolated guinea-pig ileum. Abstracts 6th International Congress on Pharmacology, p 156.

Kapadia, L. & Elder, M.G. (1978). Flufenamic acid in treatment of primary spasmodic dysmenorrhoea. Lancet 1: 348-350.

Karim, S.M.M. & Ganesan, P.A. (1974). Prostaglandins and the digestive system. Ann. Acad. Med. Singapore, 3: 286-293.

Karim, S.M.M., Carter, D.C., Bhana, D. & Ganesan, P.A. (1973). Effect of orally and intravenously administered prostaglandin 15(R)-15 methyl E_2 on gastric secretion in man. Adv. Biosci. 9: 255-264.

Kassai, T., Redl, P., Balla, E., Jecsay, G.Y. & Harangozo, E. (1979). Nippostrongylus brasiliensis in the rat: failure to induce worm rejection by prostaglandins. Abstracts 4th International Prostaglandin Conference, Washington, DC, p58.

Kauppila, A. & Ylikorkala, O. (1977). Indomethacin and tolfenamic acid in primary dysmenorrhoea. Eur. J. Obstet. Gynaecol. Reprod. Biol. 7: 59-64.

Kelly, J.D., Dineen, J.K., Goodrich, B.S. & Smith, I.D. (1974). Expulsion of Nippostrongylus brasiliensis from the intestine of rats. Int. Arch. Allergy Appl. Immunol. 47: 458-465.

Kennedy, I., Coleman, R.A., Humphrey, P.A.A., Levy, G.P. & Lumley, P. (1982). Studies on the charaterization of prostanoid receptors: a proposed classification. Prostaglandins 24: 667-689.

Khan, A.K.A., Piris, P. & Truelove, S.C. (1977). An experiment to determine the active therapeutic moiety of sulphasalazine. The Lancet 2: 892-895.

Khan, O., Hensby, C.N. & Williams, G. (1981). Prostacyclin in Prostatic disease. In: Lewis, P.G., O'Grady, J. (eds) Clinical pharmacology of prostacyclin. Raven Press, New York, pp 49-52.

Knapp, H.R., Oelz, O., Sweetman, B.J. & Oates, J.A. (1978). Synthesis and metabolism of prostaglandins E_2, $F_{2\alpha}$ and D_2 by the rat gastrointestinal tract. Stimulation by a hypertonic environment in vitro. Prostaglandins, 15: 751-757.

Konturek, S.J., Brzozowski, T., Piastucki, I., Radecki, T. & Dembinska-Kiec, A. (1983). Role of prostaglandin and thromboxane biosynthesis in gastric necrosis caused by taurocholate and ethanol. Dig. Dis. Sci. 28: 154-160.

Korman, S.M., Berant, M. & Alon, U. (1981). Review: Prostaglandins in diarrheal states. Isr. J. Med. Sci. 17: 1109-1113.

Kruidinier, J., Tao, P. & Wilson, D. (1978). The role of prostaglandins in lower esophageal sphincter pressure in man. Clin. Res. 26, 663A.

Lancaster, C. & Robert, A. (1978). Intestinal lesions produced by prednisolone: Prevention (cytoprotection) by 16,16-dimethyl prostaglandin E_2. Am. J. Physiol. 235: E703-E708.

Lieb, J. (1978). Prostaglandin synthesis inhibitors in prophylaxis of food intolerance. Lancet 2: 157.

Lieb, J. (1980). Prostaglandin synthesis inhibitors and prophylaxis of coffee intolerance. JAMA 243: 32.

Luderer, J.R., Demers, L.M., Nomides, C.T. & Hayes, A.H. Jr. (1980). Mechanism of action of castor oil: a biochemical link to the prostaglandins. Adv. Prostaglandin Thromboxane Res. 8: 1633-1635.

Lundstrom, V. (1978). Treatment of primary dysmenorrhoea with prostaglandin synthetase inhibitors - a promising alternative. Acta. Obstet. Gynecol. Scand. 57: 421-428.

Maher, J.W., Hollenbeck, J.I., Crandall, V., McGuigan, J. & Woodward, E.R. (1978). Prostaglandin E_2 effect on lower esophageal sphincter pressure and serum gastrin. J. Surg. Res. 24: 87-91.

Main, I.H.M. (1973). Prostaglandins and the gastrointestinal tract. In: Cuthbert, M.F. (ed) The prostaglandins. Pharmacological and therapeutic advances. Heinemann, London, pp 287-323.

Main, I.H.M. & Whittle, B.J.R. (1973). The effects of E and A prostaglandins on gastric mucosal blood flow and acid secretion in the rat. Br. J. Pharmacol. 49: 428-436.

Main, I.H.M. & Whittle, B.J.R. (1974). Methyl analogues of prostaglandin E_2 and gastrointestinal function in the rat. Br. J. Pharmacol. 52: 113P.

Main, I.H.M. & Whittle, B.J.R. (1974). Prostaglandin E_2 and the stimulation of rat gastric acid secretion by dibutryl cyclic 3',5'-AMP. Eur. J. Pharmacol. 26: 204-211.

Mathias, J.R., Carlson, G.M., Bertiger, G., Martin, J.L. & Cohen, S. (1977). Migrating action potential complex of cholera: a possible prostaglandin-induced response. Am. J. Physiol. 232: E529-E534.

Matuchansky, C. & Bernier, J.J. (1973). Effect of prostaglandin E_1 on glucose, water, and electrolyte absorption in the human jejunum. Gastroenterology, 64: 1111.

McCance, R.A. & Pickles, V.R. (1960). Cyclical variations in intestinal activity in women. J. Endocrinol 20: XXVII.

Mennie, A.T. & Dalley, V. (1973). Aspirin in radiation-induced diarrhoea. Lancet 1: 1131.

Mennie, A.T., Dalley, V.M., Dineen, L.C. & Collier, H.O.J. (1975). Treatment of radiation-induced gastro-intestinal distress with acetylsalicylate. Lancet 2: 942-943.

Milton-Thompson, G.J., Billings, J.A., Cummings, J.H., Newman, A. & Misiewicz, J.J. (1973). The effect of circulating prostaglandin $F_{2\alpha}$ on the function of the human small intestine. Rend. Rom. Gastroenterol. 5: 139.

Milton-Thompson, G.J., Cummings, J.H., Newman, A., Billings, J.A. & Misiewicz, J.J. (1975). Colonic and small intestinal response to intravenous prostaglandin $F_{2\alpha}$ and E_2 in man. Gut 16: 42-46.

Misiewicz, J.J., Waller, S.L., Kiley, N. & Horton, E.W. (1969). Effect of oral prostaglandin E_1 on intestinal transit in man. Lancet 1: 648-651.

Molin, L. & Stendahl, O. (1979). The effect of sulfasalazine and its active components on human polymorphonuclear leukocyte.

Function in relation to ulcerative colitis. Acta. Med. Scand. 206: 451-457.

Mukhopadhyay, A. Rattan, S. & Goyal, R.K. (1975). Effect of prostaglandin E_2 on esophageal motility in man. J. Appl. Physiol. 39, 479-481.

Mukhopadhyay, A.K., Weisbrodt, N.W., Copeland, E.D. & Johnson, L.R. (1974). Effect of prostaglandin E_2 infusion on patterns of intestinal myoelectric activity. Gastroenterology, 66: 752.

Naish, F.C. (1952). Breast feeding. In: Moncrieff, A., Thompson, W.A.R. (eds) Child health. Eyre & Spottiswoode, London, p 218.

Newman, A., DeMoraes-Filho, J.P.P., Philippakos, D. & Misiewicz, J.J. (1975). The effect of intravenous infusions of prostaglandins E_2 and $F_{2\alpha}$ on human gastric function. Gut, 16: 272-276.

Nilsson, F. & Ohrn, P.G. (1974). Duodeno-gastric reflux after administration of prostaglandin $F_{2\alpha}$. Studies of gastrointestinal propulsion in the rat. Int. Res. Commun. Serv. 2: 1558.

Nompleggi, D., Myers, L., Castell, D.O. & Dubois, A. (1979). Do endogenous prostaglandins play a role in gastric emptying and gastric secretion? Clin. Res. 27: 269A.

Nompleggi, D., Myers, L., Ramwell, P., Castell, D.O. & Dubois, A. (1980). PGE_2 involvement in the regulation of gastric emptying. In: B. Samuelsson, P.W. Ramwell, R. Paoletti (eds), Advances in Prostaglandin and Thromboxane Research, Vol 8, Raven Press, New York, pp 1587-1588.

Nylander, B. & Andersson, S. (1975). Effect of two methylated prostaglandin E_2 analogs on gastroduodenal pressure in man. Scand. J. Gastroenterol. 10: 91-95.

Nylander, B. & Mattsson, O. (1975). Effect of 16,16-dimethyl PGE_2 on gastric emptying of a barium food test meal in man. Scand. J. Gastroenterol. 10: 289-292.

O'Grady, J., Warrington, S., Moti, M.J., et al (1979). Effects of intravenous prostacyclin infusions in healthy volunteers - some preliminary observations. In: Vane, J.R., Bergstrom, S (eds) Prostacyclin. Raven Press, New York, pp 409-417.

Ohashi, S., Ohmuro, S., Sugawara, I., Kuwata, K. & Okamoto, E. (1973). Effects of prostaglandin E_1 on canine gastrointestinal motility in vivo and human isolated smooth muscle in vitro. Jpn. J. Smooth Muscle Res. 9: 69-77.

Peskar, B.M. (1978). Regional distribution of prostaglandin-metabolizing enzymes in the mucosa of the human upper gastrointestinal tract. Acta. Hepato-gastroenterol. (Stuttg) 25: 49-51.

Peskar, B.M., & Peskar, B.A. (1976). On the metabolism of prostaglandins by human gastric fundus mucosa. Biochim. Biophys. Acta. 424: 430-438.

Peskar, B.M., Seyberth, H.W. & Peskar, B.A. (1980). Synthesis and metabolism of endogenous prostaglandins by human gastric mucosa. Adv. Prostaglandin Thromboxane Res. 8: 1511-1514.

Radmanovic, B. (1972). The effect of PGE_1 on the peristaltic
    activity of the guinea-pig isolated ileum. Arch. Int.
    Pharmacodyn. Ther. 200: 396-404.
Rampton, D.S. & Sladen, G.E. (1981). Prostaglandin synthesis in-
    hibitors in ulcerative colitis: Flurbiprofen compared with
    conventional treatment. Prostaglandins 21: 417-425.
Rask-Madsen, J. & Bukhave, K. (1978). Indomethacin-responsive
    diarrhoea in irritable bowel syndrome. Gut 19: A448.
Rask-Madsen, J. & Bukhave, K. (1979). Prostaglandins and chronic
    diarrhoea: clinical aspects. Scand. J. Gastroenterol (Suppl
    53) 14: 73-78.
Robert, A. (1974). Effects of prostaglandins on the stomach and
    the intestine. Prostaglandins 6: 523-532.
Robert, A. (1975). An intestinal disease produced experimentally
    by a prostaglandin deficiency. Gastroenterology 69: 1045-1047.
Robert, A., Hanchar, A.J., Lancaster, C. & Nezamis, J.E. (1979a).
    Prostacyclin (PGI_2) and PGD_2 prevent enteropooling and diarr-
    hea caused by prostaglandins and cholera toxin. Fed. Proc.
    38: 1239.
Robert, A., Hancher, A.J., Lancaster, C. & Nezamis, J.E. (1979c).
    Prostacyclin inhibits enteropooling and diarrhoea. In: Vane,
    J.R., Bergstrom, S. (eds) Prostacyclin. Raven, New York, pp
    147-158.
Robert, A., Hanchar, A.J., Nezamis, J.E. & Lancaster, C. (1979b).
    Cytoprotection against acidified aspirin: Comparison of prosta-
    glandin, cimetidine and probanthine. Gastroenterology, 76:
    1227.
Robert, A., Nezamis, J.E. & Lancaster, C. (1976). Effect of 16,
    16-dimethyl PGE_2 on gastric emptying. In: B. Samuelsson
    and R. Paoletti (eds), Advances in Prostaglandin and Throm-
    boxane Research, Vol 2, Raven Press, New York, p 946.
Robert, A. Nezamis, J.E., Lancaster, C., Hanchar, A.J. & Klepper,
    M.S. (1976). Enteropooling assay: A test for diarrhea pro-
    duced by prostaglandins. Prostaglandins 11: 809-828.
Robert, A. & Ruart, M.J. (1982). Effects of prostaglandins on the
    digestive system. In: Prostaglandins, ed J.B. Lee, Elsevier,
    New York pp 113-176.
Ruwart, M.J., Klepper, M.S. & Rush, B.D. (1978). The beneficial
    effects of prostaglandins in post-operative ileus. Gastro-
    enterology, 74: 1088.
Ruwart, M.J., Klepper, M.S. & Rush, B.D. (1979). Regulation of
    gastric emptying, small intestinal transit and colonic transit
    in the rat. Gastroenterology 76: 1232.
Ruwart, M.J. Klepper, M.S. & Rush, B.D. (1980). Prostaglandin
    stimulation of gastrointestinal transit in post-operative
    ileus rats. Prostaglandins 19: 415-426.
Rybicka, J. & Gibinski, K. (1978). Methyl-prostaglandin E_2 analo-
    gues for healing of gastroduodenal ulcers. Scand. J. Gastro-
    enterol. 13: 155-159.

Sakato, M. (1975). Studies on the physiological role of prostaglandins in adrenergic and non-adrenergic inhibitory neurotransmission in the guinea-pig taenia coli. Folia Pharmacol.
Jpn. 71: 445-455.

Sakato, M. & Shimo, Y. (1976). Possible role of prostaglandin E_1
on adrenergic neurotransmission in the guinea-pig taenia coli.
Eur. J. Pharmacol. 40: 209-214.

Samuelsson, B., Borgeat, P., Hammarstrom, S. & Murphy, R.C. (1979).
Introduction of a nomenclature: leukotrienes. Prostaglandins,
17: 785-787.

Sanger, G.J. & Bennett, A. (1979). Fenamates may antagonise the
actions of prostaglandin endoperoxides in human myometrium.
Br. J. Clin. Pharmacol. 8: 479-482.

Sanger, G.J. & Bennett, A. (1980). Regional differences in the
responses to prostanoids of circular muscle from guinea-pig
isolated intestine. J. Pharm. Pharmacol. 32: 705-708.

Sanner, J.H. (1969). Antagonism of prostaglandin E_2 by 1-acetyl-
2-(8-chloro-10,11-dihydrobenz(b,f)(1,4)oxazepine-10-carbonyl)
hydrazine(SC-19220). Arch.Int. Pharmacodyn Ther. 180: 45-56.

Shafran, I., Maurer, W. & Thomas, F.D. (1977). Prostaglandins and
Crohn's disease. N. Engl. J. Med. 296: 694.

Shea-Donohue, P.T., Myers, L., Castell, D.O. & Dubois, A. (1980).
Effect of prostacyclin on gastric emptying and secretion in
rhesus monkey. In: B. Samuelsson, P. Ramwell, & R Paoletti
(eds), Advances in Prostaglandin and Thromboxane Research, Vol
8, Raven Press, New York, pp 1557-1558.

Shearin, N.L. & Pancoe, W.L. (1976). Effect of prostaglandin E_1
on rat gastric motility and cyclic nucleotide content. Experientia 32: 1553-1554.

Shehadeh, Z., Price, W.E. & Jacobson, E.D. (1969). Effects of
vasoactive agents on intestinal blood flow and motility in
the dog. Am. J. Physiol. 216: 386-392.

Sinar, D.R., Fletcher, R. & Castell, D.O. (1979). Differences in
the effect of arterial or venous prostaglandins E_1, E_2, or I_2
on lower esophageal sphincter pressure. Clin. Res. 27: 271A.

Sircar, J.C. (1983). Inhibition of soybean lipoxygenase by sulphasalazine and 5 ASA a possible mode of action in ulcerative
colitis. Biochem. Pharmacol. 32: 170-172.

Smejkal, V. (1969). On the action of prostaglandin E_1 on smooth
muscle of the digestive system. Cesk. Gastroenterol. Vyz.
23: 32-35.

Smythies, J.R. & Russell, R.O. (1974). Possible role of prostaglandins in idiopathic postural hypotension. Lancet 2: 963.

Soll, A.H. (1978). Prostaglandin inhibition of histamine-stimulated aminopyrine uptake and cyclic AMP generation by isolated
canine parietal cells. Gastroenterology, 72: 1146.

Sorensen, H.R., Boesby, S. & Pedersen, S.A. (1974). The effect of
prostaglandin E_1 on resting gastroesophageal sphincter pressure
in normal human subjects. Scand. J. Gastroenterol. 9 (Suppl.
27), 29.

155

Spruegel, W., Mitznegg, P., Domschke, W., Domschke, S., Wuensch, E.
     Moroder, L. & Demling, L. (1977).   Direct inhibitory effects
     of enkephalins on contractile responses in the guinea-pig
     ileum.   Gastroenterology 72: 1135.
Stamford, I.F., Bennett, A. & Greenhalf, J. (1978).   Treatment of
     diarrhoea in cattle and pigs with nucmeg.   Vet. Rec. 103:
     14-15.
Stamford, I.F. Bennett, A. & Greenhalf, J. (1980).   Treatment of
     diarrhoea in calves with nutmeg.   Vet. Rec. 106: 389.
Stenson, W.F. & Lobos, E. (1982).   Sulphasalazine inhibits the
     synthesis of chemotactic lipids by neutrophils.   J. Clin.
     Invest. 69: 494-497.
Summers, R.W., Kent, T.H. & Osborne, J.W. (1970).   Effects of drugs,
     ileal obstruction, and irradiation on rat gastrointestinal
     propulsion.   Gastroenterology. 59: 731-739.
Takai, M., Matsuyama, S. & Yagasaki, O. (1974).   Prostaglandin
     release during extension of the small intestine of the guinea-
     pig.   Jpn. J. Smooth Muscle Res. 10: 187-189.
Thompson, J.H. & Angulo, M. (1968).   Prostaglandin-induced sero-
     tonin release.   Experientia. 25: 721-722.
Vaughan-Williams, E.M. & Dohadwalla, A.N. (1969).   Diarrhoea and
     intestinal fluid accumulation in uninfected rabbits cross
     perfused with blood from donor rabbits intra-intestinally
     infected with cholera.   Nature 222: 586-587.
Waller, S.L. (1973).   Prostaglandins and the gastrointestinal tract.
     Gut, 14: 402-417.
Way, L. & Durbin, R.P. (1969).   Inhibition of gastric acid secre-
     tion in vitro by prostaglandin E_1.   Nature (London) 221:
     874-875.
Whittle, B.J.R. (1981).   Temporal relationship between cyclo-oxy-
     genase inhibition, as measured by prostacyclin biosynthesis,
     and the gastrointestinal damage induced by indomethacin in
     the rat.   Gastroenterology, 80: 94.
Whittle, B.J.R., Boughton Smith, N.K., Moncada, S. & Vane, J.R.
     (1978).   Actions of prostacyclin (PGI_2) and its product,
     6-oxo-$PGF_{1\alpha}$ on the rat gastric mucosa in vivo and in vitro.
     Prostaglandins, 15: 955-967.
Whittle, B.J.R., Kauffman, G.L. & Moncada, S. (1981).   Vasocon-
     striction with thromboxane A_2 induces ulceration of the gastric
     mucosa.   Nature, 292: 472.
Willis, A.L., Davison, P. & Ramwell, P.W. (1974).   Inhibition of
     intestinal tone, motility and prostaglandin biosynthesis by
     5,8,11,14-eicosatetraynoic acid (TYA).   Prostaglandins, 5:
     355-368.
Wilson, D.E. (1972).   Prostaglandins and the gastrointestinal tract.
     Prostaglandins, 1: 281-293.
Winship, D.H. & Bernhard, G.C. (1970).   Basal and histamine-
     stimulated human gastric acid secretion.   Lack of effect of
     indomethacin in therapeutic doses.   Gastroenterology 58:
     762-765.

Yagasaki, O., Matsuyama, S. & Takai, M. (1974). The release of prostaglandins from the passively distended wall of guinea-pig intestine. Jpn. J. Pharmacol. (Suppl) 24:31.

GALLBLADDER MOTILITY AND ITS REGULATION

John R. Wood and David R. Jenkins

Gastroenterology Unit, Glaxo Pharmaceuticals Ltd
Greenford, Middlesex, and Department of Surgery
Kings College Hospital Medical School, London, England

INTRODUCTION

Teleologically the gallbladder may be considered to act to reconcile the continuous requirements of the liver to perform excretion of various bile constituents and the periodic requirement for the delivery of concentrated bile to the intestine during digestion. Thus bile is stored in the gallbladder between meals and evacuated into the intestine during digestion.

The ability of the gallbladder to concentrate hepatic bile results from active transport processes present in its mucosal cells, a function which is considered later in this volume. The present review examines the effects of various endocrine and neurocrine mediators on gallbladder motility and their putative roles in the neurohumoral control of gallbladder filling and emptying.

ANATOMY AND INNERVATION

The gallbladder is a musculomembranous sac which rests on the inferior surface of the liver. It is variable in shape from a spherical or pear shape to a cylinder depending upon the animal species. The gallbladder wall consists of three layers: the external or serosa, the fibromuscular and the internal or mucosa. The fibromuscular layer comprises a perimuscular layer of connective tissue rich in blood vessels and lymphatics, and a muscular layer consisting of inner fibres which course longitudinally and outer fibres arranged as an oblique spiral. The distribution of gallbladder muscle is species variable.[1]

159

The gallbladder receives both a sympathetic and parasympathetic nerve supply while its vasculature appears to receive only fibres from the former. Sympathetic fibres from the thoracic spinal cord pass to the gallbladder via the splanchnic nerves and coeliac plexus after which they mingle with parasympathetic fibres from the right and left vagus and the right phrenic nerve to form the anterior and posterior hepatic plexuses. Branches enter the gallbladder from both plexuses. Its wall contains a ganglionated nerve plexus located at the outer surface of the muscle coat. Adrenergic fibres are exchanged between the ganglionated plexus and the perivascular nerves. Another nerve plexus containing adrenergic and cholinergic fibres but without ganglia lies in the lamina propria between the mucosa and the muscle coat.[2] In addition to the efferent fibres supplied by this network the vagus and splanchnic nerves contain a considerable proportion of afferent fibres of unknown function, some of which presumably mediate information from receptors in the gallbladder wall.

GALLBLADDER MOTILITY

Hormonal Effects

   Cholecystokinin and related peptides. The potent contractile effect of this hormone on the gallbladder has been extensively studied in man and animals.[3] Due to difficulties with the development of a radioimmunoassay for cholecystokinin it has only very recently been established that CCK is the principle mechanism by which a fatty meal causes gallbladder contraction.[4]

   Though the precise mechanisms by which CCK exerts its effects on the gallbladder are unknown, there is general agreement about which parts of the molecule are essential for biological activity. Studies investigating the structure-activity requirements for CCK were simplified by the finding that a C-terminal fragment of it could exhibit the cholecystokinetic activity of the entire molecule.[5] This part of the CCK molecule shows a marked sequence homology with the corresponding terminus of gastrin.

   Comparison of the biological effects of three naturally occuring peptides CCK, gastrin and caerulein, their fragments and various synthetic analogues has defined some of the features necessary for CCK activity. Sulphation of the phenolic group on the terminal tyrosine residue markedly affects the cholecystokinetic potency of these peptides.[6] Thus the C-terminal octapeptide of CCK (CCK8) was found to be some 150 times more potent at contracting the guinea pig gallbladder both in vitro and in vivo than was its unsulphated analogue. Similar findings have been reported for these peptides in the conscious cat.[7] In the isolated cat gallbladder sulphated CCK8 was even more potent (a thousand times) than the unsulphated form.[8]

The finding that the difference in activity of sulphated and unsulphated peptides is more pronounced in vitro than in vivo is also true for the cholecystokinetic effect of caerulein on the guinea pig gallbladder. Whether or not this results from in vivo sulphation of the nonsulphated form or de-sulphation of the sulphated form is unknown.

In addition to its sulphation the position of the tyrosine residue is also important for cholecystokinetic activity. CCK, caerulein and gastrin have identical C-terminal pentapeptide sequences. The two potent cholecystokinetic peptides (CCK and caerulein) have their sulphated tyrosine residue displaced from this pentapeptide sequence by an intervening amino acid. This is absent in gastrin where the sulphated residue is linked directly to the pentapeptide sequence. The importance of this arrangement has been confirmed by translocation of the sulphated tyrosine residue in CCK8 with either of the two adjacent amino acids. This change markedly reduces its CCK-like activity.[6]

Though mammalian gallbladders can distinguish CCK-caerulein type peptides from those of the gastrin type, a recent study in the salmon reported that the gallbladder of this species cannot make this distinction.[10] The sulphated peptides were however here also more potent. The cholecystokinetic effects of gastrin is less influenced by sulphation. In the conscious dog no difference was detectable between the two forms.[6] However in the guinea pig gallbladder both in vitro and in vivo[11] and in the cat gallbladder in vitro[8] sulphated gastrin was at least ten times more potent than the non-sulphated form.

Early studies documented that the spasmogenic action of CCK on the isolated gallbladder was not inhibited by atropine.[12] This response is also resistant to the effects of alpha and beta adrenergic antagonists, depolarising agents, tetrodotoxin [13,14,15] and to indomethacin.[16] The response to CCK and caerulein is augmented by blockade of inhibitory histamine H_2 receptors[17,18] as is the response to histamine by its action on stimulatory H1 receptors.[17,19]

In the isolated rabbit gallbladder, contraction stimulated by either acetylcholine or adrenergic agonists was associated with a fall in tissue cyclic AMP (cAMP) concentration.[13] Although the fall in tissue cAMP with CCK did not achieve statistical significance CCK was subsequently found to activate phosphodiesterase in rabbit gallbladder[14] and to decrease cAMP in guinea pig gallbladder muscle.[20] CCK also stimulated guanyl cyclase in rabbit gallbladder muscle acting to increase tissue cyclic GMP, an effect which preceded muscle contraction.[21] The ability of indomethacin to abolish the rise in tissue cyclic GMP concentration without affecting muscle contraction makes it unlikely that this nucleotide acts as a second messenger in gallbladder contraction induced by CCK.[16] It is also unlikely that prostaglandins mediate the CCK response despite their CCK-like actions.[22]

The level of free myoplasmic calcium ions is generally believed to regulate muscle contractile activity. Lanthanum has been reported to inhibit the cholecystokinetic effects of both cholecystokinin and acetylcholine, possibly by displacing a fraction of membrane-bound calcium or by preventing the flow of calcium ions across the plasma membrane.[23] The precise mechanism by which the activation of CCK-receptors effects changes in intra-cellular calcium and gallbladder muscle contraction remains to be elucidated.

Secretin and related Peptides. Five chemical mediators comprise the secretin family of gastrointestinal peptides: secretin, glucagon, vasoactive intestinal polypeptide (VIP), gastric inhibitory peptide (GIP) and peptide histidine isoleucine (PHI). These peptides, with the exception of GIP, have been reported to affect gallbladder motility. The actions of VIP and PHI, which are neuropeptides, are considered later.

Secretin Early studies reported that intraduodenal acid causes gallbladder contraction, an effect attributed to secretin release. It now seems likely that this effect results from release of cholecystokinin or activation of neural reflexes. In the conscious gallbladder fistula dog secretin was without effect on gallbladder pressure even at unphysiologically high doses.[24] It did however augment gallbladder contraction induced by CCK. Studies in vivo in the guinea pig[25], cat[26], and opossum[27] have reported either a lack of any cholecystokinetic activity or a relaxation of gallbladder muscle suggesting that the contractile effect seen with less pure secretin preparations is likely to result from contaminants. The augmentation by secretin of the contractile response of gallbladder muscle to CCK has also been reported for cat[8] and guinea pig[25] gallbladder. In addition secretin has been reported to significantly enhance gallbladder contractions evoked by vagal stimulation.[28]

Glucagon Glucagon administered subcutaneously or intravenously relaxed the gallbladder of the conscious dog dose-dependently.[29] In the anaesthetised guinea pig glucagon alone had no effect but augmented CCK-induced contractions.[25] No effect on gallbladder volume was detected during its infusion into the anaesthetised cat. In man glucagon increased gallbladder size when given alone or after a fatty meal.[30] This presumed relaxant effect of the peptide in vivo could not be demonstrated in vitro.[31]

<u>Gastric Inhibitory Peptide</u> Natural porcine GIP infused into anaesthetised cats relaxed the stomach but had no effect on gallbladder volume.[32] The apparent contractile effect of this peptide on the isolated guinea pig gallbladder is likely to result from contamination of natural GIP with CCK as no effect was observed with synthetic GIP.[34]

<u>Motilin</u> Motilin has been reported to cause a dose-dependent increase in gallbladder pressure in the conscious pig.[35] In decerebrate dogs this peptide also induced an increase in gallbladder intraluminal pressure in most animals studied, though no response was recorded in a few dogs.[36] This excitatory effect on gallbladder muscle was dependent upon vagal tone, being enhanced by increased vagal activity and largely diminished or abolished after vagotomy or treatment with atropine. It seems likely that the effects of motilin on gallbladder contractile function in vivo do not result from a direct effect on gallbladder muscle as in vitro studies in three species have failed to document any effect.[33,36,37] The response of the gallbladder to motilin depends upon the phase of digestion. In a recent study in the conscious dog intravenous infusions of motilin induced transient contractions of the gall-bladder during the interdigestive, but not the digestive period. The contractions occurred simultaneously with the initiation of phase two contractions in the duodenum and were inhibited by atropine.[38]

A study in fasting humans using a radioactive isotope scanning technique has reported an association between endogenous plasma motilin concentrations and spontaneous gallbladder emptying. Plasma motilin concentrations were found to invariably rise prior to, and not to occur in the absence of, gallbladder contraction.[39]

<u>Pancreatic polypeptide</u> Bovine pancreatic polypeptide (BPP) has been reported to relax the gallbladder and increase the tone in the common bile duct of the dog, effects opposite to those of chole-cystokinin. [40,41] Porcine pancreatic polypeptide however was reported to be without effect on dog, rabbit and human gallbladder strips and failed to inhibit the contraction induced by CCK8. In the conscious pig intravenous infusion of pancreatic polypeptide caused a dose related fall in gallbladder pressure.[35] Intravenous infusion of BPP into man decreased the entry of bilirubin into the duodenum, a change taken to indicate gallbladder relaxation.[43,44] A further study examined the effects of pancreatic polypeptide on gallbladder storage and emptying patterns in normal and chole-cystectomised man by a duodenal perfusion technique using indo-cyanine green as a biliary marker.[45] Infusion of BPP to achieve physiological interprandial levels (with a background infusion of secretin and caerulein to simulate the interprandial state of gastrointestinal hormone stimulation) promoted gallbladder storage of bile. Release of endogenous pancreatic polypeptide in man by

caerulein failed to antagonise the cholecystokinetic effect of the latter peptide.[46]

   Peptide tyrosine tyrosine(PYY)   Despite the structural similarity of PYY to pancreatic polypeptide it has been reported to cause a dose-dependent contraction of the gallbladder of the anaesthetised guinea pig[47] and to be without effect on gallbladder contraction caused by injection of CCK.[48]   It is conceivable that this effect may result from CCK impurity of the natural PYY used and in vitro studies with synthetic PYY are necessary to evaluate this.

Neural Effects
   Cholinergic effects   Acetylcholine and muscarinic cholinergic agonists have been known for many years as stimulants of gallbladder contraction.   The release of this neurotransmitter by electrical stimulation of the vagus nerves, while resulting in contraction of the gallbladder and increased intraluminal pressure, appears not to result in gallbladder evacuation.[49]   In man it is well established that vagotomy results in progressive enlargement of the gallbladder. This dilatation may not result simply from a reduction in muscle tone due to interference with the cholinergic innervation as the intra-luminal pressure of the gallbladder in dogs has been found to increase after complete truncal vagotomy.[50]   Though the precise physiological significance of the cholinergic innervation of gall-bladder muscle is uncertain it seems likely that vagal cholinergic fibres act to maintain muscle tone and participate in certain digestive vagal and vago-vagal reflexes considered later.

   Adrenergic effects   Bainbridge and Dale[51] as early as 1905 demonstrated that 'gallbladder relaxation was the invariable result of Faradising the right splanchnic nerve'.   It has been subsequently shown that splanchnic nerve stimulation also causes contraction of the sphincter of Oddi.[52]   It seems however that the gallbladder pressure has to be elevated (eg by cholecystokinin) before a clear-cut relaxation is consistently obtained by stimulation of the sympathetic nerve supply.   These adrenergic effects on biliary smooth muscle can be explained in terms of adrenoceptor population and functions in the gallbladder and sphincter of Oddi.   In the cat both the gallbladder and the sphincter of Oddi possess contraction-mediating alpha-receptors and relaxation-mediating beta-receptors.[53,54]   The gallbladder appears however to have only a small population of alpha-receptors as contraction to noradrenaline med-iated via these receptors was weak and could only be observed when the beta-receptors had been blocked.   The presence of postsynaptic alpha-adrenoceptors mediating contraction and beta-adrencoeptors mediating relaxation has also been reported for guinea pig gallbladder.   Studies in other species have produced variable results.   Thus though adrenaline relaxed the isolated monkey gall-bladder[55] responses to it in the intact primate gallbladder were unpredictable.56

Peptidergic Effects

Vasoactive intestinal polypeptide VIP relaxes the isolated superfused guinea pig gallbladder[57] and in the same species in vivo can antagonise the contractile effects of CCK.[25] In the anaesthetised opossum this peptide decreased basal gallbladder pressure dose dependently, eliminated spontaneous contractile activity when present and antagonised the expected pressure increase to CCK infusion.[50] Similar findings were reported using guinea pig gallbladder muscle strips and in addition VIP was found to be without effect on acetylcholine induced contraction.[59] VIP has also been reported to relax rabbit and dog gallbladder strips, to inhibit the contraction induced by CCK8,[41] to relax the gallbladder of the anaesthetised cat[60] and the conscious pig.[35]

Peptide Histidine Isoleucine (PHI) PHI has been found to relax the isolated guinea pig gallbladder.[61]

Substance P present in the gallbladder wall[62] has been reported to be without effect on the motility of rabbit,[63] dog[64] and guinea pig[65] gallbladder in vitro. Administered systemically however it contracts canine gallbladder[66] and the gallbladder in situ in guinea pigs, cats, rabbits, dogs and chickens.[67] A recent study in the cat[68] has documented the presence of neurones in the gallbladder wall containing substance P immunoreactivity. These fibres were localised around blood vessels, close to the epithelium, around ganglia and a few were noted to be in contact with smooth muscle. Whether or not these fibres are afferent, efferent or both remains to be established. Exogenous administration of substance P caused gallbladder contraction which was abolished by pretreatment with atropine.

Somatostatin In man exogenous somatostatin inhibits gallbladder contraction induced by intravenous administration of carbachol or CCK[69,70,71] and that due to oral ingestion of glucose.[72] It also has been reported to antagonise CCK-induced contraction of pig gallbladder[73] and to decrease gallbladder pressure in the chronic gallbladder fistula dog[74] and the conscious pig.[35] In the anaesthetised cat infusion of somatostatin inhibited gallbladder contraction elicited by duodenal acidification.[75] In vitro this peptide is without effect on the contractility of rabbit and dog gallbladder strips.[41] A study in the guinea pig failed to demonstrate any effect of somatostatin on gallbladder contraction due to cholecystokinin octapeptide or acetylcholine, both in vitro and in vivo.[76]

Opioid peptides have been detected in the gallbladder wall in man[77] and in the cat.[68] In the latter species enkephalin-immunoreactive nerve fibres were seen within local ganglia surrounding ganglion cells originating either from preganglionic vagal fibres or local interneurones. Intravenous infusion of leucine enkephalin in this study caused gallbladder contraction which was antagonised by naloxone or indomethacin. In the in vitro guinea pig gallbladder dynorphin, methionine enkephalin and beta-endorphin were reported to be without effect on contraction induced by transmural electrical stimulation.[78]

Bombesin Intravenous administration of bombesin to dogs and man causes gallbladder contraction.[79,80] This effect is believed to result predominantly from release of CCK as bombesin has only weak spasmogenic actions on in vitro gallbladder preparations.[79,81] The in vitro contractile effect of bombesin appears to be mediated by a mechanism independent of CCK receptors as the CCK antagonist dibutyryl cyclic guanosine 3',5' monophosphate was without effect on this response.[76] Concentrations of bombesin without effect on gallbladder contraction have been found to augment nerve mediated contraction activated by transmural electrical stimulation of the isolated perfused guinea pig gallbladder.[82] Like bombesin its mammalian counterpart gastrin releasing peptide (GRP) stimulates contraction of the isolated guinea pig gallbladder.[83]

NEUROHUMORAL CONTROL OF GALLBLADDER FILLING AND EMPTYING

Bile is stored in the gallbladder between meals and evacuated into the intestine following ingestion of food. Studies in the baboon however indicate that as much as one half of the hepatic bile output may enter the duodenum directly during fasting.[84]

Gallbladder filling occurs passively when the pressure in the common bile duct exceeds the resistance to flow offered by the cystic duct and the pressure within the gallbladder. It is assumed to occur as a back pressure produced by the flow of hepatic bile against a closed sphincter of Oddi. The precise mechanisms regulating gallbladder filling are poorly understood. The adrenergic findings described above suggest that adrenergic mechanisms play a role in gallbladder filling, promoting the entry of bile into the gallbladder by both effects on it and on the sphincter of Oddi. There is increasing evidence that vasoactive intestinal peptide (VIP) present in nerves in the gallbladder wall[85] may also act to mediate gallbladder relaxation.

Little information is available concerning gallbladder motor function between meals. Recent studies in the conscious dog[86], using surgically implanted force transducers, have examined intestinal and gallbladder contractile patterns continuously for several weeks. Though bile entry into the duodenum was not measured, these studies documented, during the interdigestive state, periodic gall-bladder contractions corresponding to approximately 80% of the force of postprandial contractions. These were associated with motor activity in the gastric antrum and duodenum and elevations in plasma motilin. Infusions of exogenous motilin during the interdigestive state have reproduced these changes which are dependent upon intact vagal function.

Gallbladder emptying occurs in response to the ingestion of food. The viscus does not empty itself entirely and thus at any time it contains a variable mixture of concentrated bile and new hepatic bile. In the 1920's Ivy and his co-workers put forward evidence to support a humoral mechanism for gallbladder emptying. Chole-cystokinin, the humoral factor responsible was additionally found to relax the sphincter of Oddi. Stimulation of the vagus also causes contraction of the gallbladder and increased intraluminal pressure. However though parasympathetic fibres may be involved in the maintenance of normal gallbladder tone they do not appear to be essential for gallbladder evacuation by cholecystokinin. Thus although vagal stimulation facilitates contraction induced by chol-ecystokinin the vagus is not required for the normal effect of this hormone as demonstrated by normal gallbladder emptying following vagotomy.

Though the physiological significance of the cholinergic nerve supply to gallbladder muscle remains to be defined the existence of vagal and vago-vagal reflexes, which can mediate cephalic, gastric and intestinal control of gallbladder motility, have recently been documented. Studies in man have shown a small decrease in gallbladder volume following vagal activation by sham feeding.[87] In the dog graded distension of the gastric antrum caused graded contraction of the gallbladder by a cholinergic pyloro-cholecystic reflex.[88] A neural reflex may also exist between the intestine and the gallbladder analagous to that reported to facilitate pancreatic amylase secretion.[89] The delay in gallbladder evacuation and the abolition of a rise in gallbladder pressure to intraduodenal fat after vagotomy provide evidence for the existence of such an enterocholecystic reflex.[90]

The studies reviewed above illustrate the early stage of knowledge of the humoral and neural mechanisms regulating gall-bladder motor function. Their relative roles have still to be defined. The recent development of a dynamic method to study gallbladder tone in an situ primate gallbladder model[91] together with new specific radioimmunoassays for cholecystokinin and other gastrointestinal regulatory peptides provide sensitive techniques to study the relative contributions of various endocrine and neural influences regulating changes in gallbladder motility.

REFERENCES

1. N. A. Michels, "Blood Supply and Anatomy of the Upper Abdominal Organs", Lippincott, Philadelphia, (1955)

2. W. Cai and G. Gabella, Innervation of the gallbladder and biliary pathways in the guinea-pig, J Anat. 136:97 (1983)

3. T. M. Lin, Actions of gastrointestinal hormones and related peptides on the motor function of the biliary tract. Gastroenterology. 69:1006 (1975)

4. I. Wiener, K. Inove, C. J. Fagan, P. Lilja, L. C. Watson and J. C. Thompson, Release of cholecystokinin in man. Correlation of blood levels with gallbladder contraction, Ann Surg. 194:321 (1981)

5. M. Vagne and M. I. Grossman, Cholecystokinetic potency of gastrointestinal hormones and related peptides, Am J Physiol. 215:881 (1968)

6. M. A. Ondetti, B. Rubin, S. L. Engel, J. Pluscec and J. T. Sheehan, Cholecystokinin-pancreozymin. Recent developments, Am J Dig Dis. 15:149 (1970)

7. L. R. Johnson, G. F. Stehling and M. I. Grossman, Effect of sulfation of the gastrointestinal actions of caerulein, Gastroenterology. 58:208 (1970)

8. J. R. Chowdhury, J. M. Berkowitz, M. Praissman and J. W. Fara, Effect of sulfated and non-sulfated gastrin and octapeptide cholecystokinin on cat gallbladder in vitro, Experientia 32:1173 (1976)

9. J. W. Fara and S. M. Erde, Comparison of in vivo and in vitro responses to sulfated and non-sulfated ceruletide, Eur J Pharmacol. 47:359-363 (1978)

10. S. R. Vigna and A. Gorbman, Effects of cholecystokinin, gastrin and related peptides on coho salmon gallbladder contractions in vitro, Am J Physiol. 232:E485 (1977)

11. M. S. Amer, Studies with cholecystokinin. II cholecystokinetic potency of gastrins I and II and related peptides in three systems, Endocrinology 84:1277 (1969)

12. F. T. Jung and H. Greengard, Responses of the isolated gallbladder to cholecystokinin, Am J Physiol. 103:275 (1933)

13. M. S. Amer, Studies with cholecystokinin in vitro. III Mechanism of the effect on the isolated rabbit gallbladder strips, J Pharmacol Exp Ther 183:527 (1972)

14. M. S. Amer, G. R. McKinney, Studies with cholecystokinin in vitro. IV Effect of cholecystokinin and related peptides on phosphodiesterase, J Pharmacol Exp Ther. 183:535 (1972)

15. W. M. Yau, G. M. Makhlouf, L. E. Edwards and J. T. Farrar, Mode of action of cholecystokinin and related peptides on gallbladder muscle, Gastroenterology. 65:451 (1973)

16. K. E. Andersson, R. G. G. Andersson, P. Hedner and C. G. A. Persson, Interrelations between cyclic AMP, cyclic GMP and contraction in guinea-pig gallbladder stimulated by chole-cystokinin, Life Sci. 20:73 (1977)

17. D. B. Waldman, A. M. Zfass and G. M. Makhlouf, Stimulatory (H_1) and inhibitory (H_2) histamine receptors in gallbladder muscle, Gastroenterology. 72:932 (1977)

18. J. Stasiewicz, W. Szalaj and A. Gabryelewicz, Motor inter-action between cimetidine and cholecystokinin related pep-tides in the gallbladder, Pol J Pharmacol Pharm. 32:643 (1980)

19. D. J. Schoetz, W. E. Wise, W. W. LaMorte, D. H. Birkett and L. F. Williams, Histamine receptors in the primate gallbladder, Gastroenterology 74:1090 (1978)

20. K. E. Andersson, R. Andersson and P. Hedner, Cholecysto-kinin effect and concentration of cyclic AMP in gallbladder muscle in vitro, Acta Physiol Scand. 85:511 (1972)

21. M. S. Amer, Cyclic guanosine 3',5'-monophosphate and gall-bladder contraction, Gastroenterology. 67:333 (1974)

22. K. E. Andersson, R. Andersson, P. Hedner and C. G. A. Persson, Parallelism between mechanical and metabolic responses to cholecystokinin and prostaglandin E_2 in extrahepatic biliary tract, Acta Physiol Scand. 89:571 (1973)

23. K. E. Andersson, P. Hedner and C. G. A. Persson, Effects of lanthanum and calcium antagonists on contractile responses of isolated guinea pig gallbladder, Acta Physiol Scand. 91:16A (1974)

24. G. F. Stening and M. I. Grossman, Potentiation of cholecysto-kinetic action of cholecystokinin by secretin, Clin Res. 17:528 (1969)

25. M. Vagne and V. Troitskaja, Effect of secretin, glucagon and VIP on gallbladder contraction, Digestion. 14:62 (1976)

26. R. Jansson and J. Svanvik, Effects of intravenous secretin and cholecystokinin on gallbladder net water absorption and motility in the cat, Gastroenterology. 72:639 (1977)

27. J. Ryan and S. Cohen, Gallbladder pressure volume response to gastrointestinal hormones, Am J Physiol. 230:1461 (1976)

28. J. S. Davison and S. Fosel, Interactions between vagus nerve stimulation and pentagastrin or secretin on the guinea pig gallbladder, Digestion. 13:251 (1975)

29. T. M. Lin, Actions of secretin, glucagon, cholecystokinin and endogenously released secretin and cholecystokinin on gall-bladder, choledochus and bile flow in dogs, Fed Proc. 33:391 (1974)

30. S. M. Chernish, R. E. Miller, B. D. Rosenak and N. E. Scholz, Effect of glucagon on size of visualised human gallbladder before and after a fat meal, Gastroenterology. 62:1218 (1972)

31. A. J. Cameron, S. F. Phillips, W. H. J. Summerskill, Effect of cholecystokinin, gastrin, secretin and glucagon on human gallbladder muscle in vitro, Proc Soc Exp Biol Med. 131:149 (1969)

32. R. Jansson, G. Steen and J. Svanvik, A comparison of glucagon, gastric inhibitory peptide and secretin on gall-bladder function, formation of bile and pancreatic secretion in the cat, Scand J Gastroenterol. 13:919 (1978)

33. J. R. Wood, L. J. Brennan, J. M. Hormbrey and T. A. McLoughlin, Effects of regulatory peptides on gallbladder function, Scand J Gastroenter. 17 suppl 78:528 (1982)

34. J. R. Wood, L. J. Brennan and T. A. McLoughlin, unpublished findings.

35. T. E. Adrian, P. Mitchenere, G. R. Sagor, N. D. Christofides and S. R. Bloom, Effect of motilin and other gut hormones on gallbladder pressure, Regulatory Peptides. Suppl 1:S1 (1980)

36. S. Nakayama, M. Mizutani, T. Neya and M. Takaki, Effect of motilin on gallbladder and gastroduodenal motility in dogs, Ital J Gastroenterol. 13:6 (1981)

37. U. Strunz, W. Domschke, P. Mitznegg, S. Domschke, E. Schubert, E. Wunsch, E. Jaeger, L. Demling, Analysis of the motor effect of 13-norleucine motilin on the rabbit, guinea pig, rat and human alimentary tract in vitro, Gastroenterology. 68:1485 (1975)

38. I. Takahashi, T. Suzuki, I. Aizawa, Z. Itoh, Comparison of gallbladder contractions induced by motilin and cholecystokinin in dogs, Gastroenterology. 82:419 (1982)

39. T. M. Lin, and R. E. Chance, Spectrum of gastrointestinal actions of bovine PP. In: 'Gut Hormones', edited by S. R. Bloom, 242-246, Churchill Livingstone, Edinburgh (1978)

40. T. M. Lin, T. C. Evans, C. J. Shaar and R. E. Chance, Physiological versus pharmacological actions of bovine pancreatic polypeptide on the pancreas, stomach, gallbladder, choledochal sphincter and intestine of dogs, In: 'Gut Peptides', edited by A. Miyoshi, 175-181 Elsevier, Amsterdam (1979)

41. J. Lonovics, P. Devitt, P. L. Rayford, and J. C. Thompson, Actions of VIP, somatostatin and pancreatic polypeptide on gallbladder tension and CCK-stimulated gallbladder, Surg Forum. 30:407 (1979)

42. I. S. Pomeranz, J. S. Davison and E. A. Shaffer, In vitro effects of pancreatic polypeptide and motilin on contractility of human gallbladder, Dig Dis Sci. 28:539 (1983)

43. G. R. Greenberg, R. F. McCloy, V. S. Chadwick, T. E. Adrian, J. H. Baron and S. R. Bloom, Effect of bovine pancreatic polypeptide on basal pancreatic and biliary outputs in man, Dig Dis Sci. 24:11 (1979)

44. T. E. Adrian, H. S. Besterman, C. N. Mallinson, G. R. Greenberg and S. R. Bloom, Inhibition of secretin stimulated pancreatic secretion by pancreatic polypeptide, Gut. 20:37 (1979)

45. O. G. Bjornsson, T. E. Adrian, J. Dawson, R. F. McCloy, G. R. Greenberg and S. R. Bloom, Effects of gastrointestinal hormones on fasting gallbladder storage patterns in man, Eur J Clin Invest. 9:293 (1979)

46. K. Tsuda, Y. Seino, H. Sakurai, S. Seino, J. Takemura, H. Kuzuya, H. Adachi and H. Imura, Cerulein-induced pancreatic polypeptide secretion, Am J Gastroent. 74:355 (1980)

47. K. Tatemoto and V. Mutt, Isolation of two novel candidate hormones using a chemical method for finding naturally occuring polypeptides, Nature. 285:417 (1980)

48. K. Tatemoto, Isolation and characterisation of peptide YY (PYY), a candidate gut hormone that inhibits pancreatic exocrine secretion, Proc Natl Acad Sci USA. 79:2514 (1982)

49. A. C. Ivy, The physiology of the gallbladder, Physiol Rev. 14:1 (1934)

50. R. D. Williams and T. T. Huang, The effect of vagotomy on biliary pressure, Surgery 66:353 (1969)

51. F. A. Bainbridge and H. H. Dale, The contractile mechanism of the gallbladder and its extrinsic nervous control, J Physiol. 33:138 (1964)

52. B. Pallin and S. Skoglund, Neural and humoral control of the gallbladder emptying mechanism in the cat, Acta Physiol Scand. 60:358 (1964)

53. C. G. A. Persson, Adrenoceptors in the gallbladder, Acta Pharmacol (Kbh). 31:177 (1972)

54. C. G. A. Persson, Dual effects on the sphincter and gall-bladder contraction induced by stimulation of the right great splanchnic nerve, Acta Physiol Scand 87:334 (1973)

55. I. S. Ravdin and J. L. Morrison, Gallbladder Function. The contractile function of the gallbladder, Arch Surg. 22:810 (1931)

56. D. J. Schoetz, D. H. Birkett and L. F. Williams, Gallbladder motor function in the intact primate: autonomic pharmacology, J Surg Res. 24:513 (1978)

57. P. J. Pper, S. I. Said and J. R. Vane, Effects on smooth muscle preparations of unidentified vasoactive peptides from intestine and lung, Nature. 225:1144 (1970)

58. J. Ryan and S. Cohen, Effect of vasoactive intestinal polypeptide on basal and cholecystokinin-induced gallbladder pressure, Gastroenterology. 73:870 (1977)

59. J. P. Ryan and S. Ryave, Effect of vasoactive intestinal polypeptide on gallbladder smooth muscle in vitro, Am J Physiol. 234:E44-46 (1978)

60. R. Jansson, G. Steen and J. Svanvik, Effects of intravenous vasoactive intestinal peptide (VIP) on gallbladder function in the cat, Gastroenterology. 75:47 (1978)

61. L. J. Brennan, T. A. McLoughlin, V. Mutt, K. Tatemoto and J. R. Wood, Effects on PHI, a newly isolated peptide, on gallbladder function in the guinea pig, J Physiol. 329:71P (1982)

62. G. Nilsson and E. Brodin, Tissue distribution of substance P-like immunoreactivity in dog, cat, rat and mouse, in: 'Substance P', US v Euler and B. Pernow, ed. Raven Press, New York (1977)

63. H. Bjurstedt, U.S.v Euler and B. Gernandt, Biological actions of substance P and its relations to cholecystokinin, Skand Arch Physiol. 83:257 (1940)

64. B. Pernow, Studies on substance P: purification, occurance and biological actions, Acta Physiol Scand. 29:Suppl 105, 1 (1953)

65. E. H. Hultman, The relation between cholecystokinin and substance P, Acta Chem Scand. 9:1042 (1955)

66. K. Starke, F. Lembeck, W. Lorenz and U. Weiss, Gallen-und pankreas secretion unter substanz P und einem physalamin-derivat, Naunyn Schmiedibergs Arch Pharmacol. 260:269 (1968)

67. F. Lembeck and H. Juan, Comparative actions of peptides on the gallbladder and the sphincter of Oddi, Adv Exp Med Biol. 21:337 (1972)

68. S. Bjorck, J. M. Lundberg, L. Jivegard and J. Svanvik, Substance P, enkephalin and VIP in the feline gallbladder: distribution of immunoreactivity and functional effects by exogenous administrtion, to be published.

69. P. G. Lankisch, R. Arnold and W. Creutzfeldt, Wirkung von somatostatin auf die betzolstumulierte pancreassekretion und gallenblasenkontraktion des menschen, Dt Med Wschr. 36:1798 (1975)

70. W. Creutzfeldt, P. G. Lankisch and U. R. Folsch, Hemmung der sekretin and cholecystokinin-pankreozyminin-duzierten saft- und enzymesekretion des pancreas und der gallenblasendontra-ktion beim menschen durch somatostatin, Dtsch Med Wschr. 100:1135-1138 (1975)

71. D. Von Kleist, M. Zschiedrich, D. Stopik and K. E. Hampel, Das verhalten der secretin-pankreozymin-stimulaierten sekretion des pankreas, der gallenblasenkontraktion und der cholerese unter somatostatin, Dt Z Verdau-U Stoffuiechselkr. 41:219 (1981)

72. C. Johansson, B. Kollberg, S. Efendic and K. Uvnas-Wallen-sten, Effects of graded doses of somatostatin on gallbladder emptying and pancreatic enzyme output after oral glucose in man, Digestion. 22:24 (1981)

73. S. R. Bloom, S. N. Joffe, and J. M. Polak, Effect of somatostatin on pancreatic and biliary function, Gut. 16:836 (1975)

74. T. M. Lin, G. F. Spray and R. H. Tuft, Actions of somatostatin (SS) on choledochal sphincter (CS), gallbladder (GB) and bile flow (BF) in dog, Fed Proc. 36:557 (1977)

75. S. Bjorck and J. Svanvik, The influences of somatostatin on gallbladder response to intraduodenal acid and autonomic nerve stimulation in the cat, Scand J Gastroent. In Press.

76. P Poitras, T. Yasmada, J. H. Walsh, Absence of effect of somatostatin in the guinea pig gallbladder, Can J Phys Pharmacol. 58:179 (1980)

77. J. M. Polak, S. R. Bloom, S. N. Sullivan, P. Facer and A. G. E. Pearse, Enkephalin-like immunoreactivity in the human gastrointestinal tract, Lancet. 1:972 (1977)

78. M. Ouchi, H. Asaoka, T. Mitsutake and M. Miyagawa, Endo-genous opioid peptide effects on the guinea pig biliary tract, Peptides. 4:125 (1983)

79. V. Erspamer, G. Improta, P. Melchiorri, N. Sopranzi, Evidence of cholecystokinin release by bombesin in the dog, Br J Pharmacol. 52:227 (1974)

80. E. Corazziari, A. Torsoli, P. Melchiorri, G. F. Delle Fave, Effect of bombesin on human gallbladder emptying, Rendic Gastroenterol. 6:227 (1974)

81. V. Erspamer, G. Erspamer, M. Inselvini, L. Negri, Occurrence of bombesin and alytesin in extracts of skin of three European discoglossid frogs and pharmacological actions of bombesin on extravascular smooth muscle, Br J Pharmacol. 45:333 (1972)

82. M. H. Al-Hassani and J. S. Davison, Interactions between intrinsic cholinergic nerve stimulation and gastrointestinal polypeptides on the guinea pig gallbladder, J Physiol (Lond). 285:24P (1978)

83. T. J. McDonald, Non-amphibian bombesin-like peptides, in: Gut Hormones, Ed. S. R. Bloom and J. M. Polak, Churchill Livingston, London (1981)

84. J. J. O'Brien, E. A. Shaffer, L. J. Williams, D. M. Small, J. Lynn and J. Wittenberg, A physiologic model to study gall-bladder function in primates, Gastroenterology. 67: 119 (1974)

85. F. Sundler, J. Alumets, R. Hakenson, S. Ingemansson, J. Fahrenkrug and O. Schaffalitzky de Muckadell, VIP innervation of the gallbladder, Gastroenterology. 72:1375 (1977)

86. Z. Itoh, I. Takahashi and T. Suzuki, Contractile patterns of the gallbladder between meals in the dog, in: 'Motility of the Digestive Tract', M. Weinbeck, ed., Raven Press, New York (1982)

87. W. E. Hansen, H. Maurer and H. Haberland, The effect of Sham-feeding on gallbladder volume and circulation of bile acids, Hepato-Gastroenterol. 29:108 (1982)

88. H. Debas and T. Yamagishi, Evidence of a pyloro-cholecystic reflex for gallbladder contraction, Ann Surg. 190:170 (1979)

89. M. V. Singer, T. E. Solomon, J. R. Wood and M. I. Grossman, Latency of pancreatic enzyme response to intraduodenal stimulants, Am J Physiol. 238:623 (1980)

90. G. M. Fried, W. D. Ogden, G. Greeley and J. C. Thompson, Correlation of release and actions of cholecystokinin in dogs before and after vagotomy, Surgery, 93:786 (1983)

HISTOPATHOLOGICAL FINDINGS RELATING TO DISORDERED MOTILITY AND SECRETION

Jeremy R. Jass

Department of Histopathology
Westminster Medical School
London SW1P 2AR. UK.

INTRODUCTION

Patterns of motility and secretion may be altered in several ways. For example, disease processes (congenital or acquired) may interfere with either neural or endocrine control mechanisms or with the musculature or connective tissue of the gut wall. The function of a particular cell is also dependent on the expression of genotype and this will be influenced by interactions between the cell and its environment. Some consideration will first be given to the ways in which motility and secretory control mechanisms become deranged, emphasizing morphological findings. Secondly, examples of altered secretory activity associated with disorders of differentiation will be presented.

MOTILITY DISORDERS

These may result from either a primary neuromuscular defect, or through a variety of secondary aetiologies. Secondary motility disorders have been ascribed to autonomic neuropathy (diabetes mellitus, porphyria, Shy-Drager syndrome, Chagas' disease, laxative abuse), thyroid disease, scleroderma, mechanical obstruction, dystrophia myotonica and endocrine tumours. Of these only the endocrine tumours will be considered further. Some primary motility disorders associated with at least partially understood anatomical lesions include achalasia, congenital pyloric stenosis, Hirschsprung's disease and diverticular disease. Primary functional motility disorders including diffuse oesophageal spasm (Vantrappen and Hellemans, 1982), chronic pseudobstruction of the intestine (Snape, 1982) and idiopathic megacolon (Morson and Dawson, 1979) will not be considered further.

Achalasia

The aetiology is unknown, but Chagas' disease may be associated with an identical clinical picture. Achalasia is characterised by the absence of peristalsis in the body of the oesophagus and the failure of the gastro-oesophageal sphincter to relax during swallowing. Stasis of food results in a progressive dilatation of the oesophagus. Histopathological lesions have been described at various levels and the changes include degeneration and disappearance of nerve cells in the dorsal vagal nucleus, Wallerian degeneration of the vagus, destruction of the myenteric plexus together with mono- nuclear cell infiltration and fibrosis and degenerative changes in the fibres of the muscularis externa (Vantrappen and Hellemans, 1982). It is possible that non-cholinergic neurons are the site of the primary lesion (Smith, 1970; Vantrappen and Hellemans, 1982). The motility disorder could thus result from the loss of an inhibitory supply to the smooth muscle (? VIP nerves) and therefore a failure of relaxation. A neurotoxic virus or an autoimmune process have been offered as underlying aetiologies.

Congenital pyloric stenosis

This condition presents between the second and fourth weeks of extra-uterine life with feeding difficulties including projectile vomiting. Macro- scopically there is concentric thickening of the pylorus due to hypertrophy of the circular muscle coat (fig. 1). The primary defect is likely to reside in the myenteric plexus. Some workers have noted the ganglion cells to degenerate and reduced in number whereas others have found one category of ganglion cell to be absent (Rintoul and Kirkman, 1961). This latter suggestion links well with the modern concept of a family of non-adrenergic, non-cholinergic neurons within the myenteric plexus.

Hirschsprung's disease

The majority of patients present in infancy with constipation, abdominal distension and episodes of intestinal obstruction. The condition is due to congenital agangliosis of a bowel segment, usually the rectum.

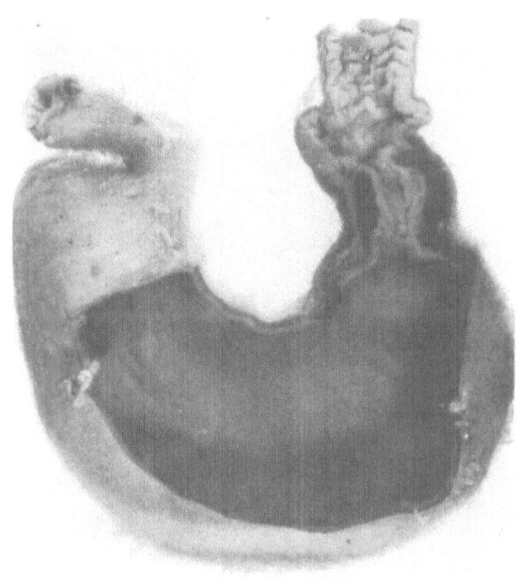

Fig. 1. Specimen of congenital pyloric stenosis.

Both myenteric and submucosal ganglia are absent. The affected segment is narrowed and is between 3-40 cm. long in 90% of patients. Long segment cases have been described which may involve the small bowel. The proximal, normally innervated bowel becomes dilated as faecal material and gas accumulate.

During embryogenesis ganglion cells normally migrate along a pathway formed by preganglionic parasympathetic fibres which have previously innervated the bowel wall. In Hirschsprung's disease the normal migration fails to occur and the extrinsic cholinergic and adrenergic fibres apparently undergo abnormal ramification. This appears as an increase in the number and size of fibres between the circular and longitudinal muscle coats and within the submucosa. Fine cholinesterase positive fibres cross the muscularis mucosae into the lamina propria (Trigg et al., 1974; Meier-Ruge, 1974) (fig. 2). This finding has been utilised in the diagnosis of Hirschsprung's disease and proved successful in the hands of paediatric pathologists (Lake, 1983). It may also be employed to document the length of the aganglionic segment (Lukas and Ludvikovsky, 1983). Providing the occasional small cholinesterase positive fibre is ignored, false positives will not occur. However false negative results have been

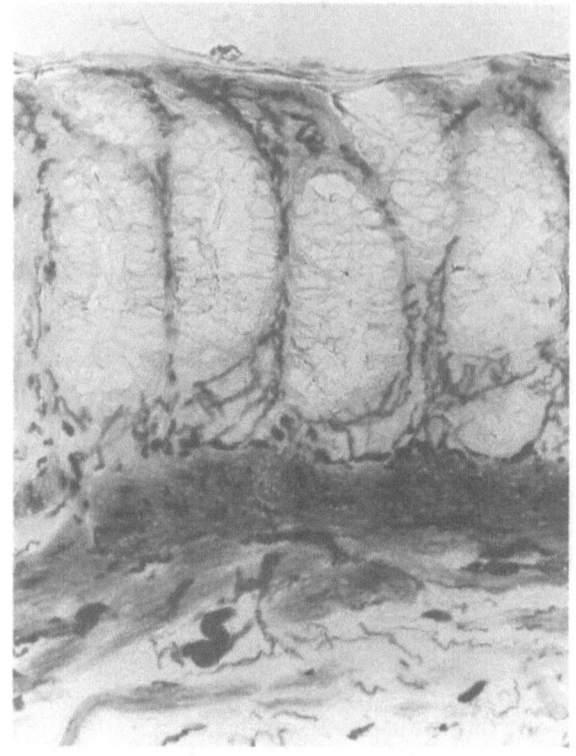

Fig. 2. Mucosal biopsy from case of Hirschsprung's
disease showing cholinesterase positive
fibres in the lamina propria, muscularis
mucosae and submucosa (X 160).

reported (Hamoudi et al., 1982).

It is now realised that Hirschsprung's disease and
related disorders cannot be explained entirely in terms
of the adrenergic and cholinergic nervous systems, but
must also implicate the non-adrenergic, non-cholinergic
nervous system. A decrease in VIP and substance P
containing nerves has been described in affected segments
(Bishop et al., 1981). A deficiency of cholinergic fibres
has been noted to occur in the adynamic bowel syndrome
(pseudo-Hirschsprung's disease) and other patients
reveal an absence of the argyrophilic myenteric plexus
(Puri et al., 1977). There are some additional congenital disorders of the myenteric plexus which require
further study including hypogangliosis (Howard et al.,
1982) and intestinal neuronal dysplasia in which there
is hypergangliosis (Scharli and Meier-Ruge, 1981).

Diverticular disease

This condition is associated with changes in the mechanical properties of the aging bowel (Eastwood et al., 1982). It is seen most commonly in countries with a western diet and is improved by increasing dietary fibre. The distinctive changes are a muscular abnormality and the formation of diverticula. The muscular abnormality is thought to be the primary event, since diverticula are not necessarily present in all cases of diverticular disease (Morson and Dawson, 1979). The changes may be due to the propulsion of small volume stools (Painter, 1975).

The disease is usually confined to the sigmoid colon though the right colon appears to be a site of predilection in Japanese. The longitudinal muscle layer of the colon is arranged in three taeniae coli. In diverticular disease these appear thickened and show a cartilage like consistency. The circular muscle coat is also thickened with a concertina-like appearance. The diverticula pierce the bowel wall in between the muscular corrugations. This takes place at weak points, where the blood vessels pass to supply the colonic mucosa. The corrugations are not formed of concentric rings of smooth muscle, but rather semilunar arcs. Although the muscle is thickened, histological examination shows no evidence of fibre hypertrophy. The pathogenesis of the muscular alterations is not understood.

The diverticula usually occur in two rows on each side of the bowel wall between the mesenteric and anti-mesenteric taeniae. The mucosal pouches are covered by an attenuated layer of longitudinal muscle and lie within the pericolic fat. The anatomical relations are consistent with a pulsion rather than a traction aetiology. Sustained muscle contraction may lead to an elevated intracolonic pressure. This would in turn facilitate mucosal herniation through the points of least resistance.

ENDOCRINE TUMOURS

These are unusual but most interesting causes of disordered motility and secretion. Endocrine tumours may be divided into two broad groups, the enterochromaffin (carcinoid) and the non-enterochromaffin (Morson and Dawson, 1979). The former are relatively common and usually follow a benign course. They may secrete peptides as well as amines. However 5HT is the predominant secretion, accounting for the characteristic histochem-

istry of the enterochromaffin cells (argentaffinity).
Most of these tumours arise in the ileum or appendix.
Two main histological patterns have been described, the
trabecular or mosaic type (A1) and the tubulo-acinar type
(A2) (Jones and Dawson, 1979). The latter is associated
extracellular mucus production. The uncommon goblet cell
carcinoid tumour features intermediate cells, with both
mucus and endocrine secretions in the same cell. The non-
enterochromaffin tumours are rare and have often meta-
stasized by the time of discovery. They arise mainly
in the stomach, pancreas, duodenum or colon. In addition
to the histological patterns noted above, ribbon formation
(type B) and poorly differentiated subtypes have been
described. Further divisions of this group according to
the type of peptide secretion have been proposed (Solcia
et al., 1981). The main gastro-intestinal sequelae are
peptic ulceration (Zollinger-Ellison syndrome due to
gastrinoma) and diarrhoea (argentaffinoma, VIPoma,
glucagonoma, somatostatinoma). One tumour frequently
secretes more than one type of peptide, so it is often
difficult to relate the various clinical effects to one
particular hormone.

CHANGES IN SECRETORY ACTIVITY ASSOCIATED WITH DISORDERS
OF DIFFERENTIATION

    Conspicuous alterations in secretory function occur
in both metaplastic and neoplastic lesions of the gastrointestinal tract. Metaplasia is defined as the replacement
of one adult tissue by another, usually as a consequence
of chronic inflammation. It probably represents a form
of tissue adaptation to a hostile environment. Metaplastic
lesions do not necessarily have a normal adult counterpart
and a less rigid definition would be simply a change in
direction of differentiation. The term neoplasia implies
a disturbance in the control of growth and differentiation
so that growth becomes autonomous. This definition does
not exclude the possibility of coincident metaplasia.

Intestinal metaplasia of the stomach

    Metaplastic foci arising in the stomach may resemble
small intestine with both the fine structural details
and histochemical characteristics of the various cell
lines all reproduced faithfully (fig. 3). However metaplastic differentiation may also be imperfect with the
Paneth cells not represented and the absorptive cells
replaced by less specialised columnar mucous cells (Jass,
1980). The latter may secrete either mainly neutral mucins
or sulphomucins (fig. 4).

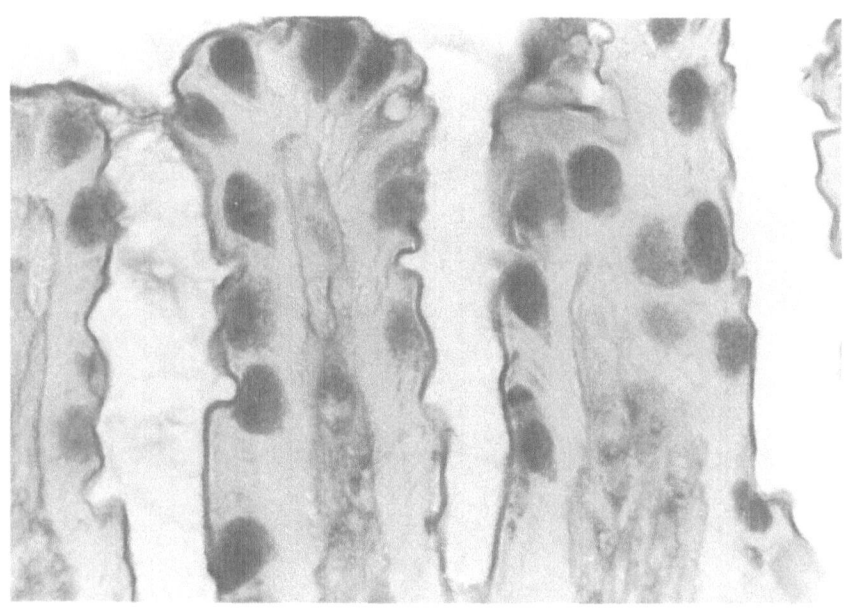

Fig. 3. Complete intestinal metaplasia of the stomach
stained with High iron diamine/Alcian blue. The
goblet cells secrete sialomucins and the intervening columnar cells show a well developed
brush border (X 600).

The relationship between intestinal metaplasia and
gastric carcinoma has been debated for many years. It is
now clear that only the imperfectly differentiated form
secreting sulphomucins (fig. 4) shows a selective association with gastric carcinoma (Jass, 1980; Sipponen et
al., 1980; Segura and Montero, 1983). Sulphomucins also
occur in benign (Jass and Filipe, 1980) and malignant
neoplasms of the stomach (Jass and Filipe, 1981).

Sulphomucins may be appropriate for cytoprotection
when gastric pH is elevated. A less acidic gastric juice
favours the colonisation of the stomach by nitrate reducing bacteria. Nitrites may react with amines to produce
carcinogenic nitrosamines (Ruddell et al., 1976). Thus
sulphomucin secretion may signal a carcinogenic microenvironment. Sulphomucins may also confer biological
advantage on emerging neoplastic clones, by contributing
to a mucous barrier able to withstand the cytotoxic
effects of pepsin (Sun, 1967) and bile salts. These
possibilities may offer some explanation for the relationship between sulphomucin production and gastric carcino-
genesis.

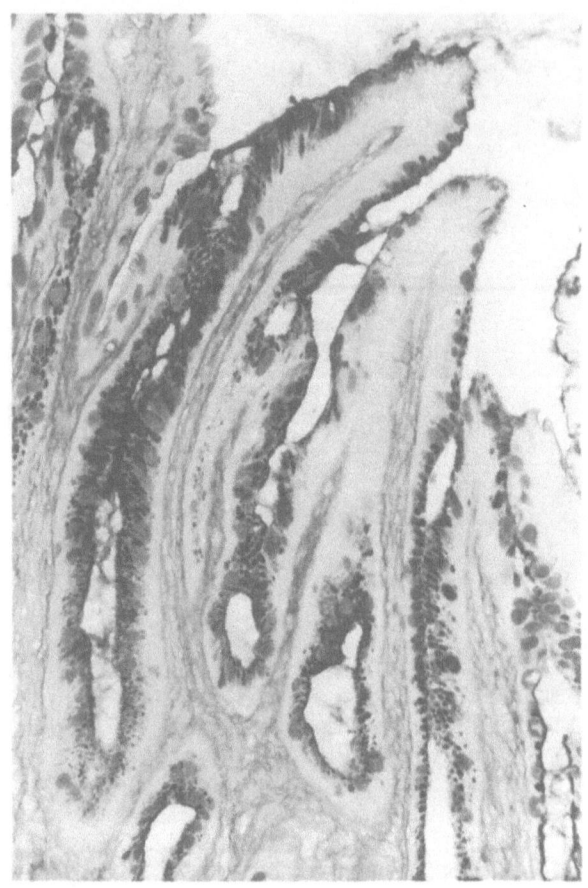

Fig. 4. Imperfectly differentiated form of intestinal
metaplasia of the stomach stained with High iron
diamine/Alcian blue. The goblet cells secrete
sialomucins and the intervening columnar cells
secrete sulphomucins (X 160).

Metaplastic polyps of the colorectum

The metaplastic polyp was so named to emphasize its
benign nature and because it appeared morphologically
different from its parent tissue. It has recently been
shown that this lesion differs from colorectal epithelium
at a functional level too. The secretory changes include
a reduced production of O-acylated sialomucin (Jass et
al., 1982), the abnormal expression of peanut lectin
binding sites (Boland et al., 1982), markedly reduced
staining for secretory component and IgA (Rognum et al.,

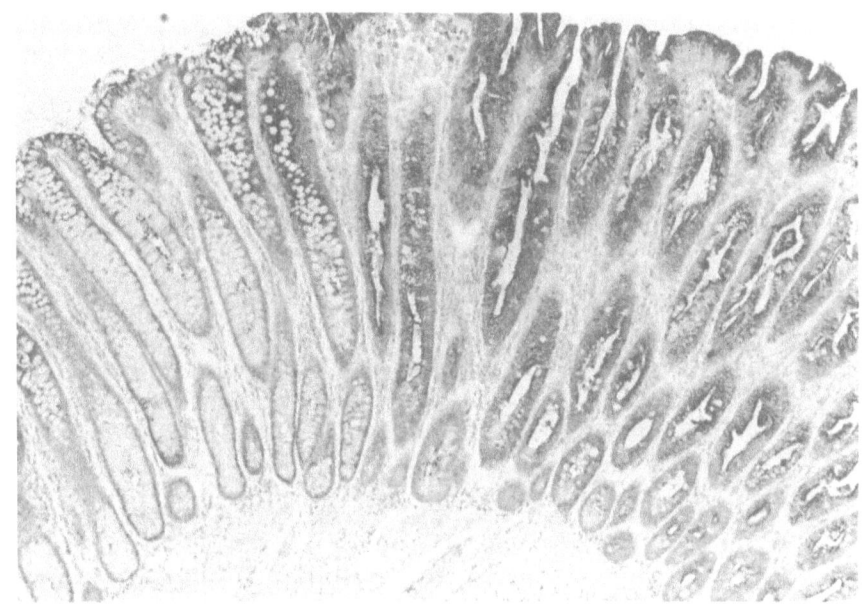

Fig. 5. Metaplastic polyp (right) and normal colorectal
mucosa (left) stained by immunoperoxidase
technique for carcinoembryonic antigen. Increased
expression of CEA by the metaplastic polyp is
evident (X 65).

1982) and increased expression of carcinoembryonic antigen (Jass et al., 1982; Rognum et al., 1982) (fig. 5).
These metaplastic phenotypes are also evidenced by colorectal carcinoma (Jass, 1983). This could be mere coin-
cidence, but may also reflect a shared predisposing factor
for both lesions (Boland et al., 1982; Jass, 1983). This
could (by analogy with the stomach) be an elevated colonic
pH (Thornton, 1981). In certain structural and functional
respects, the cells lining metaplastic crypts show
features, albeit grossly exaggerated, of normal colorectal
surface epithelial cells. These include the expression
of CEA, reduced staining for secretory component and IgA
and increased periodic acid Schiff reactivity.

REFERENCES

Bishop, A.E., Polak J.M., Lake, B.D., Bryent, M.G., and
Bloom, S.R., 1981, Abnormalities of the colonic
regulatory peptides in Hirschsprung's disease,
Histopathology, 5:679.

Boland, C.R., Montgomery, C.K., and Kim, Y.S., 1982,
        A cancer-associated mucin alteration in benign
        colonic polyps, Gastroenterology, 82:664.
Eastwood, M.A., Watters, D.A.K., and Smith, A.N., 1982,
        Diverticular disease - Is it a motility disorder?
        in: " Clinics in Gastroenterology vol 11/Number
        3, Motility and its disturbances," A.M. Connell,
        ed., Saunder Co. Ltd, London Philadelphia
        Toronto.
Filipe, M.I., 1979, Mucins of the human gastrointestinal
        epithelium: a review, Invest. Cell. Pathol.,
        2:195
Hamoudi, A.B., Reiner, C.B., Boles, E.T., McClung, H.J.,
        and Kerzner, B., 1982, Acetyl cholinesterase
        staining activity of rectal mucosa:Its use in
        the diagnosis of Hirschsprung's disease, Arch.
        Pathol. Lab. Med., 106:670.
Howard, E.R., Garrett, J.R., and Kidd, A., 1982,
        Congenital neuronal disorders of the hind-gut:
        the value of ano-rectal biopsies, Scand. J.
        Gastroenterol., (suppl) 71:151.
Jass, J.R., 1980, Role of intestinal metaplasia in the
        histogenesis of gastric carcinoma, J. Clin.
        Pathol., 33:801.
Jass, J.R., 1983, Relation between metaplastic polyp
        and carcinoma of the colorectum, Lancet, 1:28.
Jass, J.R., and Filipe, M.I., 1980, Sulphomucins and
        precancerous lesions of the human stomach,
        Histopathology, 4:271.
Jass, J.R., and Filipe, M.I., 1981, The mucin profiles
        of normal gastric mucosa, intestinal metaplasia
        and its variants and gastric carcinoma,
        Histochem. J., 13:931.
Jass, J.R., Filipe, M.I., Abbas, S., Falcon, C.A.J.,
        Wilson, Y., and Lovell, D., 1982, Altered
        expression of carcinoembryonic antigen and sialo-
        mucin in metaplastic polyps of the colorectum,
        IRCS Med. Sci., 10:678.
Jones, R.A., and Dawson, I.M.P.,1977, Morphology and
        staining patterns of endocrine tumours in the
        gut, pancreas and bronchus and their possible
        significance, Histopathology, 1:137.
Lake, B.D., 1983, Hirschsprung's disease, in: "Histo-
        chemistry in Pathology," M.I. Filipe and B.D.
        Lake, eds., Churchill Livingstone, Edinburgh
        London, New York.
Lukas, Z., and Ludvikovsky, J., 1983, Histochemical
        examination of rectal biopsies in the course
        of diagnosis and treatment of Hirschsprung's
        disease, Histochem. J. 15:323.

Meier-Ruge, W., 1974, Hirschsprung's disease. Its aet-
     iology, pathogenesis and differential diagnosis,
     Curr. Topics. in Pathol., 59:131.
Morson, B.C., and Dawson, I.M.P., 1979, "Gastrointest-
     inal Pathology," Blackwell Scientific Publications,
     Oxford.
Painter, N.S., 1975, in:"Diverticular disease of the
     colon," William Heineman Medical Books, London.
Puri, P., Lake, B.D., and Nixon, H.H., 1977, Adynamic
     bowel syndrome. Report of a case with disturbance
     of the cholinergic innervation, Gut, 18:754.
Rintoul, J.R., and Kirkman, N.F., 1961, The myenteric
     plexus in infantile hypertrophic pyloric stenosis,
     Arch. Dis. Childh., 36:474.
Rognum, T.O., Fausa, O., Brandtzaeg, P., 1982, Immuno-
     histochemical evaluation of carcinoembryonic anti-
     gen, secretory component, and epithelial IgA in
     tubular and villous large-bowel adenomas with
     different grades of dysplasia, Scand. J. Gastro-
     enterol., 17:341.
Ruddell, W.S.J., Bone, E.S., Hill, M.J., Blendis, L.M.,
     and Walters, C.L., 1976, Gastric juice nitrite.
     A risk factor for cancer in the hypochlorhydric
     stomach?, Lancet, 2:1037
Scharli, A.F., and Meier-Ruge, W., 1981, Localised and
     disseminated forms of neuronal dysplasia mimick-
     ing Hirschsprung's disease, J. Paed. Surg., 16:
     164.
Segura, D.I., and Montero, C., 1983, Histochemical
     characterisation of different types of intestinal
     metaplasia in gastric mucosa, Cancer, 52:498.
Sipponen, P., Seppala, K., Varis, K., Hjelt, L., Ihamaki,
     T., Kekki, M., and Siurala, M., 1980, Intestinal
     metaplasia with colonic type sulphomucins in the
     gastric mucosa; its association with gastric
     carcinoma, Acta. Path. Microbiol. Scand., 88:217.
Smith, B., 1970, The neurological lesion of achalasia
     of the cardia, Gut, 11:388.
Solcia, E., Capella, C., Buffa, R., Usellini, L., Fiocca,
     R., Frigerio, B., Tenti,P., and Sessa,F., 1981,
     The diffuse endocrine-paracrine system of the gut
     in health and disease: ultrastructural features,
     Scand. J. Gastroenterol., (Suppl) 70:25.
Snape, W.J., 1982, Pseudo-obstruction and other
     obstructive disorders, in: "Clinics in Gastro-
     enterology vol 11/Number 3, Motility and its
     disturbances," A.M. Connell, ed., W.B. Saunders
     and Co. Ltd., London philadelphia Toronto.

Sun, D.C.H., 1967, Effect of a synthetic sulphated poly-
    saccharide on gastric peptic activity in humans,
    Ann. N. Y. Acad. Sci., 140:747.
Thornton, J.R., 1981, High colonic pH promotes colorectal
    cancer, Lancet,1:1081.
Trigg, P.H., Belin, R., Haberkorn, S., Long, W.J., Nixon,
    H.H., Plaschkes, J., Spitz, L., and Willital, G.H.,
    1974, Experience with a cholinesterase histochem-
    ical technique for rectal suction biopsies in the
    diagnosis of Hirschsprung's disease, J. Clin .
    Pathol., 27:207.
Vantrappen, G., and Hellemans, J., 1982, Motor disorders
    of the oesophagus, in: "Topics in Gastroenterology
    vol 10," D.P.Jewell and W.S.Selby eds., Blackwell
    Scientific Publications, Oxford.

NEURO-HORMONAL CONTROL OF GASTRIC ACID SECRETION: THE ROLE

OF HISTAMINE

Stanislaw J. Konturek

Institute of Physiology
Academy of Medicine
Krakow, Poland

INTRODUCTION

The role of histamine as a physiological stimulant of gastric acid secretion has been a subject of controversy and discussion since Popielski (1920) first observed that injection of histamine causes copious gastric acid secretion. This observation initiated studies on the possible involvement of histamine in gastric secretory mechanisms. It has been suggested that the increased blood level of histamine, released from various depots in the body, could stimulate HCl secretion. Although this view was not supported experimentally, the finding of Gavin, McHenry and Wilson (1933) that histamine is abundant in the parietal cell region of the gastric mucosa, prompted Babkin (1938) and MacIntosh (1938) to propose that histamine released locally from gastric mucosal stores could stimulate parietal cells to secrete HCl. Emmelin and Kahlson (1944) presented evidence of a functional link between gastrin and mucosal histamine, in that the action of gastrin results in the appearance of histamine in the gastric juice of dogs and cats. Kahlson, Rowengren, Svahn and Turnberg (1964) reported experimental results from rats supporting the view that histamine is a physiological mediator of gastric acid secretion. The rat stomach shows a high level of histidine decarboxylase activity which catalyses the formation of histamine from histidine. This enzyme activity increases in response to gastrin, vagal stimulation and feeding, and there is a concurrent decrease in the amount of bound histamine within the mucosa. Based on these findings Kahlson et al.,(1964) hypothesized that gastrin, acetylcholine and feeding release mucosal histamine which stimulates the parietal cells; the depletion of histamine stores then triggers a feedback increase in histidine decarboxylase

189

activity resulting in the formation of new histamine.

Johnson (1971) argued that gastrin in rats may release histamine from its mucosal stores and activate histidine decarboxylase
to provide more endogenous histamine, but there is no evidence that
endogenous histamine is a physiological mediator of acid secretion.
In the presence of secretin, gastrin still releases histamine and
stimulates histamine formation due to activation of histidine decarboxylase but acid secretion does not occur.   Since secretin does
not inhibit histamine-stimulated acid secretion, it cannot be assumed
that secretin acts via histamine pathway to inhibit gastrin-stimulated secretion (Johnson and Tumpson, 1970;   Johnson, 1971).

The isolation and synthesis of gastrin (Gregory and Tracy, 1961;
Gregory, Hardy, Jones, Kenner and Sheppard, 1964) which is many times
more potent on a molar basis than histamine in stimulating gastric
acid secretion, and the failure of classical antihistamines to inhi-
but histamine-induced gastric acid secretion, cast further doubts as
to the physiological importance of histamine in the parietal cell
secretion.   Nevertheless, Loew (1947), suggested that these antihistamines have no affinity for the elements of the parietal cells
which react with histamine, while Folkow, Haeger and Kahlson (1948)
observed that histamine antagonists only partially reduced the depressor action of histamine.

These early observations led to the formal classification of
histamine receptors into the histamine H_1 type (Ash and Schild, 1966)
and the H_2 type (Black, Duncan, Durant, Ganellin and Parsons, 1972).
The discovery of histamine H_2-receptor antagonists such as burimamide,
metiamide, cimetidine and ranitidine, resulted in rapid advances in
the characterization of many responses to histamine.   Progress was
also made in the synthesis of highly selective and potent H_1- and
H_2-receptor agonists such as dimaprit and impromidine (Parsons, Owen,
Ganellin and Durant 1977).   It was found that H_1-receptors alone
are involved in the increase of vascular permeability, and contractions of airways, gut and human coronary artery muscle (Ginsburg,
Bristow, Kantrowitz, Baim and Harrison, 1981). H_2-receptors alone
mediate stimulation of gastric acid secretion and tachycardia (Black
et al, 1972), while both types mediate vasodilation (Black, Owen and
Parsons, 1975) and stimulation of adenylate cyclase in brain (Palacois and Garbare, 1978).   There are some exceptions from these
findings suggesting the heterogeneity of H_2-receptors.

HISTAMINE AND H_2-RECEPTORS IN GASTRIC ACID SECRETION

Analysis of antagonist specificity in various tissues, such as
the whole rat isolated stomach, guinea-pig atrium and rat uterus,
established burimamide as the first competitive antagonist of histamine H_2-receptors (Black et al, 1972).   Further evidence based on

190

the results obtained with other H_2-blockers such as cimetidine on isolated gastric glands and parietal cells confirmed that the histamine receptors mediating acid secretion are, indeed, like those in the heart and the uterus.

Interestingly, however, the histamine H_2-receptor antagonists were found in vivo to inhibit competitively not only histamine-stimulated acid secretion but also to reduce basal and gastrin- or vagus-stimulated acid secretion (Grossman and Konturek, 1974; Konturek, Biernat and Oleksy, 1974). Our secretory studies used two H_2-receptor antagonists; cimetidine with its basic imidazole ring that was considered necessary for antagonist activity, potency and selectivity, and ranitidine which is a substituted furan. We found that in humans either drug dose-dependently inhibited histamine-induced secretion but also caused non-competitive suppression of pentagastrin-induced secretion. These drugs also reduced acid secretion induced by sham-feeding and ordinary feeding without affecting serum gastrin responses (Konturek, 1982). The results can be interpreted as contradicing the claim for the high selectivity and specificity of H_2-antagonists, or as providing evidence for a physiological role of histamine in gastric acid secretion.

The "mediator" or "final common chemostimulator" concept of histamine involvement in gastric acid secretory mechanisms

The findings that H_2-receptor antagonists can suppress gastric acid secretion induced by various stimulants lead to the concept that histamine plays a primary role in acid secretion. MacIntosh (1938) and Code (1977) suggested that histamine is the "final local chemostimulator" of the parietal cell in response to gastrin and acetylcholine (the "mediator" hypothesis). Several findings strongly support a crucial role for histamine which, in canine and human mucosa, is stored in the numerous mast cells in the lamina propria, near to the oxyntic cells (Soll, Lewin and Beaven, 1979; Beaven, Soll and Lewin, 1982). In contrast, histamine in rats is stored in enterocrine-like cells that lie in the epithelium rather than in the lamina propria (Soll, Lewin and Beaven, 1981). Oxyntic mucosa in rats, but not in dogs or humans, contains histidine decarboxylase, which catalyses the formation of histamine from histidine.

The major degradative pathway for histamine in dog gastric mucosa is methylation of the imidazole nitrogen, a reaction catalyzed by histamine methyltransferase which is associated with the parietal cells. Inhibition of this enzyme enhances acid secretion in response to histamine (Barth, Lorenz and Troidl, 1975) or pentagastrin (Troidl, Lorenz and Barth, 1973). Finally, histamine is the most potent stimulant of the isolated parietal cells or isolated oxyntic glands as evidenced by increases in oxygen uptake, adenylate cyclase activity, aminopyrine uptake and cyclic AMP accumulation (Soll, 1978).

The H_2-receptors mediating histamine stimulation of the oxyntic cells have been characterized pharmacologically and by ^{14}C-histamine binding (Lewin, Grzelec, Cheter, Rene and Bonfils, 1979).

According to the "mediator" hypothesis (Code, 1977) histamine released from cellular stores by mechanical (distention), humoral (gastrin) and nervous (vagus) stimuli, diffuses to the parietal cells and stimulates acid secretion. Thus, whenever the secretory "drive" is accelerated, the release and synthesis of histamine should also be increased. However, it must be noted that the observations relating to the mobilization and accelerated production of gastric histamine to acid secretion are only in rats; less information is available regarding this relationship in other species, and even in rats, gastric acid secretion may not be related to the release and synthesis of histamine. For instance, following pylorus ligation and subsequent gastric distention, there is a marked rise in the acid secretion, but the release and synthesis of histamine are low (Hakanson, Hedenbro, Liedberg, Sundler and Vallgren, 1980). Conversely, following nephrectomy, the serum gastrin is increased and the production of histamine is greatly accelerated, but the acid secretion is reduced (ElMunshid, Liedberg, Rehfeld, Sundler, Larsson and Hakanson, 1976). Furthermore, some agents such as secretin or somatostatin, given in doses which completely inhibited acid response to gastrin, have little or no effect on histamine-stimulated acid secretion. In addition, these doses fail to prevent gastrin-induced release of histamine and activation of histidine decarboxylase (ElMunshid, Hakanson, Liedberg and Sundler, 1980). Thus acid secretion was inhibited even though histamine was released, suggesting that rat gastric mucosal histamine does not necessarily stimulate acid secretion and that gastrin (or acetylcholine) may stimulate the parietal cells without histamine intervention.

The histamine mediator concept explains the inhibition by H_2-blockers of vagal stimulation and gastrin action, but fails to explain why atropine inhibits gastric acid secretion induced by histamine or by gastrin (Hirschowitz and Sachs, 1969).

The "multi-messenger" concept. Potentiating interaction of secretagogues

Babkin (1938) stated that the "action of the vagus on the gastric glands causes liberation of histamine or histamine-like substances, which stimulate the parietal cells". However, the well known antisecretory effect of anticholinergics, such as atropine or pirenzepine, indicate that muscarinic cholinergic receptors are involved in gastric acid secretion (Konturek, Kwiecien, Obtulowicz, Swierczek, Kopp and Oleksy, 1982). Since both anticholinergics and H_2-blockers interfere with cholinergically induced or gastrin-stimulated acid secretion, the question arose whether the parietal

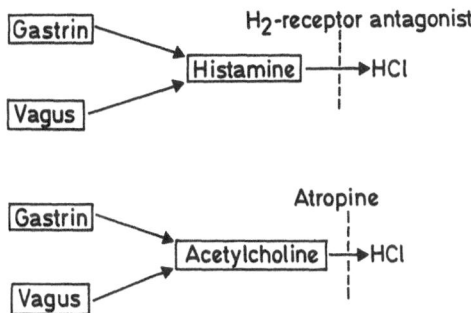

Figure 1   The concept of "final common chemostimulator" is supported
            by the fact that H_2-receptor antagonists block the re-
            ponse of the parietal cells to all kinds of stimuli (top)
            but fails to explain the inhibition of this response by
            antimuscarinic agents (below).

cells are equipped with separate receptors for histamine, acetylcholine and gastrin, and whether the interaction of these secretagogues in vivo can be explained by special properties of the parietal
cell receptors.

    The question has been partly answered in studies on the isolated
parietal cells, whose stimulation can be evidenced by changes in
oxygen consumption, aminopyrine accumulation or morphological transformation.   Soll (1978) found that such cells responded well to
histamine and carbachol and, to a smaller extent, also to gastrin.
The specificities of the receptors involved were assessed by studying
the effects of H_2-blockers and anticholinergics on the stimulation
by these secretagogues. H_2-blockers inhibited the response to histamine, but not to carbachol or gastrin.   Atropine inhibited the response to carbachol but not to histamine or gastrin.   These findings
suggest that parietal cells are equipped with separate receptors for
histamine (H_2-receptors), and cholinergic agents (muscarinic receptors) and that gastrin acts via a third receptor type.   Although
gastrin is a weak stimulant of the canine parietal cells and fails

to stimulate the amphibian parietal cells or rabbit gastric glands, there is little doubt that gastrin receptors exist. There is a potentiating interaction of gastrin with histamine, and ^{3}H-gastrin binds to rat enriched parietal cells.

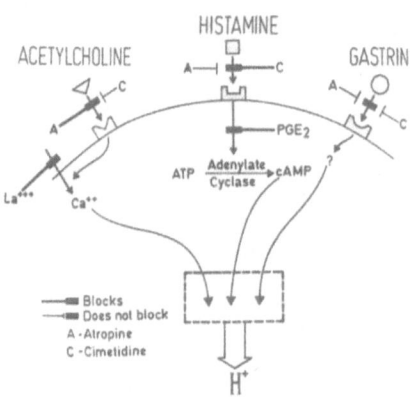

Figure 2   A proposed model for the action and interaction of secretagogues and blockers on parietal cells. Histamine stimulation of adenylate cyclase and the proposed site of action of PGE_2 are indicated (Soll, 1978).

In vivo, the interdependence of secretagogue action on the parietal cells is evident in the apparent nonspecificity of the effects of anticholinergics and H_2-blockers on gastric acid secretion. This can be explained by the potentiating interaction between secretagogues. Soll (1978) showed that the response to gastrin or carbachol was potentiated by histamine, but there was little potentiation between gastrin and carbachol. However, the addition of a small amount of histamine to gastrin plus carbachol produced a greatly potentiated response, suggesting a three-way potentiation between these stimulants. In the presence of anticholinergics, this potentiated response was reduced to that achieved with histamine plus gastrin; the addition of H_2-blockers reduced the response to that found with carbachol plus gastrin, and adding both the H_2-blocker and anticholinergic reduced the response to that seen with gastrin (Soll, 1978).

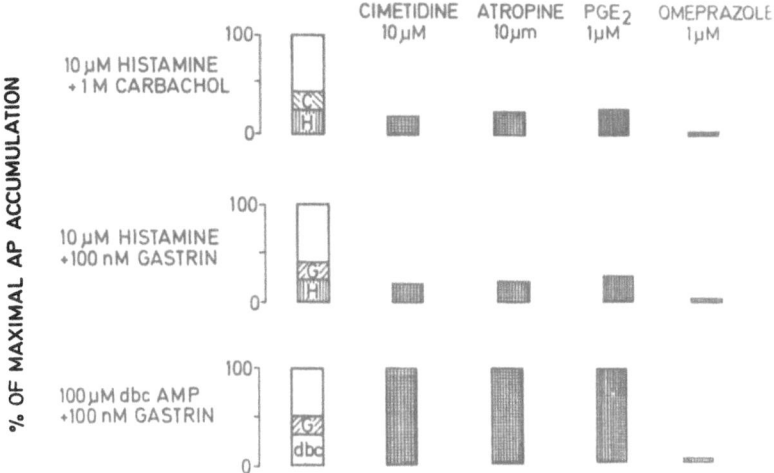

Figure 3   Potentiating interaction between parietal cell stimulants
and the effect of inhibitors.   C carbachol,   H histamine,
G gastrin,   dbc dibutyryl cyclic AMP.

In vivo, the parietal cells appear to remain under tonic influences from endogenous histamine, gastrin and acetylcholine, which
act as a potentiating background.   In addition, acetylcholine and
gastrin may be released phasically in response to vagal stimulation,
eg by sham- or ordinary feeding.   Activation of vagal reflexes during
the cephalic and gastric phases of the response to eating is assumed
by cause a substantial increase in the delivery of acetylcholine to
the parietal cells.   Phasic increase in gastrin release which occurs
postprandially is well documented.   In the case of histamine, there
is strong evidence that histamine is delivered to the parietal cells
as a continuous basal background, but there is no convincing evidence
that a phasic increase in histamine release occurs during stimulation
by the gastrin released by food or exogenous secretagogues.

THE RELEASE OF HISTAMINE BY GASTRIN AND VAGAL STIMULATION

The problem of histamine release by various secretagogues has
been carefully studied both in animals and man.   It was reported
that following pentagastrin stimulation there was increased gastric
acid output accompanied by increased amounts of histamine in gastric
juice and plasma (Man, Saunders, Ingoldby and Spencer, 1981).   The
association between histamine and gastric acid secretion was considered as compatible with the hypothesis that pentagastrin acts on

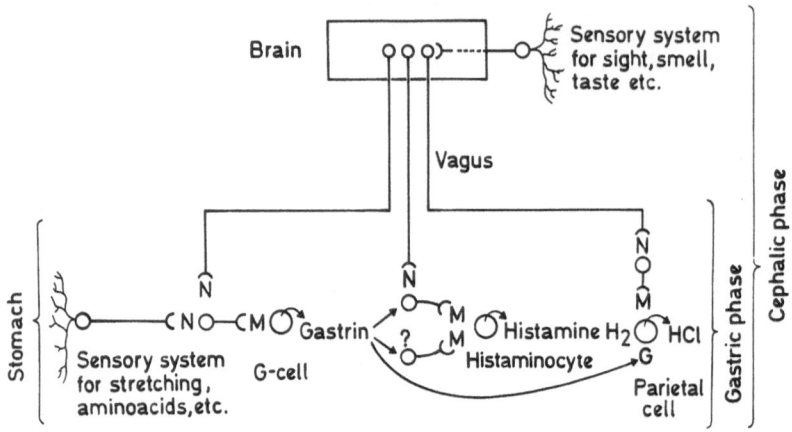

o—c = Nerve cell. N and M indicate nicotinic acid and muscarinic
cholinergic transmission respectively.

Figure 4   A proposed model for the mediation of histamine in the
stimulation of the parietal cells during cephalic and
gastric phases of acid secretion

the parietal cells indirectly, by releasing histamine in the gastric
mucosa.

Since gastrin is only a weak stimulant of the isolated parietal
cells or gastric glands (Berglindh, Helander and Obrink, 1976), the
powerful in vivo acid stimulation by this secretagogue may be explained by the release of histamine from histaminocytes.   According
to Chew and Hersey (1982), the most important component of the parietal cell stimulation is released histamine.   Less important are
direct gastrin stimulation (H_2-antagonist insensitive) and an interaction of histamine and gastrin on the parietal cells.   Evidence
supporting this interaction comes from the powerful inhibition of
gastrin- and pentagastrin-induced responses by H_2-blockers.   In the
presence of an H_2-antagonist, the dose-response curve for pentagastrin is shifted to the right.   There is also a decreased maximal
response (non-competitive antagonism), presumably because the release
of histamine by pentagastrin cannot be raised sufficiently to compete
with the H_2-antagonist.

The release of histamine by gastrin suggests that histamine

cells have hormonal receptors, and there are other receptors responsible for the release of histamine by vagal stimulation and acetylcholine.   Using luminally perfused mouse isolated stomach (Angus,
1982; Angus and Black, 1982), which is devoid of any interaction
with circulating gastrin, electrical field stimulation of acid secretion was inhibited by atropine, hexamethonium or tetrodotoxin, as
well as by H_2-receptor antagonists.   It is of interest that the
gastric response to carbachol, but not to the stable muscarinic antagonist bethanechol, was reduced by H_2-blockers (Angus and Black, 1982).
In the presence of hexamethonium, however, the response curve to carbachol was unaltered by H_2-blockers.   This could be interpreted as
a stimulation by carbachol of nicotinic receptors on vagal ganglia,
releasing gastrin.   Thus, vagal stimulation delivers transmitter
directly to muscarinic receptors of histamine-containing cells near
the parietal cells (Angus, 1982).   In this way histamine-containing
cells, which are outnumbered by the parietal cells, act as biological
amplifiers for transmission of both gastrin- and vagal-stimulation
to acid secretion (Soll et al., 1982; Soll et al., 1981).   The fact
that H_2-blockers fail to affect bethanechol-induced secretion could
be interpreted as a direct action on muscarinic receptors of the
parietal cells without any contribution from histamine released via
stimulation of vagal ganglia.   The presence of such receptors on
the parietal cells has been shown by binding of ^{3}H-quinuclidinyl
benzilate to these cells but the receptor population was rather
sparse (Yamamura and Snyder, 1974).

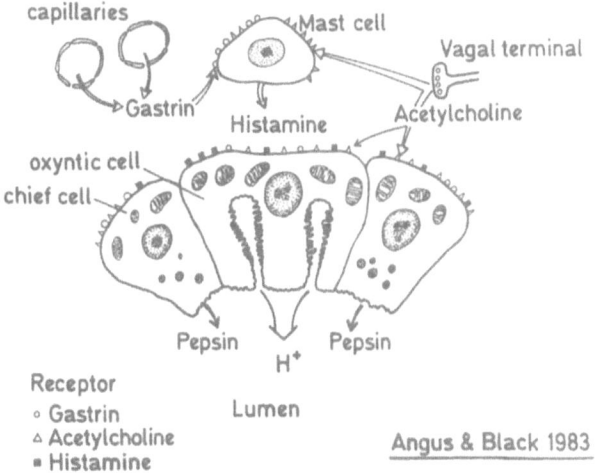

Fig 5. Circulating gastrin and vagal acetylcholine release mast
       cell histamine which then stimulates the parietal cells
       (these have relatively few muscarinic and gastrinic
       receptors, Angus, 1982).

197

ROLE OF HISTAMINE IN PEPTIC ULCER DISEASE

Histamine has long been known to be a potent gastric secreta-gogue in humans, and its potential significance in the pathophysio-logy of ulcer disease has been emphasised by recent findings that histamine H_2-receptor antagonists such as cimetidine or ranitidine reduce gastric acid secretion (Konturek, 1982) and accelerate the healing of peptic ulcer (Schiller and Feldman, 1981).

Using highly sensitive fluorometric-fluoroenzymatic methodology for measuring histamine (Rohde, Lorenz and Troidl, 1980), it has been reported that gastric mucosa of normal subjects has an astonishingly high histamine content of about 40µg/g (Troidl, Rohde, Lorenz, Hafner and Hamelmann, 1978). Duodenal ulcer patients, however, were found to store about 30% less histamine than control healthy subjects. After complete selective vagotomy (Troidl et al, 1978) and cimeti-dine treatment (Barth, Troidl and Lorenz, 1977), the levels of hista-mine in the mucosa returned to normal or above normal. The increase in mucosal histamine storage was related to the fall in acid output observed after vagotomy. In patients with incomplete vagotomy and recurrent duodenal ulcer the mucosal histamine was as low as that in duodenal ulcer patients without operation.

It is of interest that gastric mucosa of duodenal ulcer patients exhibits less activity of gastric mucosal methyltransferase (HMT), a principal histamine-metabolising enzyme (Lorenz, Parkin, Rohde, Barth, Troidl, Thon, Hinterland, Weber, Albrecht and Roher, 1981; Lorenz, Mohri, Reimann, Troidl, Rohde and Barth, 1981). These findings have been confirmed recently by Peden, Callachan, Shepherd and Wormsley, 1982), who also observed that cigarette smokers showed significantly lower levels of fundic histamine (but not HMT) than did non-smokers. Since there was a preponderance of cigarette smokers among patients with duodenal ulcer, it has been suggested that smoking may cause the lower content of mucosal histamine in ulcer patients. Lorenz's group (Lorenz et al.,1981) postulated that in patients with duodenal ulcer an increased vagal drive results in gastric acid hypersecretion due to increased histamine release and decreased inactivation, quite apart from other actions of the vagal nerves on the stomach. Thus, patients with peptic ulcer have de-pleted gastric mucosal histamine stores and this abnormality may be a major feature of peptic ulcer disease. Vagotomy abolishes the vagal drive, decreases histamine release and enhances histamine in-activation resulting in the reduction in gastric acid secretion. Histamine H_2-receptor antagonists block the effect of released hista-mine at the parietal cells and also speed up histamine inactivation. Further studies are required to examine the possible role of hista-mine in the pathophysiology of peptic ulcer disease, by monitoring storage of histamine in mast cells and parietal cells during secre-tory responses to various agonists and antagonists.

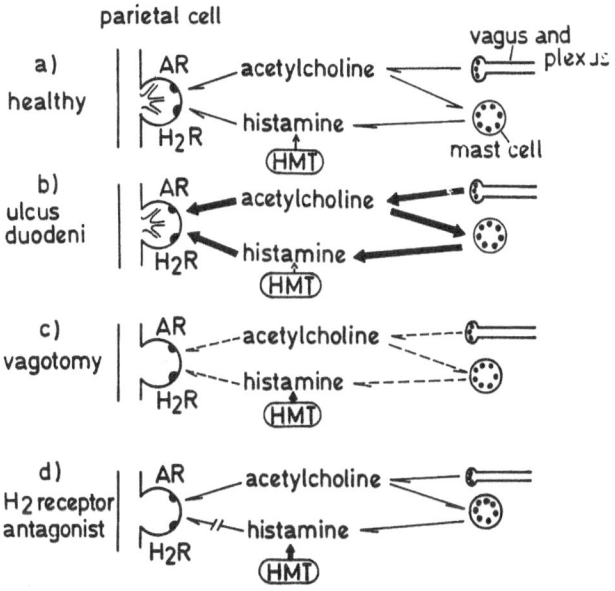

Figure 6. Mechanisms for stimulation of gastric acid secretion
in normal subjects and in duodenal ulcer patients
after vagotomy and histamine H_2-receptor treatment.

enhanced effect
normal effect
diminished effect.

AR = muscarinic receptor. H_2R = histamine H_2
receptor (Lorenz et al., 1981).

SUMMARY

The physiological role of histamine in gastric secretion has
been controversial since Popielski demonstrated that histamine stimulates this secretion.   The results using H_2-receptor antagonists,
together with the findings that histamine is produced and stored in
the fundic mucosa and released upon vagal or hormonal stimulation,
indicate that this amine is the major physiological stimulant of the
parietal cells.   The concepts of histamine as a 'final common chemostimulator' of parietal cells, and as part of a 'multi-messenger'
potentiating interaction of various hormonal secretagogues on parietal
cells, have both been proposed to explain the involvement of histamine in gastric secretory mechanisms.   Histamine may also be an important factor in the pathogenesis of gastric hypersecretion and
peptic ulcer disease since its mobilization from gastric mucosal
stores is accelerated in peptic ulcer disease, and since treatment
with vagotomy or H_2-receptor antagonists decreases histamine release
and increases its degradation in the gastric mucosa.

REFERENCES

Angus, J.A., 1982, Histamine receptors - their classification and
role in gastric acid secretion, in: Receptor Update; Proceedings.
Excerpta Medica, Geneva, 29.
Angus, J.A., and Black, J.W., 1978, Production of acid secretion in
the isolated stomach by electrical field stimulation, Br.J. Pharmacol.
62: 460P.
Angus, J.A., and Black, J.W., 1982, The interaction of choline esters,
vagal stimulation and H_2-receptor blockade on acid secretion in
vitro, Eur. J. Pharmacol. 80: 217.
Ash, A.S.F., and Schild, H.O., 1966, Receptors mediating some actions
of histamine, Br. J. Pharmacol. 27: 427.
Babkin, B.P., 1938, The abnormal functioning of the gastric secretory
mechanisms as possible factor in the pathogenesis of peptic ulcer,
J. Can. Med. Assoc. 38: 421.
Barth, H., Lorenz, W., and Troidl, H., Effect of amodiquin on gastric
histamine methyltransferase and histamine-stimulated gastric secretion, Br. J. Pharmacol. 55: 321.
Barth, H., Troidl, H., and Lorenz, W., 1977, Histamine and peptic
ulcer disease: histamine methyltransferase activity in gastric
mucosa of control subjects and duodenal ulcer patients before and
after surgery, Agents and Actions 6: 75.
Beaven, M.A., and Lewin, K.J., 1982, Histamine synthesis by intact
mast cells from canine fundic mucosa and liver, Gastroenterology
82:254.
Berglindh, T., Helander, H.T., and Obrink, K.J., 1976, Effect of
secretagogues on oxygen consumption, aminopyrine accumulation and
morphology of isolated gastric glads, Acta Physiol. Scand. 97: 401.
Black, J.W., Duncan, W.A.M., Durant, C.J., Ganellin, C.R., and

Parsons, M.E., 1972, Definition and antagonism of histamine H$_2$-receptors, Nature (Lond.) 236: 385.

Black, J.W., Owen, D.A.A., and Parsons, M.E., An analysis of the depressor responses to histamine in the cat and dog: involvement of both H$_1$- and H$_2$-receptors, Br. J. Pharmacol. 54: 319.

Chew, C.S., and Hersey, S.J., 1982, Gastrin stimulation of isolated gastric glands, Am. J. Physiol. 242: G504.

Code, C.F., 1977, Reflections on histamine, gastric secretion and H$_2$-receptors, New Engl. J. Med. 296: 1459.

Effects of various gastrointestinal peptides on parietal cells and endocrine cells in the oxyntic mucosa of the rat stomach, J. Physiol. 305: 249.

ElMunshid, H.A., Lieberg, G., Rehfeld, J.T., Sundler, P., Larsson, L.I., and Hakason, R., 1976, Effect of bilateral nephrectomy on serum gastrin concentration, gastric histamine content, histidine decarboxylase activity and acid secretion in the rat, Scand. J. Gastroenterol. 11:87.

Emmelin, N., and Kahlson, G.S., 1944, Histamine as a physiological excitant of acid gastric secretion, Acta Physiol. Scand. 8: 289.

Folkow, B., Haeger, K., and Kahlson, G.S., 1948, Observations on reactive hyperaemia as related to histamine, on drugs antagonising vasodilation induced by histamine and on vasodilator properties of adenosine triphosphate, Acta Physiol. Scand, 15: 264.

Gavin, G., McHenry, W.E., and Wilson, M.J., 1933, Histamine in canine gastric tissue, J. Physiol. 79: 234.

Ginsburg, R., Bristow, M.R., Kantrowitz, N., Baim, D.S., and Harrison, D.C., 1981, Histamine provocation of clinical coronary artery spasm: implications concerning pathogenesis of variant angina pectoris. Am. Heart J. 102: 819.

Gregory, R.A., and Tracy, H.J., 1961, The preparation and properties of gastrin. J. Physiol, 156: 523.

Gregory, H., Hardy, P.M., Jones, D.S., Kenner, G.W., and Sheppard, R.C., 1964, The antral hormone gastrin I. Structure of gastrin, Nature (Lond.) 204:931.

Grossman, M.I., and Konturek, S.J., 1974, Inhibition of acid secretion in dog by metiamide, a histamine antagonist acting on H$_2$-receptors. Gastroenterology 66: 517.

Hakanson, R., Hedenbro, J., Liedberg, G., Sundler, F., and Vallgren, S., 1980, Mechanism of gastric acid secretion after pylorus and oesophagus ligation in the rat. J. Physiol. 305: 139.

Johnson, L.R., 1971, Control of gastric secretion: no room for histamine? Gastroenterology 61: 106.

Johnson, L.R., and Aures, D., 1970, Evidence that histamine is not the mediator of acid secretion in the rat, Proc. Soc. Exp. Biol. Med. 134: 880.

Johnson, L.R., and Tumpson, D.B., 1970, Effect of secretin on histamine stimulated secretion in the gastric fistula rat, Proc. Soc. Exp. Biol. Med., 133: 125.

Kahlson, G.S., Rowengren, E., Svahn, D., and Thurnberg, R., 1964, Mobilization and formation of histamine in the gastric mucosa as related to acid secretion, J. Physiol. 174: 400.

Konturek, S.J., 1982, Pharmacology and clinical use of ranitidine, Mt Sinai J. Med. 49:370.

Konturek, S.J., Biernat, J., and Oleksy, J., 1974, Effect of metiamide, a histamine H_2-receptor antagonist on gastric response to histamine, pentagastrin, insulin and peptone meal in man, Dig. Dis. Sci. 19: 609.

Kopp, B., and Oleksy, J., 1982, Muscarinic control of gastrin release in duodenal ulcer patients, in: Symposium Advances in Gastroenterology with the Selective Antimuscarinic Compound Pirenzepine, Excerpta Med. 31.

Konturek, S.J., Obtulowicz, W., Kwiecien, N., Kopp, B., and Oleksy, J., 1981, Dynamics of gastric acid inhibition by ranitidine in duodenal ulcer patients, Digestion 22: 119.

Lewin, M.J.M., Grzelec, F., Cheter, A.M., Rene, E., and Bonfils, S., Demonstration and characterization of histamine H_2-receptor on isolated guinea-pig gastric cell, in: Hormone Receptors in Digestion and Nutrition, G. Roselin, B. Fromageat, S. Bonfils, eds, Elsevier/North Holland, Amsterdam 1979, 383.

Loew, E.R., 1947, Pharmacology of antihistamine compounds, Physiol. Rev., 27: 542.

Lorenz, W., Mohri, K., Reimann, H.J., Troidl, H., Rohde, H., and Barth, H., 1981, Intramucosal mechanisms: relevance of the mast cell concept, in: Advances in Ulcer Disease, K.H. Holtermuller, J.R. Malagelada, eds, Excerpta Medica, Amsterdam.

Lorenz, W., Parkin, J.V., Rohde, H., Barth, H., Troidl, H., Thon, K., Hinterland, E., Weber, D., Albrecht, R., and Roher, H., 1981, Histamine in gastric secretory disorders: The relevance of the mucosal histamine content and the origin of histamine in gastric aspirate, in: Gastric Secretion. Basic and Clinical Aspects. S.J. Konturek, W Domschke, eds, Thieme-Stratton Inc., New York, 29.

MacIntosh, F.C., 1938, Histamine as normal stimulant of gastric secretion, Q.J. Exp. Physiol. 28:87.

Man, W.K., Saunders, J.H., Ingoldby, C., and Spencer, J., 1981, Effect of pentagastrin on histamine output from the stomach in patients with duodenal ulcer, Gut 22: 916.

Man, W.K., Saunders, J.H., Ingoldby, C., and Spencer, J., 1981, Effect of cimetidine on the amounts of histamine in the gastric mucosa of patients with gastric or duodenal ulcers. Gut 22: 923.

Palacois, J.M., and Garbare, M., 1978, Pharmacological characterization of histamine receptors mediating the stimulation of cyclic AMP accumulation in slices from guinea-pig hippocampus, Mol. Pharmacol. 14: 971.

Parsons, M.E., Owen, D.A.A., Ganellin, C.R., Durant, F.J., 1977, Dimaprit- S- 3 - N,N-dimethylamine isopyl (isothiourea), a highly specific histamine H_2-receptor agonist. Part 1. Pharmacology. Agents and Actions, 7: 31.

Peden, N.R., Callachan, H., Shepherd, D.N., and Wormsley, K.G., 1982, Gastric mucosal histamine and histamine methyltransferase in patients with duodenal ulcer, Gut 23: 58.

Popielski, L., 1920, Beta-imidazolylathylamin und die Organ Extrakte; Beta-Imidazolylathylamin als machtiger Erreger der Magendrusen. Pflug. Arch. Physiol. 178: 214.

Rohde, H., Lorenz, W., and Troidl, H., 1980, Histamine and peptic ulcer: influence of sample-taking on the precision and accuracy of fluorometric histamine assay in biopsies of human gastric mucosa, Agents and Actions, 10: 175.

Schiller, L.R., and Feldman, M., 1981, Medical therapy of peptic ulcer disease, in: Foregut. Gastroenterology 1, J.H. Baron, F.G. Moody, eds, Butterworths.

Soll, A.H., 1978, The action of secretagogues on oxygen uptake by isolated mammalian parietal cells. J. Clin. Invest. 61: 370.

Soll, A.H., 1978, The interaction of histamine with gastrin and carbamylcholine on oxygen uptake by isolated mammalian parietal cells, J. Clin. Invest. 61: 381.

Soll, A.H., Lewin, K.J., and Beaven, M.A., 1979, Isolation of histamine-containing cells from canine fundic mucosa, Gastroenterology 77: 1283.

Soll, A.H., Lewin, K.J., and Beaven, M.A., 1981, Isolation of histamine-containing cells from rat gastric mucosa: Biochemical and morphological differences from mast cells, Gastroenterology 80: 717.

Troidl, H., Lorenz, W., and Barth, H., 1973, Augmentation of pentagastrin stimulated gastric secretion in the Heidenhain pouch dog by amodiaquin. Inhibition of histaminemethyltransferase in vivo, Agents and Actions 3: 157.

Troidl, H., Rohde, H., Lorenz, W., Hafner, H., Hamelmann, H., 1978, Effect of selective gastric vagotomy on histamine concentration in gastric mucosa of patients with duodenal ulcer, Brit. J. Surg. 65: 10.

Yamamura, H.I., and Snyder, S.J., 1974, Muscarinic cholinergic receptor binding in the longitudinal muscle of the guinea-pig ileum ^{3}H quinuclidinyl benzilate. Mol. Pharmacol. 10: 861.

GASTROINTESTINAL MUCUS

A. Allen, N. Carroll, A. Garner,* D.A. Hutton
and C.W. Venables†

Departments of Physiological Sciences and †Surgery
University of Newcastle upon Tyne, U.K. and
*Bioscience Department, I.C.I. Pharmaceuticals Division
Alderley Park, Macclesfield, Cheshire, U.K.

FUNCTIONS OF MUCUS

Mucus occurs throughout the gastrointestinal tract as a water insoluble gel adherent to the mucosal surface and as soluble or suspended mucus in the lumen. The principal function ascribed to mucus is protection of the underlying mucosa from the harmful factors in the lumen.[1,2] In the stomach and duodenum the adherent gel together with the mucosal bicarbonate secretion provides an environment for neutralisation of luminal acid, maintaining a near neutral pH at the mucosal surface[3,4] (Fig. 1). Acid from the lumen readily diffuses through the mucus cover,[6,7] but it is neutralised in the stable, unstirred layer within the mucus by bicarbonate secreted from the surface epithelial cells. In this way the adherent mucus gel limits the mixing of the bulk of luminal acid with the smaller quantity of mucosal bicarbonate secretion. Recent evidence for such a protective mechanism has come from studies of gastroduodenal epithelial bicarbonate secretion;[4,8] the structure of mucus[9,10] measurements of pH gradients adjacent to the mucosal surface[11,12,13,14] and observations on the adherent mucus gel layer in situ.[15,16] Although permeable to hydrogen and bicarbonate ions, mucus is not permeable to large molecular weight pepsins.[10] A hydraulic pressure is created in the gastric glands and rapid secretion of H^+ and pepsin will enable them to gain access to the stomach lumen through the thin cover of surface mucus. The annealing properties of mucus will allow it to reseal when secretion has ceased. Once in the lumen of the stomach, pepsin cannot diffuse back through the adherent gel and attack the underlying mucosal cells. Mucosal defence against pepsinolysis is further complicated by the fact that pepsin solubilises

205

the mucus gel to produce soluble degraded mucus in the gastric juice. [10,17,18] Therefore mucus will only provide an effective barrier against pepsin if proteolytic degradation at its luminal surface is balanced by secretion of new mucus gel.

The protective properties of mucus discussed above clearly depend on the thin, continuous cover of adherent mucus gel over the mucosa. Soluble mucus found in the lumen consists of a mixture of proteolytically degraded and native glycoprotein. It is the result of degradation of the adherent mucus layer at its luminal surface by pepsin and abrasion. Pepsin, while not permeating the mucus gel, can degrade mucus by hydrolysis of the polymeric glycoprotein components which form the gel, to release soluble degraded glycoprotein subunits.[10,17] Some soluble mucus, e.g. that released following prostaglandin administration[19] is likely to be a direct secretion from the mucosa rather than degradation of the adherent mucus. The glycoprotein content of the luminal juice will therefore bear little relation to the amount of the functional mucus gel on the mucosal surface and is not an index of secretion of mucus as previously suggested by some authors (see Allen, 1981,[9] for discussion). The functions of soluble mucus are not clear but it certainly does not appear to play a part in mucosal protection. A function of both the adherent and soluble mucus is that of lubrication, facilitating the passage of solid material through the gut and preventing epithelial damage from the shear forces of digestion.[2] Other functions proposed for mucus are (i) the binding of ions, e.g. iron and calcium;[20] (ii) as a protective barrier against pathogenic organisms in the gut[9,20] and (iii) as a nutrient source for the endogenous anaerobic bacteria.[21]

MUCUS STRUCTURE

Mucus gels are weak, viscoelastic gels with properties well suited to forming a continuous protective cover over the mucosal surface. Rheological studies of the intact native gastric mucus show that it is a gel and not a super viscous liquid.[22,23] However, in contrast to rigid gels (e.g. strong agar) mucus will slowly flow and anneal if sectioned. Mucus is sticky and adheres to the surface of cells, another important feature if the mucus layer is not to be washed away during digestion. The mucus gel is formed by non-covalent interactions between large, highly hydrated glycoprotein molecules which occupy the whole solution volume. Physical methods, e.g. strong shear forces (homogenisation in a blender for 1 min or sonication) will break the non-covalent bonds between the glycoprotein molecules and dissolve the gel. By this method a soluble glycoprotein is obtained which apparently possesses full rheological properties and can form a gel with the same structural characteristics as the original native mucus.[22] Thus the purified glycoproteins from pig gastric duodenal mucus at concentrations similar to that found in the native mucus (55 mg ml^{-1}, 50 mg ml^{-1}, for gastric and duodenal respectively) also possess the characteristic rheological profile of the native gastroduodenal mucus gel.[24] The high concentration of glycoprotein in gastric and duodenal mucus will result in a particularly good unstirred layer within the gel matrix.

When the native mucus gels or the reformed gels from all regions of the gastrointestinal tract are treated with proteolytic enzymes (e.g. pepsin, trypsin, Pronase or papain) there is a complete collapse of gel structure. The proteolytically digested mucus has a rheological profile characteristic of a viscous liquid, and the gel-forming properties of the isolated glycoprotein are lost. The same collapse of gel structure occurs if mucus is incubated for 24 hours at 4°C in 0.2M mercaptoethanol. This collapse of the mucus gel structure is the result of breakage of the covalent structure of the protein core of the component glycoproteins by proteolysis or splitting of the disulphide bridges.[17,25,26]

The mucus gel is resistant to a wide variety of agents that break non-covalent bonds. For example, the rheological profile of fresh pig gastric mucus is unchanged after exposure to 0.2M NaCl, 2M NaCl, 6M guanidinium chloride, at 4°C.[8] Similarly exposure of the fresh gastric mucus to undiluted pig gall bladder bile (pH 2.6 and 8 for 18 hr) or to 0.1M acid (4°C for 4 hr) did not disrupt the gel structure.

Glycoproteins of high molecular weight are the functional components of mucus secretions and are responsible for its viscous and gel-forming properties.[9,27,28] The mucus will also contain, besides the glycoproteins, material from sloughed off epithelial cells, bacteria, digested food, plasma proteins, digestive enzymes, secretory IgA, bile and electrolytes.[20] In the lumen the situation is further complicated by degradation and dilution of the mucus secretion by other fluids so that the glycoprotein is only a minor component of the total luminal contents and is frequently degraded. Major technical problems are associated with isolating pure and undegraded mucous glycoproteins from the other components. To overcome this a wide variety of different procedures have been used resulting in the isolation of mucous glycoproteins ranging in size from 2×10^5 to 40×10^6 mol. wt. Included in the lower size range will be proteolytically degraded glycoproteins while the upper end of the size range will reflect non-covalent aggregates of the native glycoproteins.[29] To study the relationship between mucus structure and physiological properties it is necessary to isolate a glycoprotein that retains the viscous and gel-forming properties of the adherent gel.[17] The basic structure of mucous glycoproteins from the gastrointestinal and other tracts of the body is well established and demonstrates that they are a distinct class of molecules with clear structural differences from other related substances (e.g. serum or membrane glycoproteins and the proteoglycans of connective tissue). Recently substantial amounts of lipid have also been shown to be strongly bound to purified mucous glyco-protein preparations.[30]

Mucous glycoproteins are characterised by a high carbohydrate composition (often over 80% by weight of the molecule) which is composed of the following sugars: galactose, fucose, N-acetylgluco-samine, N-acetylgalactosamine and sialic acids. Only traces, if any, of mannose and no uronic acids are found in these glycoproteins which distinguishes them from serum glycoproteins and proteoglycans respec-tively.[27,28] The sugars are present as hundreds of oligosaccharide chains (an average of 500 and 600 chains per molecule of 1 or 2 million molecular weight for pig submaxillary[11] and gastric mucous glycoproteins[1] respectively) attached to a central protein core. This is often referred to as a bottle brush structure where the bristles represent the carbohydrate chains and the wire support the protein core (Fig. 2). The carbohydrate chains vary in size accord-int to the origin of the mucus, but they can range from a maximum of 2 or 5 sugars per chain (submaxillary mucus,[11 25]) to complex chains with a maximum of 19 sugars per chain (gastric mucus,[39,41]). The physical and chemical data for the pig gastrointestinal mucous glycoproteins is shown in Table I and are characteristic of gastro-intestinal mucous glycoproteins generally, including those of man.[31,32,33,34] The pig is a good animal model with a plentiful supply of mucus. In the pig gastrointestinal tract there are clear structural differences in the carbohydrate chains of the mucous glycoproteins from different regions of the gastrointestinal tract. The mucous glycoproteins from all secretions of the gastrointestinal tract in man (ABH secretors) and pig (A&H) have blood group substance activity and have the blood group antigenic structures at the ends of their completed carbohydrate chains.[35,36] Why mucous glycoproteins should possess these antigenic structures, characteristic of the erythrocyte surface, is unknown.

Mucous glycoproteins are negatively charged. This arises from 3 sources: (i) the sialic acid residues in terminal positions on the carbohydrate chains, (ii) the ester sulphate residues which in pig gastric mucus occur deeper down within the sugar units, (iii) from the amino acid analysis of which shows a net excess of negatively charged amino acids in the protein core, but it is not known how many of these carboxyl groups are in the form of the amide. The average amounts of sialic acid or ester sulphate, and therefore negative charge, vary from one mucous glycoprotein to another. These negatively charged moieties provide the basis for the stain-ing characteristics of mucus secretions with Alcian blue and high iron diamine.[37]

The carbohydrate chains are attached by N-acetylgalactosamine at the reducing end of the oligosaccharide chain in an O-glycosidic linkage to threonine or serine residues in the protein core.[38] The carbohydrate chains are tightly packed together forming a

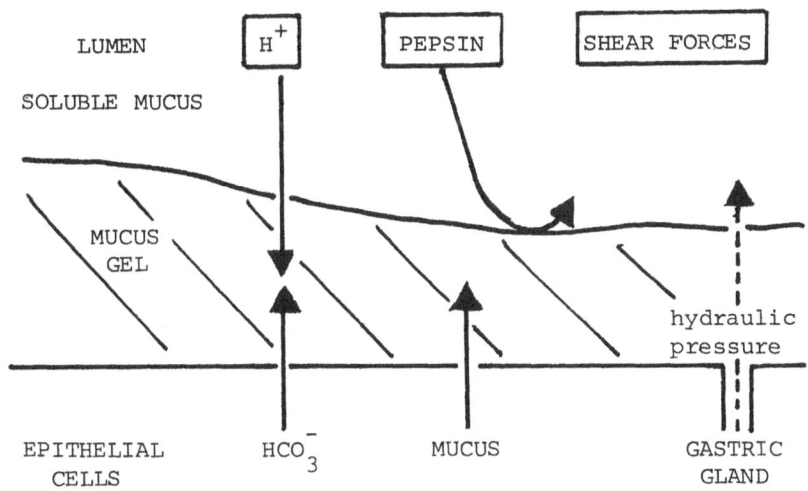

Figure I.   The role of gastroduodenal mucus in protection

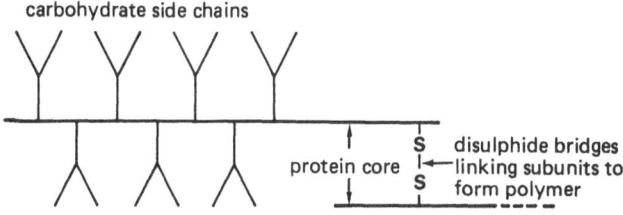

Figure II. A diagrammatic representation of a mucous
           glycoprotein subunit

TABLE I. COMPOSITION OF PIG GASTROINTESTINAL MUCOUS GLYCOPROTEIN

Constitutents	Mucous secretion	
	Gastric	Small intestinal
	Composition: % dry weight glycoprotein	
Native Glycoprotein		
Carbohydrate	82.9	77.5
Ester sulphate	3.2	2.8
Protein	13.3	19.6
	Molar ratio	
N-acetylgalactosamine	1	1
N-acetylglucosamine	2.8	0.6
Galactose	2.9	0.7
Fucose	1.9	0.3
Sialic acid	0.2	0.5
	Physical properties	
Mol. wt.	2×10^6	1.8×10^6
Intrinsic viscosity ml gm^{-1}	320	500
Blood group antigens	A & H	A & H
Proteolytically digested glycoprotein		
Protein	6.7	12.5
Mol. wt.	5.3×10^5	2.4×10^5

Data from Scawen and Allen, (1977)[25] (gastric); Mantle and Allen, (1981)[47] (small intestinal).

sheath that protects the central protein core from proteolysis -
"the bottle brush section". However there are other parts of the
protein core that are non-glycosylated and are hydrolysed by a
variety of proteolytic enzymes (Fig. 2).[25],[39] Thus after proteolytic digestion, gastric mucous glycoprotein showed two marked
differences compared to the native glycoprotein (Table I).
Firstly, there is a loss of a large portion of the protein core
(51% by weight of the total protein, 6-7% by weight of the total
glycoprotein, with pig gastric mucous glycoprotein) and with no
detectable loss of carbohydrate. The second change associated with
proteolysis is the marked reduction in molecular weight of the
glycoprotein. Detailed structural studies have shown that this
large reduction in molecular weight of the mucous glycoprotein
results from the destruction of a polymeric structure where glycoprotein subunits are joined together by disulphide bridges.[17],[27]
These disulphide bridges are located in regions of the protein core
which are free of carbohydrate (non-glycosylated) and accessible to
proteolytic attack; consequently either proteolysis of the peptide or
reduction of the interchain disulphide bridges themselves splits the
glycoprotein into subunits. In the case of pig gastric mucous
glycoprotein each native glycoprotein molecule is split into ~4 subunits on proteolysis or reduction.[25],[26] Such covalent fission of the
glycoprotein polymer into subunits results in loss of the gel-
forming properties of the molecule and explains the solubilisation
of the mucus gel following proteolysis or disulphide bond reduction.
There is evidence that polymeric structures similar to that found in
pig gastric mucus occur in glycoproteins from other mucus secretions,
e.g. human stomach,[31] pig small intestinal mucus,[40] pig colonic mucus
[41] and rat small intestinal mucus.[42]

MUCUS IN VIVO

The presence of the polymeric structure of the mucous glycoproteins is critical to gel-forming ability and thereby the function
of the mucus.[17],[26] Two examples where variations in this polymeric
structure have implications in vivo are (1) the maintenance of the
mucus gel cover in response to its solubilisation by luminal pepsin,
(2) a decrease in the amount of glycoprotein that is polymeric in
adherent antral mucus from patients with peptic ulcer disease.
Evidence for the pepsinolysis of the adherent mucus gel in man comes
from studies in duodenal ulcer (DU) patients. Analysis of gastric
juice washouts from these patients showed that the rise in glycoprotein following insulin stimulation (0.2 unit kg^{-1}) is predominently of lower molecular weight degraded glycoprotein (average 76%
of the total glycoprotein). This rise in lower molecular weight
glycoprotein (defined as material included on Sepharose 2B) paralleled a rise in pepsin. These changes were absent in vagotomised
patients following insulin infusion.[18] Incubation of pig gastric
mucus with gastric juice from D.U. patients produces a marked fall in
its viscosity with a corresponding increase in lower molecular

weight degraded glycoprotein, further evidence for pepsinolysis in vivo of the gel forming degraded mucous glycoprotein subunit.[31]

In contrast to the luminal mucous glycoprotein, that from the mucus gel adherent to histologically normal human gastric mucosa, is predominently of undegraded polymer.[31,34] Thus surface mucus gel from the normal antral mucosa of patients with cancer of the head of the pancreas, contained a mean of 67% polymeric glyco-protein, the remainder being lower molecular weight material, included on a Sepharose 2B column. In contrast the surface mucus from patients with peptic ulceration contained significantly less higher molecular weight polymeric glycoprotein (50% for DU, 35% for GU). This fall in the amount of polymeric mucous glycoprotein in peptic ulcer patients would implicate a weaker gel structure and thereby a poorer protective cover. The cause of this increase in the proportion of lower molecular weight glycoprotein in the adher-ent gastric mucus of peptic ulcer patients is not known. It is unlikely that it can be explained entirely by a higher degree of peptic degradation of the mucus. There may be a fault at the muco-sal level, the known gastritis in these patients may be associated with a release of lysosomal enzymes (proteases) capable of degrad-ing mucus.[34] Alternatively there may be incomplete biosynthesis of the glycoprotein by the mucosal cells.

It is important to be able to measure the amount and continuity of the gel cover. Erosion of the mucus gel produces mucous glyco-protein in the lumen and therefore the latter is not a direct meas-ure of mucus secretion by the mucosa (Fig. 3). Recently we have developed a method whereby the adherent mucus gel can be observed directly on unfixed sections of gastric and duodenal mucosa.[16] The mucus is seen as a thin layer of transluscent gel, optically dist-inct from the mucosa and bathing solution, forming a continuous cover over the rat gastroduodenal and human gastric mucosal surface. The mucus layer does not flow during the period of observation (60 min at 20°C) and validation experiments show that the sectioning procedure does not distort the gel. The thickness of the mucus layer, taken as the distance between the solution-mucus interface and the mucosa-mucus interface, varies markedly. In rat, values between 5-200 μm and occasionally up to 400 μm were observed over a single mucosa with 2 fold variations in mean thickness between individuals (stomach or duodenum). Such wide variations are to be expected for what is a water insoluble gelatinous secretion. Despite this variation, mucus thickness between control groups of starved rats (a minimum of 6 animals in each group) was not statis-tically different. Mean thickness of the adherent mucus gel in the rat stomach was 77 μm, in the rat duodenum 81 μm and in human stomach it was 192 μm.[19,43]

We have used the mucosal sectioning technique to study the effects of mucosal damaging agents on mucus gel thickness in vivo

Figure III. Maintenance of the adherent mucus gel layer on the gastric mucosa

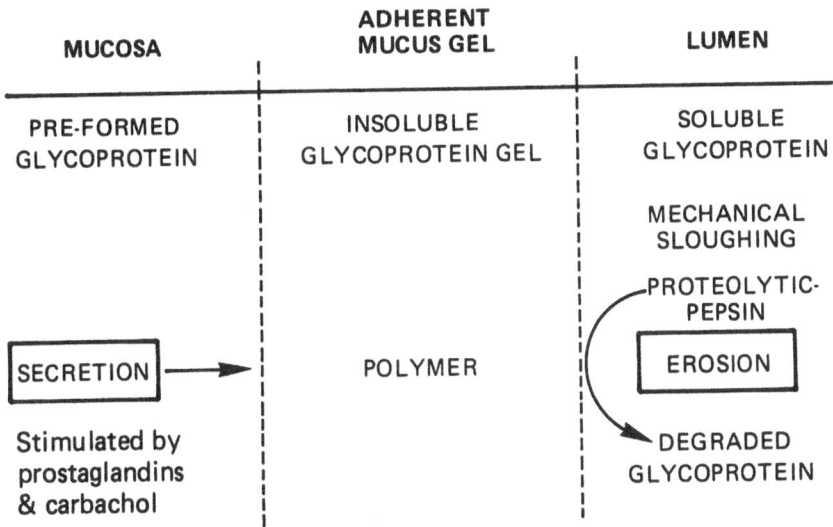

and in vitro. These studies, which are described in detail else-where[16],[19],[43] show rat gastric mucus thickness in vivo to be essentially unchanged following administration of topical damaging agents, e.g. 2M NaCl, absolute ethanol, O.6M HCl, indomethacin (30 mg/kg), 80mM taurocholate; except specifically at the site of "lesions" where breakdown of the mucus cover was observed. Topical administration to rats 1 hour previously of 0.5 ml of 60% ethanol, absolute ethanol, O.6M HCl, 80mM sodium taurocholate or indomethacin 30 mg/kg (or 15 mg/kg 24 hours previously) all resulted in the form-ation of gastric lesions visible as bands of overt haemorrhage. However the mucus layer showed resistance to these agents since there was little change in overall group mean gel thickness despite clear mucosal damage. While mean thickness of the surface mucus gel was essentially unaffected, the mucus layer was clearly disrupted at the site of lesions, identifiable by overt bleeding. Covering the focal lesions was a heterogeneous mixture of mucus and cells, and in places the mucus gel layer was absent, contrasting with the normal transluscent mucus gel covering the rest of the surface. Thus breakdown of the protective mucus cover following oral administration of damaging agents only occurs at specific sites which coincided with focal areas of severe damage.

MUCUS AND PROTECTION

Studies on the adherent mucus gel layer show that it forms a stable, continuous layer over the mucosa. The gel however varies considerably in thickness, e.g. in the rat between 5-200 μm (occasionally up to 400 μm) and in man about 2 fold greater.[16] The depth of this mucus layer is thinner than previously supposed. Thus it is to be expected that the adherent mucus does not seriously retard the diffusion of H^+ through its matrix but acts primarily as a mixing barrier in the form of a stable, unstirred layer close to the mucosal surface. Surface neutralisation in vivo would be expected to occur primarily in the mucus layer and therefore be restricted close to the mucosal surface. In addition to small ions, mucus is readily permeated by solutions of aspirin and ethanol. Thus damaging agents will gain rapid access through the mucus gel to the underlying epithelial cells. However, in vivo the mucus gel is clearly resistant to chemical abuse by ethanol, acid and bile salts so that its continued presence will result in a protective barrier over the mucosal surface even if the underlying cells are damaged. Therefore in the short term the mucus layer will restrict mixing of the buffered contents of disrupted cells and interstitial fluid with bulk acid in the lumen, maintain a permeability barrier to pepsin, and delay further disruption of the epithelium. Were the mucus layer not there it could be anticipated that damage from these agents would be more severe. Retention of the surface gel may also provide a suitable protective environment for the rapid re-epithelialisation of the mucosa following acute damage.[44] While the mucus layer remains intact it will provide a protective barrier against pepsinolysis of the epithelial cells. However, erosion of the mucus layer by pepsin and abrasion will continue and, unless this is balanced by continued mucus secretion from viable cells, breakdown of the mucus barrier will occur.

Prostaglandins and carbachol act on the mucus barrier by approximately doubling the mean thickness of the functional adherent mucus gel and increasing the amount of soluble mucus present in the lumen.[15,16,19] A thicker mucus gel will ensure continuity of its cover, provide a more effective barrier to pepsin, a more extensive stable unstirred layer in which acid is neutralised by the increased HCO_3^- output (prostaglandin stimulated) and a barrier that is more resistant to abrasion. However in view of the thickness of the adherent mucus layer on the normal mucosa, as small as 5 μm in places, it would seem that continuity of the gel layer rather than its depth is the critical factor.

So long as a continuous mucus cover is maintained between the lumen and the epithelial cells the latter should be protected from proteolytic attack by luminal pepsin. The first line of defence against acid is considered to be afforded by the neutralisation of luminal acid within the mucus gel by metabolism dependent bicarbonate transport.[3,4,8,12] Indirect support for this comes from the fact that bicarbonate transport can be stimulated by antiulcer agents and inhibited by ulcerogens. The gastric mucus gel, by virtue of its structure and ability to act as a mixing barrier at the luminal surface, can ensure that the relatively small rate of bicarbonate transport will effectively neutralise the vast excess of luminal H^+ by preventing mixing between these two components.[10] Such an interaction would be expected to generate a pH gradient at the mucosal surface as recognised originally by Heatley.[6]

Findings of a pH gradient adjacent to gastric and duodenal epithelia[11,13,14] provide direct evidence of the role for the mucus bicarbonate barrier in protection against luminal acid. Further, findings of a neutral microenvironment at the luminal surface suggest that the site of neutralisation is extracellular. However, calculation suggests that the rate of gastric bicarbonate transport, stimulated by low luminal pH, would only provide effective protection at luminal pH values down to about 2.[3] Indeed, dissipation of the pH gradient and a fall in pH at the luminal membrane occurs when luminal pH is maintained at 1.5-1.8.[13,14] It would appear that further defence mechanisms against acid must exist at the level of the epithelial cells. Mucosal acid-base balance and blood flow would also seem crucial in overall mucosal protection in the stomach (and duodenum). Thus gastric mucosal tolerance to high luminal acid concentrations is enhanced by blood (nutrient) bicarbonate either administered exogenously or generated endogenously as a result of the "alkaline tide" resulting from the H^+ secretory process of parietal cells.[4] In both stomach and duodenum, repair of damage is augmented by the rapid proliferative rate of the epithelia. In the former tissue, ability of the mucosa to re-epithelialise following acute damage[44] is likely to provide yet a further mechanism of protection. In this respect, resilience of the surface mucus gel layer as reflected by its resistance to ulcerogenic agents may be important. Thus continued presence (and hence functionality) of the adherent mucus coat following exposure of the mucosa to damaging agents would provide an environment in which repair of the underlying epithelia can occur.[19] Overall, gastric mucosal protection appears to be a multicomponent process. In the duodenum, however, rates of bicarbonate secretion seem sufficient to account for disposal of H^+ and mucosal protection against acid by a mechanism of extracellular neutralisation within the mucus, even at the lowest pH values encountered within the duodenal bulb.[4,8] For reviews of the current concepts in mucosal protection the reader is referred to books edited by Harmon (1981)[45] and Allen et al. (1983).[46]

REFERENCES

1. F. Hollander, The two-component mucus barrier, Arch. Intern. Med. 93:107 (1954).
2. H. Florey, Mucin and the protection of the body, Proc. R. Soc. Lond. (B). 143:144 (1955).

3. A. Allen, and A. Garner, Mucus and bicarbonate secretion in the stomach and their possible role in mucosal protection, Gut 21:249 (1980).

4. G. Flemström and A. Garner, Gastroduodenal HCO_3 transport characteristics and proposed role in acidity regulation and mucosal protection, Am. J. Physiol. 242:G183 (1982).

5. H.W. Davenport, Physiological structure of the gastric mucosa, in: Handbook of Physiology, Alimentary Canal II, C.F. Code, ed., American Physiological Society, Washington D.C. (1967).

6. N.G. Heatley, Mucosubstance as a barrier to diffusion, Gastroenterology 37:313 (1959).

7. S.E. Williams, and L.A. Turnberg, Retardation of acid diffusion by pig gastric mucus: a potential role in mucosal protection, Gastroenterology 79:299 (1981).

8. A. Garner, G. Flemström, and A. Allen, Gastroduodenal alkaline and mucus secretions, Scand. J. Gastroenterology, 18 Suppl. 87:25 (1983).

9. A. Allen, The structure and function of gastrointestinal mucus, in: Physiology of the Gastrointestinal Tract, L.R. Johnson et al., eds., Raven Press, New York (1981).

10. A. Allen, The structure and function of gastrointestinal mucus, in: Basic Mechanisms of Gastrointestinal Mucosal Cell Injury and Protection, J.W. Harmon, ed., Williams and Wilkins, Baltimore and London (1981).

11. G. Flemström, and E. Kivilaakso, Demonstration of a pH gradient at the luminal surface of rat duodenum in vivo and its dependence on mucosal alkaline secretion, Gastroenterology 84:787 (1983).

12. W.D. Rees, and L.A. Turnberg, Mechanisms of gastric mucosal protection: a role for the 'mucus-bicarbonate' barrier, Clin. Sci. 62:343 (1982).

13. I.N. Ross, H.M.M. Bahari, and L.A. Turnberg, The pH gradient across mucus adherent to rat fundic mucosa in vivo and the effect of potential damaging agents, Gastroenterology 81:713 (1981).

14. K.D. Takeuchi, D. Magee, J. Critchlow, and W. Silen, Role of pH gradient of mucus in protection of gastric mucosa, Gastroenterology 84:331 (1983).

15. M. Bickel, and G.L. Kauffman, Gastric mucus gel thickness: effect of distension, 16,16-dimethyl prostaglandin E_2 and carbenoxolone, Gastroenterology 80:770 (1981).

16. S. Kerss, A. Allen, and A. Garner, A simple method for measuring thickness of the mucus gel layer adherent to rat, frog and human gastric mucosa: influence of feeding, prostaglandin, N-acetylcysteine and other agents, Clin. Sci. 63:187 (1982).

17. A. Allen, Structure of gastrointestinal mucus glycoproteins and the viscous and gel-forming properties of mucus, Br. Med. Bull. 34:28 (1978).

216

18. F. Younan, J.P. Pearson, A. Allen and C.W. Venables, Gastric mucus degradation in vivo in peptic ulcer patients and the effects of vagotomy, in: Mucus in Health and Disease II, E. Chantler, J. Elder, and M. Elstein, eds., Plenum Press, New York (1982).

19. S. McQueen, D. Hutton, A. Allen and A. Garner, Gastric and duodenal surface mucus gel thickness in rat: effects of prostaglandins and damaging agents, Am. J. Physiol. 8:388 (1983).

20. J.F. Forstner, Intestinal mucins in health and disease, Digestion 17:234 (1978).

21. L. Hoskins, Degradation of mucus glycoproteins in the gastro-intestinal tract, in: The Glycoconjugates Vol. II, H.I. Horowitz, and W. Pigman, eds., Academic Press, New York, (1978).

22. A. Bell, A. Allen, E. Morris, and D.A. Rees, Rheological studies on native pig gastric mucus gel, in: Mucus in Health and Disease II, E.L. Chantler, J. Elder, and M. Elstein, eds., Plenum Press, New York (1982).

23. F.A. Meyer, and A. Silberberg, Rheology and organisation of epithelial mucus, Birheology 17:163 (1980).

24. L.A. Sellers, A. Allen, E. Morris, and S. Ross-Murphy, Rheological studies on pig gastrointestinal mucous secret-ions, Trans. Biochem. Soc. 11:763 (1983).

25. M. Scawen, and A. Allen, The action of proteolytic enzymes on the glycoprotein from pig gastric mucus, Biochem. J. 163:363 (1977).

26. D. Snary, A. Allen, and R.H. Pain, Structural studies on gastric mucoproteins. Lowering of molecular weight after reduction with 2-mercaptoethanol, Biochem. Biophys. Res. Commun. 40:844 (1970).

27. J.R. Clamp, ed., Mucus, Br. Med. Bull. 34 (1978).

28. M.I. Horowitz, and W. Pigman, eds., Purification of glyco-proteins and criteria of purity, in: The Glycoconjugates, Vol. I., Academic Press, New York (1977).

29. D. Hutton, A. Allen, and R.H. Pain, Isolation of mucous glyco-proteins, the use of guanidinium chloride and proteolytic inhibitors, Trans. Biochem. Soc. 11:764 (1983).

30. H. Witas, B.L. Slomiany, E. Zdobska, K. Kohima, Y.H. Liou, and A. Slomiany, Lipids associated with dog gastric mucus glycoprotein, J. Applied Biochem. 5:16 (1983).

31. J.P. Pearson, R. Ward, A. Allen, and C.W. Venables, Studies on gastric and biliary mucous glycoproteins, in: Mechanisms of Mucosal Protection in the Upper Gastrointestinal Tract, A. Allen, A. Garner, G. Flemström, W. Silen and L.A. Turnberg, eds., Raven Press, New York (1983).

32. J. Schrager, and M.D.G. Oates, The isolation and partial characterization of a glycoprotein isolated from human gastric aspirates and from extracts of gastric mucosa, Biochim. Biophys. Acta 372:183 (1974).

33. D. Waldron-Edward, and S.C. Skoryna, Studies on human gastric gel mucin, Gastroenterology 59:671 (1970).

34. F. Younan, J.P. Pearson, A. Allen, and C.W. Venables, Changes in the structure of the mucus gel on the mucosal surface of the stomach in association with peptic ulcer disease, Gastroenterology 82:827 (1982).

35. E.F. Hounsell, and T. Feizi, Gastrointestinal mucins, Med. Biol. 60:227 (1982).

36. W.M. Watkins, Blood group substances, Science 152:172 (1966).

37. M.I. Filipe, Mucins in the human gastrointestinal epithelium: A review, Invest. Cell Pathol. 2:195 (1979).

38. D.M. Carlson, Chemistry and biosynthesis of mucin glycoproteins, in: Mucus in Health and Disease, M. Elstein and D.V. Parke, eds., Plenum Press, New York (1977).

39. A.S.R. Donald, The products of pronase digestion of purified blood group-specific glycoproteins, Biochim. Biophys. Acta 317:420 (1973).

40. M. Mantle, D. Mantle, and A. Allen, Polymeric structure of pig small intestinal mucus glycoprotein, Biochem. J. 125:277 (1981).

41. T. Marshall, and A. Allen, Isolation and characterisation of the high molecular weight glycoproteins from pig colonic mucus, Biochem. J. 173:569 (1978).

42. P.E.F. Fahim, G.G. Forstner, and J.F. Forstner, Heterogeneity of rat goblet cell mucin before and after reduction, Biochem. J. 209:117 (1983).

43. A. Allen, D. Hutton, S. McQueen, and A. Garner, Dimensions of gastroduodenal surface pH gradients exceed those of adherent mucus gel layers, Gastroenterology 85:463 (1983).

44. K. Svanes, S. Ito, K. Takeuchi, and W. Silen, Restitution of the surface epithelium of the in vitro frog gastric mucosa after damage with hyperosmolar sodium chloride morphologic and physiologic characteristics, Gastroenterology 82:1409 (1982).

45. J.W. Harmon, ed., Basic Mechanisms of Gastrointestinal Mucosal Cell Injury and Protection, Williams and Wilkins, Baltimore, (1982).

46. A. Allen, A. Garner, G. Flemström, W. Silen, and L.A. Turnberg, eds., Mechanisms of Mucosal Protection in the Upper Gastrointestinal Tract, Raven Press, New York (1983).

47. M. Mantle, and A. Allen, Isolation and characterisation of native glycoprotein from pig small intestine. Polymeric structure of pig small intestinal mucus glycoprotein, Biochem. J. 195:267 (1981).

INTESTINAL ABSORPTION AND SECRETION

OF FLUID AND ELECTROLYTES

Henry J. Binder

Department of Interal Medicine
Yale University School of Medicine
New Haven, Conn. 06510
U.S.A.

Knowledge of the mechanisms that regulate small and large intestinal fluid and electrolyte movement has greatly expanded during the past decade. Detailed examination of individual transport processes present in the intestinal epithelia has provided insight into the control of both absorptive and secretory events. Studies of man have emphasized that the fluid load to the intestine is considerably greater than that previously appreciated and that diarrhea is almost always secondary to changes in fluid and electrolyte movement. Finally, the heterogeneity of various segments of the intestine has become increasingly evident and must be appreciated in the development of models to explain the overall control of fluid and electrolyte movement in health and disease.

There are significant differences in the function of the small and large intestine[1] (Table 1). The fluid load to the human small intestine is considerably greater than dietary intake in that approximately 8 liters of fluid enter the small intestine daily. The small intestine absorbs approximately 75% of this load as ileocecal flow is approximately 2 liters per day. Although the colon absorbs much less fluid than the small intestine, the efficiency of colonic fluid absorption is about 90%. Nutrient (i.e. glucose and amino acids) stimulated fluid absorption occurs in the small intestine but not in the colon. In contrast, sodium absorption is aldosterone-sensitive in the colon but not in the more proximal intestine. Large differences in mucosal permeability also exist between proximal and distal intestine; the jejunum has greater mucosal permeability than the colon. These differences are manifest by a lower potential difference (PD), a higher sodium equili-

Table 1: Comparision of Small Intestine and Colonic Function

	Small Intestine	Colon
Active Nutrient Absorption	present	absent
Active Na Absorption		
Stimulated by Aldosterone	no	yes
Inhibited by Amiloride	no	yes
Stimulated by Glucose	yes	no
Active Potassium Transport	absent	present
Mucosal Permeability		
Resting Potential Difference	-3 to -8mV	-15 to -25mV
Na Equilibrium Concentration	133 to 75 mEq/L	∼30 mEq/L
Pore Size	7Å to 3Å	2.3Å
Passive NaCl Movement	modest	minimal
Fluid Load per day	∼8L	∼2L
Efficiency of Fluid Absorption	∼75%	∼90%

brium concentration and greater rates of passive sodium-chloride absorption in the jejunum than in the colon.

Since water movement is secondary to solute transfer, it will be important to review the mechanism of active intestinal sodium, chloride and potassium transport as the basis for understanding changes in fluid movement. Several transport processes are responsible for sodium absorption (Table 2). Na-K-ATPase or the so-called sodium pump which is located at the basolateral membrane is central to most, though not all, active intestinal transport processes. Sodium extrusion by the sodium pump across the basolateral membrane into the intercellular space results in a reduced intracellular sodium concentration and a negative intracellular PD. As a result, the energy for sodium entry into the intestinal epithelial cell across the apical membrane is derived from the existing electrochemical concentration gradient. Metabolic energy is required for sodium extrusion (in order to maintain the electrochemical concentration gradient), not for sodium entry. This type of sodium transport is often referred to as electrogenic since it

Table 2: Mechanisms of Intestinal Sodium Absorption

1. Electrogenic Na Absorption

2. Neutral NaCl Absorption

    a) coupled cotransport
    b) dual ion exchanges (Na/H and Cl/HCO₃)

3. Glucose-stimulated Na absorption

4. Solvent drag

is associated with the development of a transepithelial potential difference.

Glucose (and other actively transported monosaccharides and amino acids) increase sodium absorption and PD. Glucose uptake across the apical membrane is also driven by the existing sodium gradient (see above). Sodium dependent nutrient absorption is dependent upon basolateral Na-K-ATPase and represents an example of so-called secondary active transport[2]. Ouabain inhibits glucose uptake by virtue of its inhibition of Na-K-ATPase with the resulting obliteration of the sodium gradient rather than a direct effect on sodium uptake.

In addition to electrogenic sodium absorption and glucose-stimulated sodium absorption, there is also chloride dependent sodium absorption or neutral sodium-chloride absorption (Figure 1). In this type of transport removal of sodium inhibits chloride absorption and lack of chloride impairs sodium absorption. This linkage of sodium and chloride absorption may be as a result of 1) coupling via the development of an electrical potential; 2) coupling via a common apical membrane transport process (i.e. cotransport); or 3) coupling via intracellular pH of dual ion exchanges.

The mechanism of sodium chloride cotransport is very similar to glucose-stimulated absorption in that chloride uptake across the apical membrane is also linked to the sodium gradient[3]. Initial studies suggested that neutral sodium chloride absorption primarily represented coupled sodium chloride cotransport. During the past few years it has become increasingly likely that neutral sodium chloride absorption may in fact represent (at least in many situations) the close coupling of dual ion exchange[4] (Na/H and Cl/HCO₃ or Cl/OH) (Figure 1). Regardless of the specific cellular mechanism responsible for neutral sodium chloride absorption, cyclic AMP, increased intracellular calcium (and possible cyclic GMP) inhibit neutral NaCl absorption. Studies of the distal tubule have identified a Na-K-Cl cotransport process[5], and it is

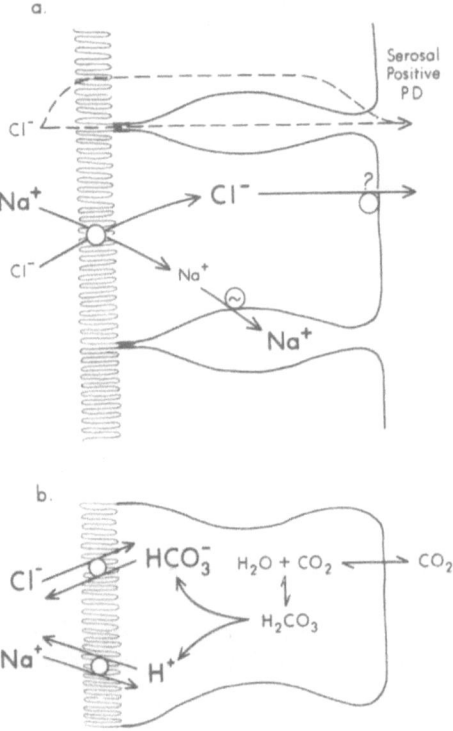

Fig. 1. Three modes of intestinal Cl absorption. Neutral NaCl absorption may represent either coupled NaCl cotransport in
which Cl movement across the apical membrane is closely
linked to Na entry or dual ion exchanges (Na/H and
Cl/HCO₃). It is likely that either process or both are
present in intestinal epithelia. Cl absorption may also
be coupled to Na absorption via electrical potential which
is most likely generated by electrogenic Na absorption.

likely that a similar transport mechanism may also exist in the
mammalian intestine.

Studies in the human jejunum support the concept that a significant fraction of sodium absorption in the proximal small intestine is secondary to solvent drag[6]. That is sodium absorption is
augmented by volume flow so that glucose stimulation of sodium absorption may be secondary to changes in water movement and not to

glucose-sodium coupled transport. Solvent drag may account for a significant component of glucose stimulated sodium absorption in the jejunum but not in the ileum or colon.

There are also several intestinal chloride transport processes, and both active and passive chloride absorptive mechanisms have been identified (Figure 1 and Table 3). <u>Potential-dependent chloride absorption</u> represents its linkage to sodium absorption by the generation of the PD by sodium movement. It is not known whether potential-dependent chloride absorption occurs via a transcellular or a paracellular route. We have already discussed <u>neutral sodium chloride absorption</u> which may represent either coupled sodium chloride cotransport or dual ion exchanges[4,5]. In addition, HCO_3-dependent Cl absorption is present in the distal intestine not always associated with Na/H exchange. It is not surprising that Cl/HCO_3 exchange is often inhibited by acetazolamide, an inhibitor of carbonic anhydrase.

Central to an understanding of the development of diarrhea and intestinal electrolyte secretion is the mechanism of <u>active chloride secretion</u>[7]. It has frequently been suggested that absorptive processes are located in villous cells and secretory processes in the crypt. Although this formulation may well be correct and represents an extremely attractive hypothesis, direct confirmation of this organizational arrangement is at present lacking. An attractive model to explain active chloride secretion is presented in Figure 2. It must be emphasized that as attractive a model as this formulation is, experiments that directly establish several of its salient features are still required to provide unequivocal confirmation of this proposal. As outlined, chloride entry into the cell across the basolateral membrane is coupled to sodium movement, which in turn is driven by an existing sodium gradient maintained by sodium extrusion by the basolateral sodium pump. As a result, the intracellular chloride concentration is greater than that predicted by the observed electrochemical concentration gradients. Normally, little chloride is secreted across the apical membrane since the apical membrane has limited chloride

Table 3: Mechanisms of Intestinal Chloride Absorption

1.   Potential-dependent Cl absorption

2.   Na-dependent Cl absorption (or neutral NaCl absorption)

        a)   Dual ion exchanges
        b)   Coupled NaCl cotransport

3. HCO_3-dependent Cl absorption

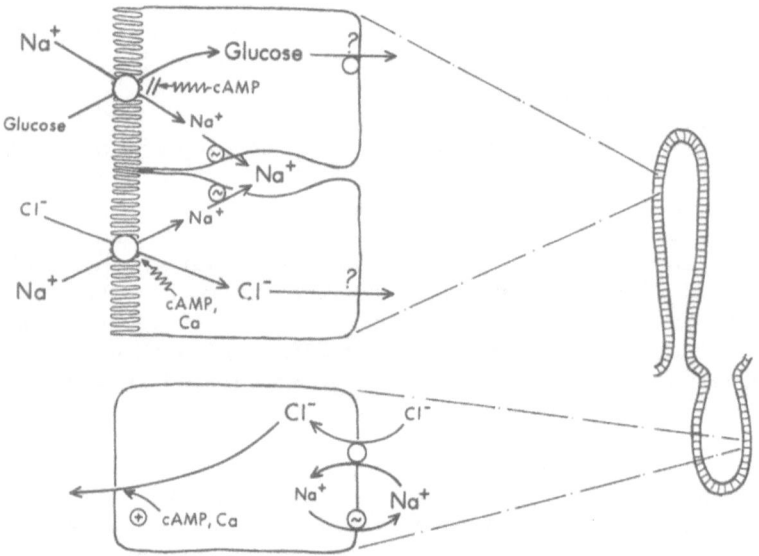

Fig. 2.   Models of sodium and chloride absorption. An attractive
           hypothesis is that absorptive processes are located in
           villous cells and secretory ones in crypt cells. Cyclic
           AMP and increased cytosolic calcium inhibit neutral NaCl
           absorption and stimulates active Cl secretion but do not
           alter glucose-stimulated Na absorption.

permeability. This model proposes that either increases in intracellular calcium or increased mucosal cyclic AMP produces active
chloride secretion by increasing apical membrane chloride conductance. Support for this attractive hypothesis[7] is based on the
observations that cyclic AMP-mediated secretion is inhibited by
1) the removal of serosal sodium, 2) the addition of serosal
furosemide (which usually inhibits sodium chloride coupled transport), 3) the addition of serosal ouabain or 4) the removal of
serosal potassium (the latter two experimental maneuvers presumably
act by inhibiting Na-K-ATPase).

The mechanism by which cyclic AMP induces chloride secretion
is also not known, but it has been proposed that cyclic AMP raises
intracellular calcium by mobilizing intracellular calcium stores.
As a result, the common mediator for the induction of active
chloride secretion is increased intracellular calcium activity. A
reasonable postulate is that increased intracellular calcium may
increase apical chloride conductance via calmodulin and/or protein
phosphorylation (Figure 3).

It has been suggested that there are three (or four) intracellular mediators of active anion secretion. In addition to
cyclic AMP and increased intracellular calcium, cyclic GMP has also
been incriminated[8]. The mechanism by which cyclic GMP alters intestine transport processes is largely unknown. There is considerable evidence that prostaglandins are also secretagogues.
Prostaglandins stimulate adenylate cyclase and thus produce an increase in mucosal AMP. However, recent studies indicate that
prostaglandins may be synthesized intracellularly[9]; the exact
mechanism by which newly synthesized intracellular prostaglandins
modulate secretion requires clarification.

Although cyclic AMP is frequently discussed as a secretagogue,
it is important to recognize that cyclic AMP (and changes in intracellular calcium) have two important effects on intestinal electrolyte transport: in addition to stimulating active chloride secretion, cyclic AMP also inhibits neutral sodium chloride absorption. Although inhibition of sodium chloride absorption contributes to fluid secretion, it must be emphasized that cyclic AMP
alters absorptive processes in addition to stimulating secretory
events.

There has been considerable uncertainty regarding intestinal
potassium transport. With regard to small intestinal potassium
movement, there is general agreement that active potassium transport does not occur and that potassium movement in the small intestine is determined by the existing electrochemical concentration
gradients.

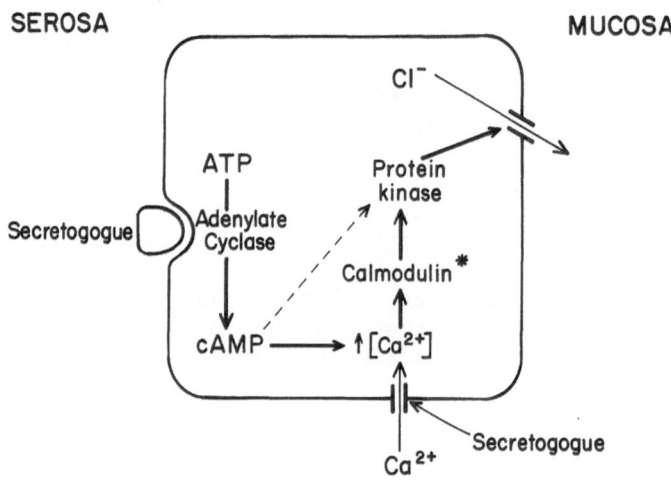

Fig. 3.   Speculative model linking both cyclic SMP and calcium-
dependent secretagogues (e.g. serotonin, cholinergic
agonists) to active Cl secretion.

Net potassium secretion occurs in the *in vivo* colon. Since the colon manifests a significant lumen negative PD (approximately 15 to 25 mV), there has been uncertainty until recently whether this basal PD is responsible for all of observed net potassium secretion. Recent studies clearly indicate that active potassium secretion is also present in the normal colon in most species and both cyclic AMP and aldosterone stimulate active potassium secretion[10]. Further, it has also been recently established that an active potassium absorptive process is also present which, if not appreciated, may obscure the demonstration of active potassium secretion[11]. In any event, the presence of oppositely-directed active potassium transport in the colon indicates that the large intestine participates in the modulation of overall potassium balance.

REFERENCES

1. H.J. Binder, Absorption and secretion of water and electrolytes by small and large intestine, in: "Gastrointestinal Diseases", M.H. Sleisenger and J.S. Fordtran, eds., W.B. Saunders Co., Philadelphia, (1983).

2. P.S. Aronson, Identifying secondary active solute transport in epithelia, Am. J. Physiol., 9: F1 (1981).

3. H.N. Nellans, R.A. Frizzell, and S.G. Schultz, Brush-border processes and transepithelial Na and Cl transport by rabbit ileum, Am. J. Physiol., 226: 1131 (1974).

4. C.M. Liedtke and U. Hopfer, Mechanism of Cl-translocation across small intestinal brush-border membrane. I. Absence of Na^+-Cl^-cotransport, Am. J. Physiol., 242: G263 (1982).

5. R.F. Gregor and E. Schlatter, Coupled transport of 2 Cl^-, 1 Na^+ and 1 K^+ at the luminal membrane of the rabbit cortical thick ascending limb of Henle's loop (CTAL), Proc. Am. Soc. Nephrol., 14: 147 (1981).

6. J.S. Fordtran, Stimulation of active and passive sodium absorption by sugars in the human jejunum, J. Clin. Invest., 55: 728 (1975).

7. K. Heintze, C.P. Stewart, and R.A. Frizzell, Sodium-dependent chloride secretion across rabbit descending colon, Am. J. Physiol., 244: G357 (1983).

8. S. Guandalini, M.C. Rao, P.L. Smith, and M. Field, cGMP modulation of ileal ion transport: in vitro effects of Escherichia coli heat-stable enterotoxin, Am. J. Physiol., 243: G36 (1982).

9. M.A. Balaa and D.W. Powell, Prostaglandin synthesis by isolated rabbit small intestinal enterocytes, <u>Gastroenterology</u>, 84: 1098 Abstract (1983).

10. E.S. Foster, G.I. Sandle, J.P. Hayslett, and H.J. Binder, Cyclic AMP stimulates active potassium secretion in the rat colon, <u>Gastroenterology</u>, 84: 324 (1983).

11. E.S. Foster, J.P. Hayslett, and H.J. Binder, Regulation of active potassium absorption and secretion in rat distal colon, <u>Gastroenterology</u>, 84: 1157 Abstract (1983).

GALLBLADDER FLUID TRANSPORT

John R. Wood and Joar Svanvik

Gastroenterology Unit, Glaxo Pharmaceuticals Ltd
Greenford, Middlesex, England and Department of
Surgery 1, University of Goteborg, Goteborg, Sweden

INTRODUCTION

One of the principal physiological functions of the
gallbladder is to store bile during interdigestive periods. By
virtue of its ability to concentrate bile, it can process and
store volumes of hepatic bile which considerably exceed its own
relatively small capacity. This transformation of 'hepatic bile'
into 'gallbladder bile' results from active transepithelial
transport of electrolytes with the associated passive movement of
water. The present review examines some aspects of the transport
processes involved and their physiological control.

PHYSIOLOGICAL CHANGES IN TRANSPORT

Classical physiology views the gallbladder mucosa as
continuously absorbing water. Several studies, however, suggest
that gallbladder transport is subject to physiological regulation. In 1932 Johnston and coworkers[1] found that the hourly
absorption of water by dog gallbladder was three times greater
during the day than at night during sleep. In a recent study [2] the
influence of fasting and feeding on the concentrating function of
the gallbladder was studied in conscious monkeys. During the day
fasting animals had a net hourly absorption rate corresponding to
one third of the fasting gallbladder volume. Feeding resulted in
a reversal of the direction of gallbladder transport from a net
absorption to a net secretion into the gallbladder
lumen. This study also confirmed the finding that compared with
the awake fasting state net water absorption from the gallbladder
was reduced at night during sleep.

TRANSPORT MECHANISMS

Transport of Sodium and Chloride

Sodium enters gallbladder epithelial cells from bile across the luminal membrane down an electrochemical gradient maintained by its extrusion across the basolateral membrane by a sodium pump. Ion replacement studies in rabbit gall bladder have revealed that active Na absorption does not occur when luminal Cl is replaced by a variety of non-transported cations.[3] The passive permeability of the luminal cell membrane to Na has been found to be too low to account for the observed transepithelial active sodium flux by diffusional Na entry.[4] On the basis of influx studies in rabbit gallbladder[5] non-diffusional Na entry has been postulated to occur by a one to one electrically neutral coupled entry mechanism for Na and C1. Such a carrier mediated mechanism would facilitate charge neutralisation with C1 entry against an electrochemical gradient.[6]

Na exit against its electrochemical gradient is facilitated by a Na, K, ATPase whose activity correlates directly with the rate of fluid transport[7]. The mechanism of the sodium extrusion at the basolateral membrane is uncertain and both electrogenic (rheogenic)[8,9] and non-electrogenic[10,11] mechanisms have been proposed.

Fluid Absorption

The gallbladder mucosa like numerous other epithelia is able to perform 'isotonic' fluid transport. That is, it can transport solute and water between equiosmolar bathing media so as to maintain equal tonicities of the bulk media.[12] Movement of water is passive and secondary to active solute movement resulting from osmotic equilibration of transported solute within the epithelium. The mechanism and site of the coupling of solute and water fluxes by this and other epithelia is unsolved and remains a central problem of current epithelial research.

In 1967 Diamond and Bossert[13] proposed the standing gradient osmotic flow theory to explain the intraepithelial osmotic coupling. According to this, solute is pumped into the long narrow spaces between adjacent epithelial cells. This creates a hypertonic compartment into which cellular water is drawn by osmosis resulting in flow towards the serosal end of the lateral intracellular space and a standing osmotic gradient within the space under steady state conditions.

The rate of NaCl and fluid absorption is enhanced by bicarbonate[14] Recent studies suggest that HCO_3 is required for the maintenance of intracellular H which in turn maintains a Na/H exchange. This mechanism is compatible with the presence of a double ion exchange mediating parallel counter-transport of Na-H and Cl-HCO$_3$ in the apical membrane.[15,16] In addition to their transcellular movement ions also traverse the gall bladder epithelium by a paracellular pathway, a route accounting for most of the passive ion permeation.

Fluid Secretion

Gallbladder secretion was reported as early as 1887 in two patients who had undergone cholecystotomy.[17] The secretion was clear to slightly opalescent, almost colourless, slightly alkaline and contained a high proportion of mucin. It was not, however, until 1969 that further evidence for water and electrolyte secretion by the gall bladder was presented. Instillation of a crude vibrio cholerae extract into the dog gall bladder reversed the direction of transport from a net absorption to a net secretion of clear, viscid alkaline fluid rich in bicarbonate.[18] Purified cholera toxin can inhibit fluid absorption by the isolated guinea pig gall bladder[19] reversing it to a net secretion. Prostaglandins,[20,21] prostacyclin,[22] and gastro-intestinal hormones[22-25] are also secretagogues in the guinea pig gall bladder in vitro. Secretion has been reported in vivo in the anaesthetised cat after intravenous infusions of gastrointestinal hormones[26,27] and local intra-arterial infusion of prostaglandin E$_2$.[28] Gallbladder secretion after feeding has been observed in the conscious monkey.[2]

The secretion of water and electrolyte by the gallbladder mucosa is dependent on active transport process[29]. The ionic events occurring during secretion have been studied only in the guinea pig gallbladder. Here under non-secretory control conditions bicarbonate is secreted into the gallbladder lumen in exchange for chloride.[14] This transport continues and is enhanced during prostaglandin-induced secretion where it is associated with a considerable reduction in chloride absorption and a reversal of sodium and potassium absorption to a net secretion. Secretion is abolished by omission of bicarbonate from the bathing solution and is independent of the external calcium concentration. These findings suggest that bicarbonate is secreted electrogenically into the gallbladder lumen.[30]

HUMORAL AND NEURAL REGULATION OF TRANSPORT

Various endocrine and neurocrine factors affect the rate of gall- bladder NaCl and water transport both in vivo and in vitro. Some of these may regulate gallbladder water and electrolyte

transfer under physiological conditions by modification of NaCl
Na extrusion, and/or junctional permeability. Cyclic AMP has
been proposed as a second messenger for the effects of several
such mediators and has been found in rabbit[15] and Necturus
bladder[31] to inhibit the NaCl coupled influx, the rate limiting
step for transepithelial Na transport. In addition to effects on
luminal membrane function cAMP may also regulate transport by
influencing tight junction permeability.[32]

Gastrointestinal Peptides

Experiments using the isolated guinea pig gallbladder have
shown that natural porcine secretin, synthetic secretin, PHI
(peptide histidine isoleucine) and natural porcine VIP (Vasoactive intestinal polypeptide) are potent concentration-depend-
ent inhibitors of fluid absorption and that each can reverse the
direction of transport from net absorption to net secretion.[23-25]

Studies in vivo in the anaesthetised cat have provided similar
results. VIP infused intravenously reversibly inhibited gallbladder water and electrolyte transport and reversed its direction
to a net secretion.[26] Similar findings were reported with natural
porcine secretin though the secretory effect was less consistent.
Natural porcine cholecystokinin was without effect on transport.[27]

VIP and secretin have been found to increase cAMP production
by isolated epithelial cells of human and guinea pig gallbladder.[33] VIP was a potent stimulant of cAMP production by human
gallbladder cells with half maximal and maximal stimulation at 0.2
and 10 nM respectively. Secretin was also a potent stimulant of
cAMP formation by guinea pig but not human gallbladder. The
effects of VIP and secretin on fluid transport by human
gallbladder have yet to be reported. VIP-ergic nerves are present
in the gallbladder wall of several species[34] and may release VIP to
act on receptors on the serosal surface of gallbladder epithelial
cells and thereby modify the direction and rate of transmucosal
fluid transport. It seems unlikely that other members of the
secretin family of peptides (ie GIP and glucagon) modify gallbladder fluid transport under physiological conditions. A variety
of other gastrointestinal peptides have been studied in the
isolated guinea pig gallbladder. Neurotensin, bombesin, motilin,
cholecystokinin, caerulein, and somatostatin were all without
effect on absorption.[35]

The gallbladder mucosa is subject to a complex series of neural
and endocrine-paracrine regulatory influences during digestion.
Of the above regulatory peptides whose effects have been studied
only VIP and secretin are able to modify gallbladder fluid

transport at concentrations which may be considered physiological. Peptides without effect on transport in vitro when administered alone may, however, act to potentiate or inhibit the effects of these candidate peptides and other as yet unrecognised regulatory factors. Thus, for example, though somatostatin had no effect on basal transport it completely reversed the inhibitory effect on absorption of VIP, secretin[36] intraduodenal acid and activation of noncholinergic vagal neurones.[37]

Influence of the Autonomic Nervous System

Adrenergic, cholinergic and peptidergic nerve fibres have been shown in gallbladder. Nerve fibres with noradrenergic immuno-fluorescence have been visualised in the gallbladder wall using histological techniques.[38] Cholinergic nerve fibres have also been shown in the gallbladder wall by histological methods. The possible role of nerve fibres immunoreactive to VIP has already been considered.

The adrenergic nerve supply to the gallbladder travels in the splanchnic nerves but as adrenergic fibres have also been visual-ised in the vagus nerve[39] a part of the adrenergic nerve supply may take this route. Cholinergic fibres are received from the vagus nerves.[40] Peptidergic fibres have been found in the vagus.

Noradrenaline increased net water absorption by the everted human gallbladder,[47] the gallbladder of the anaesthetised cat,[42] but not by the isolated guinea pig gallbladder.[43] Acetylcholine had no effect on water transport by the guinea pig gallbladder[43] in vitro or the cat gallbladder[44] in vivo in doses causing gall-bladder contraction. Of other possible neurotransmitters gastrin has been reported to reduce net water absorption by the dog gallbladder in vitro[45] and VIP has potent effects considered above.

It has been recently found that electrical stimulation of the splanchnic nerves increases the rate of water absorption by the gallbladder of the anaesthetised cat, an effect which can be abolished by alpha-adrenergic receptor blockade. The precise site of action of the sympathetic nerves on net water transport by the gallbladder is unknown. Apart from a possible direct effect on mucosal cells, sympathetic nerves may act on local ganglia to inhibit release of a neurotransmitter which inhibits water ab-sorption. A possible neuro-transmitter set free by local reflexes is VIP.

In a recent study[44] electrical stimulation of the cervical vagus nerves in the cat failed to influence the rate of fluid transport in the gallbladder measured by a pefusion technique.

Using the same technique vagal stimulation significantly reduced the net water absorption in atropinised animals. Electrical stimulation of the vagus nerves can influence the gallbladder directly. A complex of the direct effects of the nerve fibres might, however, be masked by secondary effects because of released gastrointestinal peptides and other blood borne factors. Evidently there seems to be a non-cholinergic vagal mechanism capable of reducing net water absorption by the gallbladder.

REFERENCES

1. C. G. Johnston, I. S. Ravdin, J. H. Austin, and J. L. Morrison, Studies of gallbladder function. V. The absorption of calcium from the bile-free gallbladder, Am. J. Physiol., 99:648 (1932).

2. J. Svanvik, B. Allen, C. Pellegrini, R. Bernhoft, and L. Way, Net water transport in the gallbladder of the conscious monkey, Gastroenterology, 77:A42 (1979).

3. J. M. Diamond, Transport mechanisms in the gallbladder, in: "Handbook of physiology. The alimentary canal", C. F. Code, and W. Herder, eds., Williams and Wilkins, Baltimore (1968).

4. J. Graf, and G. Giebisch, Intracellular sodium activity and sodium transport in Necturus gallbladder epithelium, J. Membr. Biol., 47:327 (1979).

5. R. A. Frizzell, M. C. Dugas, and S. G. Schultz, Sodium chloride transport by rabbit gallbladder. Direct evidence for a coupled NaCI influx process, J. Gen. Physiol., 65:769 (1975).

6. M. E. Duffey, K. Turnheim, R. A. Frizzell, and S. G. Schultz, Intracellular chloride activities in rabbit gallbladder : direct evidence for the role of sodium-gradient in energising "uphill" chloride transport, J. Membr. Biol., 42:229 (1978).

7. Os C. H. Van, and J. F. G. Slegers, Correlation between (Na^+-K^+) activated ATPase activities and the rate of isotonic fluid transport of gallbladder epithelium, Biochim Biophys. Acta., 241:89 (1971).

8. R. C. Rose, and D. L. Nahrwold, Electrolyte transport in Necturus gallbladder : the role of rheogenic Na transport, Am. J. Physiol., 238:6358 (1980).

9. R. C. Rose, Electrolyte absorption by gallbladder. Is the pump rheogenic? in: "Macknight," J. P. Leader, ed., Raven Press, New York (1981).

10. L. Reuss, Mechanisms of sodium and chloride transport by gallbladder epithelium, Fed. Proc., 38:2733 (1979).

11. L. Reuss, Mechanisms of the mucosa-negative transepithelial potential produced by amphotericin B in gallbladder epithelium, Fed. Proc., 40:2206 (1981).

12. J. M. Diamond, Transport of salt and water in rabbit and guinea pig gallbladder, J. Gen. Physiol., 48:1 (1964).

13. J. M. Diamond, and W. H. Bossert, Standing-gradient osmotic flow. A mechanism for coupling of water and solute transport in epithelia, J. Gen. Physiol., 50:2061 (1967).

14. K. Heintze, K. U. Petersen, P. Olles, S. H. Saverymuttu, and J. R. Wood, Effects of bicarbonate on fluid and electrolyte transport by the guinea pig gallbladder : a bicarbonate-chloride exchange, J. Membr. Biol., 45:43 (1979).

15. K. Heintze, K. U. Petersen, and J. R. Wood, Effects of bicarbonate on fluid and electrolyte transport by guinea pig and rabbit gallbladder : stimulation of absorption, J. Membr. Biol., 62:175 (1981).

16. K. U. Peterson, J. R. Wood, S. G. Schultze, and K. Heintze, Stimulation of gallbladder fluid and electrolyte absorption by butyrate, J. Membr. Biol., 62:183 (1981).

17. D. B. Burch, and H. Spong, The secretion of the gallbladder, J. Physiol., 8:378 (1887).

18. D. E. Schafer, D. M. Nicoloff, D. F. Gleason, and T. J. Carlson, Gallbladder secretion induced by an enterotoxin-like fraction fo crude V.Cholerae supernatant, Gastroenterology, 56:1195 (1969).

19. S. H. Saverymuttu, and J. R. Wood, Inhibitory effect of cholera toxin on gallbladder fluid absorption and its reversal by 2,4,6-triaminopyrimidine, J. Physiol., 266:68 (1977).

20. K. Heintze, W. Leinesser, K. U. Petersen, and Heidenreich, Triphasic effect of prostaglandins E1,E2,F2 on the fluid transport of isolated gallbladder of guinea pigs, Prostaglandins, 9:309 (1975).

21. S. H. Saverymuttu, J. R. Wood, and I. K. M. Morton, Animal maturity influences prostaglandin effects on gallbladder fluid transport and smooth muscle, Eur. J. Pharmacol., 60:7 (1979).

22. A. B. Ashbrooke, and J. R. Wood, Inhibition of gallbladder fluid absorption by prostacyclin, J. Physiol., 318:66P (1981).

23. I. K. M. Morton, S. J. Phillips, S. H. Saverymuttu, and J. R. Wood, Secretion and vasoactive intestinal peptide inhibit fluid absorption and induce secretion in the isolated gallbladder of the guinea pig, J. Physiol., 266:65 (1977).

24. J. R. Wood, L. J. Brennan, and J. M. Hormbrey, Comparison of the effects of VIP, secretin, GIP and glucagon on gall-bladder function, Regulatory Peptides, 3:169 (1982).

25. L. J. Brennan, T. A. McLoughlin, V. Mutt, K. Tatemoto, and J. R. Wood, Effects of PHI, a newly isolated peptide, on gallbladder function in the guinea pig, J. Physiol., 329:71P (1982).

26. R. Jansson, G. Steen, and J. Svanvik, Effects of intravenous vasoactive intestinal peptide (VIP) on gallbladder function in the cat, Gastroenterology, 75:47 (1979).

27. R. Jansson, and J. Svanvik, Effects of intravenous secretin and cholecystokinin on gallbladder net water absorption and motility in the cat, Gastroenterology, 72:639 (1977).

28. E. Thornell, J. Svanvik, and J. R. Wood, Effects of intraarterial prostaglandin E_2 on gallbladder fluid transport, motility and hepatic bile flow in the cat, Scand. J. Gastroenterol., 16:1083 (1981).

29. K. Heintze, R. Goetz, H. Koerlings, and J. R. Wood, Characterisation of the prostaglandin induced secretion in the isolated gallbladder of guinea pig, Naunyn Schmiedebergs Arch Pharmacol., 293:Suppl R34 (1976).

30. C. P. Stewart, R. Goetz, and K. Heintze, Electrogenic HCO_3 secretion by guinea pig gallbladder, in: "Electrolyte and water transport across gastrointestinal epithelia, " R.M. Case, A. Garner, and L.A. Turnberg, eds., Raven Press, New York (1982).

31. A. Diez de los Rios, N. E. DeRose, and W. Mc. D. Armstrong, Cyclic AMP and intracellular ionic activitie in Necturus gallbladder, J. Membr. Biol., 63:25 (1981).

32. M. E. Duffey, B. Hainau, S. Ho, and C. J. Bentzel, Regulation of epithelial tight junction permeability by cAMP, Nature, 294:451 (1981).

33. C. Dupont, J. P. Broyart, Y. Broer, B. Chenut, M. Laburthe and G. Rosselin, Importance of the vasoactive intestinal peptide receptor in the stimulation of cyclic adenosine 3'.5'-monophosphate in gallbladder epithelial cells of man. Comparison with the guinea pig, J. Clin. Invest., 67:742 (1981).

34. F. Sundler, J. Alumets, R. Hakansson, S. Ingemansson, J. Fahrenkrug, and O. Schaffalitzky de Muckadell, VIP innervation of the gallbladder, Gastroenterology, 72:1375 (1977).

35. J. R. Wood, L. J. Brennan, J. M. Hormbrey, and T. A. McLoughlin, Effects of regulatory peptides on gallbladder function, Scand, J. Gastroenterol., 17:suppl 78:528 (1982).

36. J. R. Wood , T. A. McLoughlin, and L. J. Brennan, VIP and secretin-induced inhibition of gallbladder fluid absorption. Reversal by somatostatin, Gastroenterology, 82:1213 (1982).

37. S. Bjork, J. Svanvik, Blocking effects of somatostatin on gallbladder response to intraduodenal acid and vagus nerve stimulation in the cat, Gastroenterology, 89:1108 (1983).

38. K. Kyosola, and Penttila, Adrenergic innervation of the human gallbladder, Histochemistry, 54:209 (1977).

39. J. M. Lundberg, H. Ahlman, A. Dahlstrom et al., Catecholamine containing nerve fibres in the human abdominal vagus, Gastroenterology, 70:516 (1976).

40. W. F. Alexander, The innervation of the biliary system, J. Comp. Neurol., 72:357 (1940).

41. G. R. Onstad, L. J. Schoenfield, and J. A. Higgin, Fluid transfer in the everted human gallbladder, J. Clin. Invest., 46:606 (1969).

42. S. Bjorck, R. Jansson, and J. Svanvik, The adrenergic influence on concentrating function in the feline gallbladder, Gut, 23:1019 (1983).

43. L. J. Brennan, J. M. Hormbrey, and J. R. Wood, Effects of methionine enkephalin, substance P and other chemical messengers on gallbladder fluid transport, J. Physiol. 319:104 (1981).

44. S. Bjorck, R. Jansson, and J. Svanvik, The influence of electrical vagal stimulation and acetylcholine on the function of the feline gallbladder, Scand. J. Gastroenterol. 18:129 (1983).

45. G. W. Peskin, G. M. G. DaCruz, and L. Kaplan, Hormonal regulation of bile fluid and electrolyte composition, Surg. Forum, 19:346 (1968).

RELATIONSHIPS AMONG INTESTINAL MOTILITY, TRANSIT AND ABSORPTION

Sidney F. Phillips

Director, Gastroenterology Unit, Mayo Clinic
Professor of Medicine, Mayo Medical School
Rochester, MN 55905, U.S.A.

1. INTRODUCTION

That relationships exist among motor events, transit of chyme and absorption in the intestine has an intuitive appeal. However, although the subject has been addressed experimentally, the development of adequate methodological approaches has not been easy. These difficulties are due, in part, to the interconnected or even parallel controls of absorptive and motor functions. Common modulating factors which need to be considered include integration of motility, transit and absorption by the central and enteric nervous systems, by local or systemic regulatory peptides, as well as by local physical conditions within the gut. Thus, neural stimuli, local chemo-regulators and pharmacologically active agents may evoke simultaneously a response from intestinal smooth muscle, from mucosal tissues and from the abdominal vasculature[1]. At another level of control, there appear to exist chronobiological rhythms which influence motor function, secretion and absorption together. It has even been proposed that these apparently diverse functions of the gut constitute a single effector system--a concept first expounded by Boldyreff early in the century[2,3]. Moreover, impaired absorption is able to influence per se the motor properties of the bowel. Malabsorption can lead to the accumulation of chemical stimuli within the lumen (e.g. fat, bile acids) which affect both absorption and motility[4,5], and distention of the bowel by unabsorbed fluid can alter motor patterns. These difficulties are compounded by our still rudimentary understanding of those motor events which facilitate the other fundamental functions of the bowel. Any or all of the motor events which promote intraluminal mixing, modify propulsion along the bowel, control the movement of villi, or which aid lymphatic or venous

drainage could constitute key events in absorption. At this time,
the subject can only be approached piece-meal, from clinical
observations of pathophysiological states and from fragmentary
experimental observations. However, the general argument can be
made that, when integrated transit of chyme is disturbed,
absorptive mechanisms are often impaired. This review will then
examine a number of phenomena, but no conclusions are possible
currently. More specific experimental approaches must be applied
if we wish to elucidate better these associations.

2. MOTILITY AND TRANSIT

Contractions of muscle in the tunica muscularis constitute the
most dramatic motor events in the bowel. The most obvious
relationships among contractile events, transit and absorption
should be the ways in which contractions of the muscularis move
chyme along the gut. Although the processes which link fluid
mechanics, gastrointestinal flow, and movements of the bowel wall
(as produced by muscular contractions) appeal as being of
fundamental importance, they have received little attention. Few
integrating or simplifying hypotheses have been established.
Moreover, "motility" is a generic term, covering phenomena which
include the electrophysiology of smooth muscle, contractions,
movements of the bowel wall, intraluminal pressure recordings, and
the propulsion or retropulsion of contents. In this sense, transit
of chyme can be considered as part of, as well as a consequence of,
"motility".

Macagno and Christensen have examined the complex relationships
between muscular contraction, movement of the bowel wall and flow;
their studies are summarized in a comprehensive review.[6] In a
series of dynamic models, these authors divided movements of the
bowel wall into those produced by longitudinal muscle ("sleeve
contractions") and circular muscle ("ring contractions"); a further
subdivision might include events which are static or which move.
Finally, a classification could be made on the basis of time; thus,
contractions might be solitary (transient), rhythmic or prolonged
(tonic). They conclude that longitudinal contractions produce an
exchange of fluid between the centriluminal core and the periphery
of the conduit, but result in minimal propulsion. Circular
contractions produce longitudinal displacement (transit,
propulsion, or retropulsion) but minimal exchange between the core
and periphery of contents.

Weems[8] tested the ability, in dynamic terms, of isolated
intestinal segments to propel fluid from their lumens. He measured
the movements of fluid, ejected by the bowel into attached
reservoirs, and recorded the amount of work needed to affect these
transits of fluid. Whilst concluding that "knowledge of propulsive
behaviour and its control is still in its infancy," his studies

suggest that a) external systems of control can alter the propulsive state of any given region, and b) that different intestinal loci have vastly different intrinsic capacities to propel. In particular, the ileum appeared unusually well adapted to develop propulsive forces.

In attempting to relate any of these underlying contractile events to transit of chyme, and to absorption, it is perhaps intuitive to equate greater levels of activity (e.g. more myoelectrical "spikes", or greater motility indices) with more rapid transit. In turn, the simplest possible view relates rapid transit with a decrease in absorption. That this is not always the case was first stated explicitly by Connell, who coined the term "paradoxical motility"[9].   By this he meant that a greater number of phasic waves or greater levels of intraluminal pressure, in the colon, were not necessarily associated with more rapid transit. Thus, more motor activity, faster transit and impaired absorption did not always lead to diarrhea. In fact, from Connell's results, the reverse often applied--constipated patients often had more active colons (more "motility" if one wishes to so define it) and patients with diarrhea often had "quiet" colons! Thus, the motor phenomena which we measure should be considered from both aspects; they might be equally important for any retardation of flow they produce, since retropulsive pressures could promote mixing and perhaps facilitate absorption. A major gap still exists in our capacity to designate which specific patterns of motility are propulsive and which are not.

The basic organizational patterns of motility in the small intestine were unclear until recent years[10]. Only then there emerged a description of the electrical patterns which control intestinal smooth muscle and of a temporal cycling in the small bowel of the migrating myoelectrical complex--the MMC[10]. The principles of this phenomenon and its neurochemical control have been reviewed recently[3,11]. In the past decade, studies of small bowel motility have been directed in particular to the MMC. This phenomenon constitutes a series of recurrent, regular, electrical and contractile events that occur at the maximum frequency of the basic electrical rhythm (BER, "slow waves") for each intestinal locus. These bursts of electrical activity and the resultant contractions, lasting 5 to 15 minutes, migrate aborally from stomach to ileum; they recur continuously during fasting each 60-120 minutes, though marked species and intra-individual variations have been noted.

The original concept was that when one sequence terminated in the ileum another commenced in the stomach. The sequence is interrupted dramatically by a meal, to be replaced by a continuous pattern of irregular spiking and contraction, the "fed pattern". Code[12] coined the term "interdigestive housekeeper" for the MMC,

proposing that its motility "front" (phase 3) sweeps clear the
small bowel of interdigestive secretions, shed cells and other
assorted debris. The concept is an attractive one, and the
hypothesis is deserving of further testing. What is still
uncertain is the exact quantitative role played by the MMC in the
propulsion of contents. What other contractile events might also
be responsible for transit of secretions during fasting and how is
chyme moved postprandially, when MMCs are inhibited? Further, in
what ways are any of these propulsive events related to absorption?

3. TRANSIT AND THE MMC

     Several lines of evidence suggest that "all that is propulsive
is not the MMC". Most obvious is the fact that MMCs are, by
definition, absent postprandially and yet meals are moved along the
small bowel. Clearly, we need a better definition of the
relationship between patterns of motility and the transit of chyme
after meals. But, all is not clear even during fasting. Mucus was
expelled from the canine small bowel when phase 3 of an MMC was
present in the bowel immediately orad to a stoma[13], but Bueno[14]
showed in the sheep that content moved most rapidly in response to
phase 2 contractions, or to the transition period between phases 2
and 3. These studies of the relationships between phases of the
MMC and transit appeared to culminate in Code's experiments[12] in
which barium was cleared rapidly only during phase 3, that is, when
the "housekeeper" was sweeping clean the bowel. However, recent
studies of the canine terminal ileum in our laboratory raise
additional questions. We record regularly from the canine ileum a
single, high pressure, propulsive contraction which sweeps rapidly
through the distal bowel and which propels ileal contents into the
colon[15]. Does this dramatic "high pressure wave" contribute more
to transit in the ileum than does the MMC (phase 3)? We have
noticed (Borody and Phillips, unpublished observations) that phase
3 becomes disorganized in the terminal ileum of healthy man. Does
phase 3 "die" immediately proximal to the ileocecal junction?

     In man, Kerlin and Phillips[16] showed that although about
one-half of ileal flow was related to phase 3 of MMCs, about
one-half was not. Moreover, flow was appreciable even during
periods of motor quiescence (phase I of the interdigestive cycle).
Thus, their conclusion was in accord with Connell's observations
that the most dramatic intraluminal pressures do not necessarily
induce the most flow. The subject has also been addressed
(personal communication) by Ruppin and Soergel. Their data suggest
that phase 3 of the MMC, though the most striking element of
interdigestive motility, is not the primary force for transit.
Rather, they believe phase 3 acts mainly to prevent orad transit
("reflux"), an event that might otherwise result from propulsive
forces which are not vectored solely in the aborad direction. In
other words, is phase 3 only a "backstop" force? Others[17-21] have

described patterns of neuromuscular activity which also appear to
be propulsive, but which do not qualify as MMCs. Most important
appear to be the frequent, "minute rhythms," which progress rapidly
in an aboral direction, but only over short distances. These are
common in the terminal ileum (personal observations) and jejunum[20]
of healthy man, and are even more prominent during mechanical
obstruction of the bowel[20]. In experimental diarrhea, the concepts
become even more complex. Abnormal myoelectrical patterns are
described in diarrheogenic conditions[22,23], and they are presumed
to produce rapid transit and to impair absorption.

Interpretation of motility tracings is complicated by the
imprecise, and at times subjective, terms which have been applied
to the groups of contractions which are recorded. The MMC is a
reasonably clear event, though even its definition is not crystal
clear; however, various observers have designated the other
patterns of motility as "clusters" of contractions and "propulsive
or retropulsive events". Doubtless, other descriptions will be
proposed. What are lacking are any systematic approaches to the
simple phenomenology of motility, transit and absorption. At this
time, the conclusions must be that, apart from the MMC, no other
motor pattern is sufficiently reproducible to be agreed upon;
further, the functional consequences with respect to transit or
absorption/secretion are still quite unclear.

Another observation which could be pertinent to any
relationships between motility and absorption is the close temporal
association between the secretion of digestive enzymes by the
stomach and pancreas and the MMC cycle. In experimental animals
and man[24,25], gastric, pancreatic and biliary secretions cycle in
parallel with motor events in the proximal bowel. Passage of motor
"fronts" through the antroduodenal region bears a close temporal
relationship to cyclic fluctuations of gastric and
pancreaticobiliary secretions. These phenomena recall the
observations of Boldyreff, who ultimately related a broad spectrum
of biological functions to the same chronobiology[2]. Perhaps even
more germaine are the intriguing observations of Read and Levin[26].
They might offer a clue as to how epithelial transport fluctuates
in relation to the MMC cycle. These authors recorded continuously
the mucosal electrical potential difference (PD) in the jejunum and
the cycles of fasting motility. Concomitant with passage of an MMC
through the bowel, there was a change in the transmucosal PD.
Their hypothesis, which begs further study, was that, concomitant
with the MMC, there was altered absorption-secretion of
electrolytes.

4. MODIFICATIONS OF TRANSIT AND ABSORPTION: FURTHER EXPERIMENTAL
   OBSERVATIONS

Currently, the tentative conclusion must be that the motor

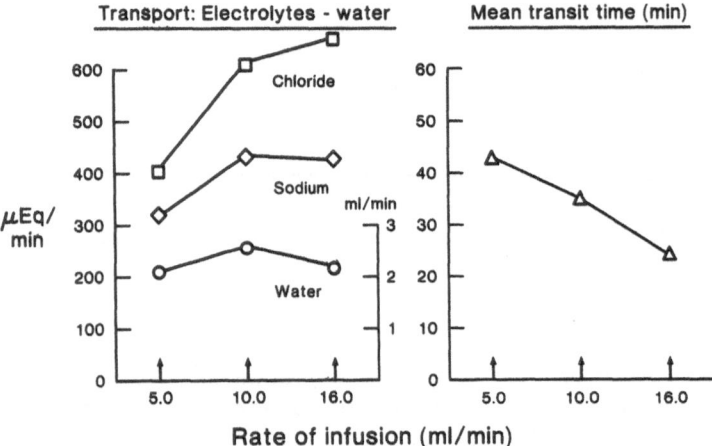

Fig. 1. Results from perfusion of the healthy human colon at three rates, 5, 10 and 16 ml min[-1]. The left panel shows that absorption reached a plateau at high rates of perfusion; transit time decreased concomitantly (right panel). See reference 27 for details.

patterns which produce transit of chyme cannot be defined completely and, moreover, that the relationships between absorption and transit are perhaps even less clear. However, might additional insights be shed by a systematic alteration of transit, with a concomitant assessment of absorption? Perfusion of the bowel in vivo offers one such approach. We and others[27,28] have perfused the human bowel at different rates--in general, the results are comparable among these and a number of other similar studies. As rates of perfusion are increased progressively, the volume of the bowel does not accommodate to the increase; the most rapid flows are handled by a decrease in transit time. We perfused the colon at 5, 10 and 16 ml min[-1]; at the fastest rate, transit time was reduced and absorption reached a plateau (Fig. 1). We concluded that a hypothetical "exposure time", of content to the absorptive surface, was important. This approach was utilized most carefully and exhaustively by Johansson in a series of major publications in 1974[29]. She studied the upper gastrointestinal tract of man, utilized test meals and sophisticated methods of measuring transit and absorption. An important conclusion was "the absorptive capacity of the investigated segment was not exceeded for any component of the meals, due to compensatory mechanisms by which the

244

gastric emptying rate was inhibited and the transit time through the segment prolonged." In other words, the intact bowel has compensatory mechanisms which counteract the perturbations of flow imposed upon it.

However, this hydrodynamic explanation is possibly simplistic; it certainly ignores other important considerations, such as the influence of flow rates upon the effective depth of unstirred layers in vivo. This concept is discussed further below. Moreover, the circumstances of luminal perfusion at rapid rates in vivo are somewhat artificial; faster rates of perfusion appear to augment only the centriluminal laminar flow, without changing juxta-mucosal conditions. It is perhaps of even greater importance that techniques of intraluminal perfusion at rapid rates mimic more the intestine during diarrhea, rather than during any "normal" state.

More recently, small bowel transit in the intact bowel has been correlated with absorption, by the use of markers of mouth to anus transit time. These methods have been augmented at times by more sensitive techniques, such as gamma-camera scintigraphy, and breath hydrogen excretion which monitors transit of a meal to the cecum. Read[30] described an ingenious approach which demonstrated that, after ingestion of a test meal, total stool weights were inversely related to whole gut transit times, but not to transit through the small bowel. He suggested that increased fecal bulk (diarrhea) resulted more from a lack of colonic accommodation than from a rapid and ineffective transit through the small bowel. However, in another group of patients with irritable bowel syndrome[31], small bowel transit was briefer in those with diarrhea. On the other hand, Molla et al[32] could find in patients with infectious diarrhea no significant relationship between whole gut transit times and the capacity to absorb macronutrients. Though the approach to these relationships in intact man has much appeal, the number of uncontrolled variables is great, and the methods are gross, though elegant. The question of how transit times relate to absorption of a test meal is still subjudice.

5. RETROGRADE PACING

One provocative relationship between transit and absorption concerns the effects of "pacing" the intestine by electrical stimuli. Electrical pulses can be applied to the canine bowel in a retrograde fashion[33] such that myoelectrical control activity of the intestine can be "paced backwards". Myoelectrical signals progress in an abnormal, orad direction, transit is slowed, and absorption is increased.[34] These experiments cannot be interpreted easily; the electrical stimuli which evoke retrograde signals and which slow transit might have a variety of other physiological effects. Thus, in one set of studies[34] forward pacing also

245

augmented absorption--though not to the same degree as did the retrograde stimulus. Nevertheless, changes in absorption are quite striking; glucose, sodium and water absorption was doubled and there was an associated slowing of transit, which increased by a factor of 3 to 4. The observations may have practical implications of considerable magnitude. Might it be possible to apply this approach clinically to patients with short bowel syndrome?

The system described above[33,34] featured an isolated loop of bowel. In another experiment, Gladen and Kelly[35,36] paced the shortened, but intact, bowel of puppies (Fig. 2). In this model, also, retrograde pacing increased absorption of water, glucose and sodium from the small bowel and decreased the loss of potassium. In five dogs, the distal two-thirds of the small bowel was removed and a jejunocolostomy was created to mimic short bowel syndrome. A comparison was made between test periods of 2 weeks, in which retrograde pacing accompanied each feeding, and control periods without pacing. Weight loss was slowed by retrograde pacing.[36]

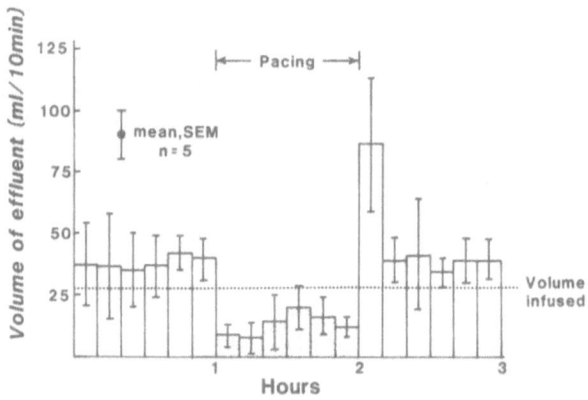

Fig. 2. Effect of retrograde pacing on the volume of effluent from a perfused segment of small intestine. The test solution was infused at 29 ml/10 min (dotted line). There was some storage of fluid during pacing, as shown by "rebound" when pacing was stopped, but net absorption was increased by pacing. Reproduced by permission from the authors and publishers, H.E. Gladen and K.A. Kelly, Surgery 88:281, 1980, C.V. Mosby Co.

6. EFFECTS OF DRUGS

The final example is also an observation that, though as yet unexplained mechanistically, also raises questions pertinent to relationships between motility and absorption. These are the pharmacologic effects of the opiates. Traditional use of opiates as antidiarrheal agents has established beyond doubt their clinical efficacy. If the assumption is made that antidiarrheals act, in the final analysis, by augmenting absorption, the question becomes how do opiates achieve this? Direct enhancement of mucosal function is possible[37]. Whether or not opiates have a direct effect on mucosal function, they also delay transit[38], and also evoke a pattern of motility which, on the surface, is very similar to phase 3 ("fronts")--even postprandially[39]. An explanation is thus needed for what role these motility "fronts" play in the anti-diarrheal effects of opiates. An important question needs to be posed; how do we equate the stimulation of motility fronts (presumed to be highly propulsive) by a class of therapeutic agents (i.e. opiates) which reduces diarrhea?

7. INTEGRATED PATTERNS OF MOTILITY AND INTESTINAL ABSORPTION

Though motility, transit and absorption are not well related mechanistically along any single segment (e.g. small intestine or colon), transit between adjacent segments of the gut has a more clearly defined influence on absorption. Thus, the gastric motor response to food, including the integrated control of emptying, has been subject to intense investigation for decades. Sufficient has been learned of these functions to establish the concept that the' pyloric region regulates gastric emptying exquisitely and that the proximal small intestine has the ability to modify the delivery of materials to it from the stomach[40,41]. Thus, duodenal receptors trigger an exquisitely sensitive "brake" on gastric emptying. Moreover, abundant experimental and clinical literature attests to the disorders of intestinal function that occur when gastric emptying is perturbed, especially by surgery[41]. Although the small intestine possesses considerable reserves of function, its ability to compensate can be stressed, and often overcome, when transit from stomach to duodenum is uncontrolled. More subtle alterations in the rate of gastric emptying can also impair absorption. In a study comparing identical meals, eaten in the solid or homogenized forms[42], it was shown that the proximal small bowel absorbed fat more efficiently (81 versus 48%) from a solid meal, which emptied at a slower rate (half time for lipid emptying 3 hr versus 1 hr), than from the same meal in homogenized form.

Another locus where integrated motor function might influence absorption is at the ileocecal sphincter. By analogy with the pylorus, this segment might act to modulate transit between the ileum and colon (Fig. 3). We have examined the motor

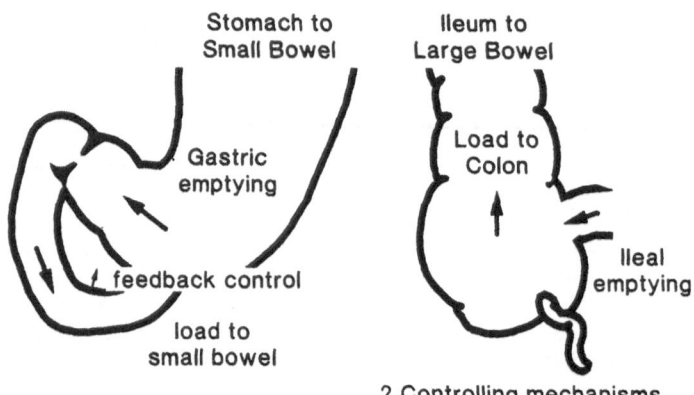

Stomach to
Small Bowel

Ileum to
Large Bowel

Gastric
emptying

Load to
Colon

feedback control

Ileal
emptying

load to
small bowel

? Controlling mechanisms

Fig. 3.   Examples of transit of chyme influencing the contact of
nutrients with critical segments of gut. Disordered
gastric emptying can lead to impaired absorption from the
upper small bowel; the fine control of gastric emptying
influences these events. By analogy, comparable control
should exist at the ileocolonic junction. Reproduced by
permission of the publishers, in Gastroenterology. New
Trends in Pathophysiology and Therapy of the Large Bowel,
Elsevier Biomedical Press.

characteristics of the ileocecal sphincter where a zone of high
pressure can be demonstrated in the dog and man[43,44]. The segment
has the characteristics, physiological and anatomical, of a
sphincter. Our initial observations have focused on the
participation of the ileocecal sphincter in the phases of
interdigestive motility and its responses to feeding. Using a
"sleeve sensor"[45], which could be maintained reproducibly across
the ileocolonic sphincter, we confirmed a zone of high pressure at
the canine sphincter. The sphincteric segment in the dog contracts
continuously in a phasic fashion; the region also participates in
the interdigestive cycle[46]. Phase III activity produces prolonged,
high pressure contractions in the sphincter. The relative
contributions of this high pressure zone to a restriction of flow
(perhaps allowing for storage in the ileum) or to propulsion of

chyme (by developing peristaltic forces in the ileum for the propulsion of solids into the cecum) remains to be determined. Techniques have been developed whereby the functions of this area can be studied predictably in intact man[47].

This concept, that the ileocecal sphincter might also act as an intestinal "brake", needs extension. We need to define the transit of chyme from ileum to colon. Logical questions to pose are, does the junctional zone retard the movement of chyme, how is this achieved, and does the terminal ileum exhibit any storage functions?

8. THE MOVEMENT OF INTESTINAL VILLI

We now move from macroscopic levels of scrutiny to motor events which could influence absorption greatly but which need to be examined at a much finer level.

Movements of intestinal villi were reported first by anatomists in the 19th century, but detailed descriptions awaited the reports of Hambleton[48] and King and Arnold[49]. Hambleton described two distinct movements: a) "lashings", which "might aid mixing and absorption", and b) alternating retraction and extension, "possibly of special aid to the absorption via lacteals"[48]. Kokas and her colleagues[50] extended these observations and noted that, whereas the finger shaped villi of some species exhibited "pumping" movements (retraction and elongation), the leaf-like villi, which are normal in other species, did not. Figure 4 is taken from the work of Kokas and it summarizes one possible association between villous motility and absorption.

Smooth muscle within the villous core forms an interrupted coat around lacteals and has been described by some as being separate from the muscularis mucosae. Villous movement is also thought to be independent of "peristalsis[48-50]. King and Arnold[49] described a third mucosal movement, also of unknown function, "ridging, grooving or pitting" of the mucosal surface. Kokas used cross-circulation and transplantation techniques to incriminate a humoral control of villous motility and extracted from intestinal mucosa a small, acidic peptide designated "villikinin"[51]. Compared to other purified or semipure gastrointestinal hormones, villikinin was a much more potent stimulus of villous movement[52]. Little new has appeared in this area for the past decade, and unanswered questions, which are plausible and of great potential significance, can be posed. Does villous "pumping" facilitate absorption, what is villikinin, what influence do the newer neuropeptides have on villous movement, and do they alter absorptive performance by such a mechanism?

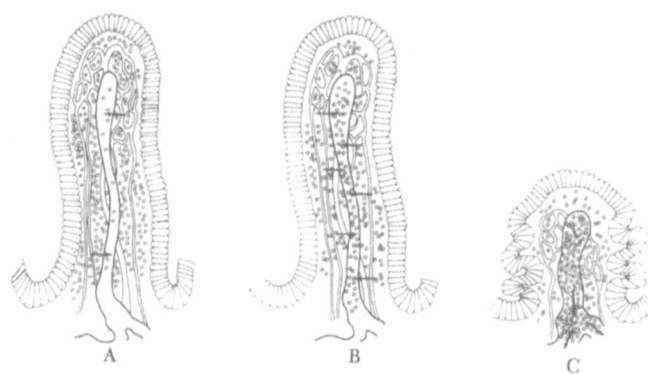

Fig. 4. Diagramatic representation of retractile motility of the intestinal villi (C). In A and B, arrows postulate the movement of absorbed solute into the vessels draining the villus. Reproduced by permission from the author and publishers, in Progress in Gastroenterology, Grune and Stratton, 1968.

The microvilli of enterocytes also exhibit movement and a relationship between motility of microvilli and absorption of nutrient solutions has an intuitive appeal. Small intestine from the chick fetus, in organ-culture, shows rapid coordinated movements of the microvilli, proposed by some to facilitate stirring and absorption[53]. In addition, the filamentous structures in the cores of microvilli contain actin-like proteins and the terminal web region contains myosin and tropomyosin[54]. Microvilli are thought not to undergo retractile movement ("pumping") but rather to splay apart in a fan-like motion[55,56]. However, there is still uncertainty as to how, if at all, such movements are related to absorptive processes. These facets of subcellular composition and structure are reviewed in detail by Trier and Madara[57].

9. MUSCULARIS MUCOSAE

This thin (3 to 10 strands of smooth muscle), but well defined band, also awaits a functional role. Participation in the process

of absorption-secretion is an attractive hypothesis. Despite the
absence of observations of its functional implications, the smooth
muscle of the mucosa can be studied effectively in vitro.[58,59]
Neural and peptidergic systems of its control have been described
(Figs. 5 and 6); for instance, vasoactive intestinal polypeptide
(VIP) fulfills the criteria of an inhibitory transmitter at two
levels of the canine bowel.[58] Substance P is a direct agonist of
contraction, whilst bombesin appears to act via the neural release
of substance P. The neuropeptidergic control of the tunica
muscularis has received more attention, but additional analogies
with the muscularis mucosae seem probable. Perhaps these delicate
strands of muscle deserve more attention. Are they modifiers of
absorption-secretion? Might they be the force for villous
motility? Might VIP, by inhibiting the muscularis mucosae, alter
villous motility and, thereby, influence absorption?

The "unstirred layer" is accepted as an aqueous barrier to
diffusion between the centriluminal compartment and the juxta
mucosal layer; it is proposed to be a rate limiting step for the
absorption of solutes exhibiting less than free diffusion in
water.[60] Though well accepted conceptually, the physical make-up
of this unstirred layer is less clear. Its definitions and
dimensions are purely operational. The diffusive barrier could, on
one hand, be a watery one and of a given thickness; on the other
hand, it could represent a more stringent, chemical or physical,
barrier of considerably smaller physical dimensions. Could it be
that the physical separation of villi controls the access of solute
to the absorptive surface? Might villous proximity or separation,
as determined by their motility, thus act as a variable "unstirred
layer". This concept is addressed by Lee in some simple but
ingenious experiments.[61]

10. CONCLUSIONS AND FUTURE STUDIES

Motor functions and the absorption of nutrients are likely to
be related closely, perhaps inextricably. Problems still exist in
identifying the specific patterns of motility which promote transit
of contents and which, therefore, spread out chyme along the bowel.
However, in this way, contact between chyme and the absorptive
surface should be modified. Of equal importance with propulsive
forces may be those pressure events which impede the flow of chyme.
Of unknown importance are the finer, more microscopic, aspects of
motility; that is, those forces which move villi, or even the
microvilli. But at a grosser level are the macroscopic movements
of contents, phenomena which govern the movement of chyme into
areas critical for absorption. These are most obvious at the major
junctions (e.g. pylorus, ileocecal sphincter). Overriding these
considerations is the likelihood of a common neurohumoral control
for the parallel functions, mucosal absorption and muscular

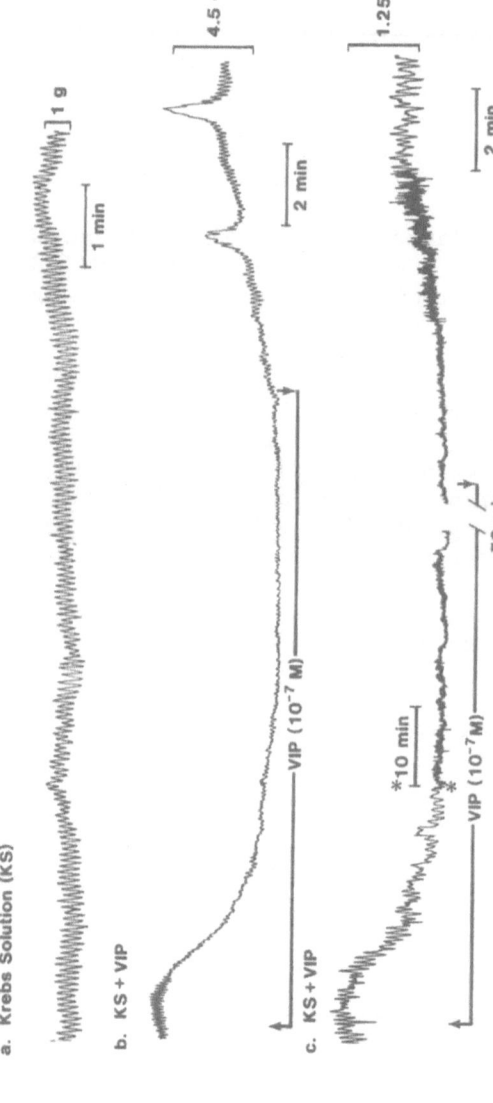

Fig. 5. Inhibitory effect of vasoactive intestinal polypeptide (VIP) on spontaneous mechanical activity of canine muscularis mucosae. In tracing (a) spontaneous activity is shown in Krebs solution. In (b) and (c), inhibition by VIP (10^{-7}M) lasted for duration of superfusion. In (c), return to control activity needed 60 minutes of wash-out. Reproduced with permission from the authors, F. Angel, et al., Journal of Physiology, in press.

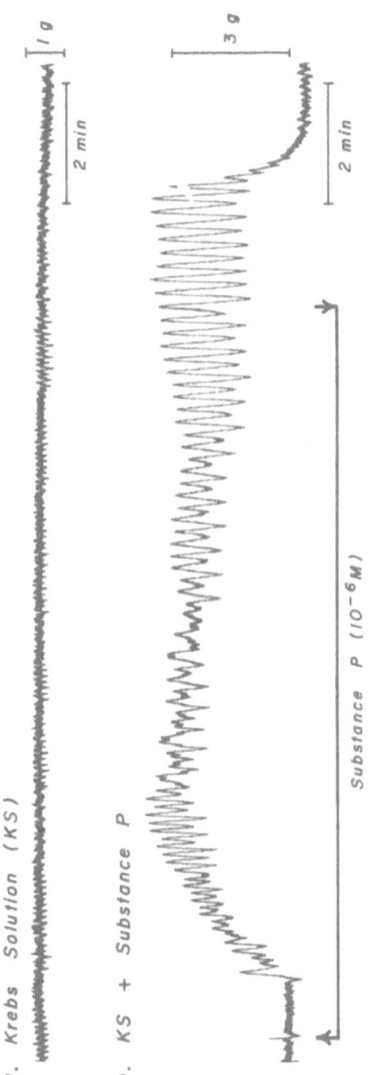

a. Krebs Solution (KS)

b. KS + Substance P

Substance P (10⁻⁶M)

Fig. 6. Stimulatory effect of substance P (10^{-6}M) on mechancal activity of canine muscularis mucosae. Reproduced by permission from the authors, F. Angel, et al, Journal of Physiology, in press.

motility. The "gastrointestinal" peptides, neuropeptides and novel pharmacological approaches have given a first insight into this parallelism. Some areas are undergoing active investigation but refined, or even new methodologies, will need to be applied. Some promising leads, particularly these pertaining to "micro motility", seem worth of a revival.

REFERENCES

1. M. D. Gershon and S. M. Erde. The nervous system of the gut. Gastroenterology, 80:1571 (1981).
2. V. N. Boldyreff. Various papers from 1902 onwards; for a review of these, see reference 3.
3. D. L. Wingate. Backwards and forwards with the migrating complex. Dig. Dis. Sci., 26:541 (1981).
4. S. F. Phillips and T. S. Gaginella. Intestinal secretion as a mechanism in diarrheal disease. Progress in Gastroenterology, In G. B. J. Glass (ed.). Grune & Stratton, New York (1977).
5. G. Van Trappen, J. Janssens and T. L. Peeters. The migrating motor complex. Med. Clin. North Am., 65:1311 (1981).
6. E. O. Macagno and J. Christensen. Fluid mechanics of gastro-intestinal flow. Physiology of the Gastrointestinal Tract, L. R. Johnson (ed.), Raven Press, New York (1981).
7. J. Christensen and E. O. Macagno. Small intestinal motility: the problems of relating contractions to flow. Frontiers of Knowledge in the Diarrheal Diseases, H. Janowitz, D. B. Sachar (ed.). Upper Montclair NJ Projects in Health, (1979).
8. W. A. Weems. The intestin as a fluid propelling system. Ann. Rev. Physiol., 43:9 (1981).
9. A. M. Connell. Motor action of the large bowel. Handbook of Physiology, Section 6, Volume 4, C. F. Code (ed.), American Physiological Society, Washington, D.C. (1968).
10. J. H. Szurszewski. A migrating motor complex of the canine small intestine. Am. J. Physiol., 217:1757 (1969).
11. D. L. Wingate. Motility of the small intestine. In Small Intestine, V. S. Chadwick and S. F. Phillips (eds.). Butterworths, London (1982).
12. C. F. Code and J. F. Schlegel. The gastrointestinal interdigestive housekeeper. In Proceedings of the 4th International Symposium on Gastrointestinal Motility, Mitchell Press, Vancouver, (1974).
13. D. A. Reinke, A. H. Rosenbaum and D. R. Bennett. Patterns of dog gastrointestinal contractile activity monitored in vivo with extraluminal force transducers. Am. J. Dig. Dis., 12:113 (1967).
14. L. Bueno, J. Fioramonti and Y. Ruckebusch. Rate of flow of digesta and electrical activity of the small intestine in dogs and sheep. J. Physiol. (London), 249:69 (1975).

15. W. Kruis and S. F. Phillips. High pressure propulsive forces of the canine ileum. Clin. Res., in press.

16. P. Kerlin, A. Zinsmeister and S. F. Phillips. Relationship of motility to flow of contents in the human small intestine. Gastroenterology, 82:701 (1982).

17. C. F. Code. Diarrheogenic motor and electrical patterns in the bowel. Frontiers of Knowledge in the Diarrheal Diseases, H. D. Janowitz and D. B. Sachar (eds.), Upper Montclair, NJ: Projects in Health, (1979).

18. J. A. Marlett and C. F. Code. Effects of celiac and superior mesenteric ganglionectomy on interdigestive myoelectrical complexes in the dog. Am. J. Physiol., 237:E432 (1979).

19. P. Fleckenstein. Migrating electrical spike activity in the fasting human small intestine. Dig. Dis. Sci., 23:769 (1978).

20. R.W. Summers, S. Anuras and J. Green. Jejunal manometry patterns in health, partial obstruction, and pseudoobstruction. Gastroenterology, in press.

21. N.S. Duskieker and R. W. Summers. Longitudinal and circumferential spread of spike bursts in canine jejunum in vivo. Am. J. Physiol., 239:G6311 (1980).

22. J.R. Mathias, G. M. Carlson, J. L. Marlin, R. P. Shields and S. Farnal. Shigella dependence. I. Enterotoxin: Proposed role in pathogenesis of Shigellisis. Amer. J. Physiol., 239:G382 (1980).

23. J. R. Mathias, J. L. Marlin, T. W. Burns, G. H. Carlson and R. P. Shields. Ricinoleic acid effects on the electrical activity of the small intestine in rabbits. J. Clin. Invest., 61:640 (1978).

24. E.P. DiMagno, J. Hendricks, V. L. W. Go and R. R. Dozois. Relationship among canine fasting pancreatic and biliary secretions, pancreatic duct pressure and duodenal phase III activity: Boldyreff revisited. Dig. Dis. Sci., 24:689 (1979).

25. G. Van Trappen, T. L. Peeters and J. Janssens. The secretory component of the interdigestive migrating motor complex in man. Scand. J. Gastroenterol., 14:663 (1979).

26. N. W. Read. The migrating motor complex and spontaneous fluctuations of transmural potential difference in the human small intestine. In Gastrointestinal Motility, J. Christensen (ed.). Raven Press, New York (1980).

27. G. J. Devroede and S. F. Phillips. Studies of the perfusion technique for colonic absorption. Gastroenterology, 56:92 (1969).

28. R. L. Dillard, H. Eastman and J. S. Fordtran. Volume-flow relationships during the transport of fluid through the human small intestine. Gastroenterology, 49:58 (1965).

29. C. Johansson. Studies of gastrointestinal interactions. Scand. J. Gastroent., (Suppl 28), 9:1 (1974).

30. H. W. Read, C. A. Miles, D. Fisher, A. M. Holgate, N.D. Kime, M. A. Mitchell, A. M. Reeve, T. B. Roche and M. Walker. Transit of a meal through the stomach, small intestine and colon in normal subjects and its role in the pathogenesis of diarrhea. Gastroenterology, 79:1276 (1980).

31. P. A. Cann, N. W. Read, C. Brown, N. Hobson and C. D. Holdsworth. Irritable bowel syndrome: relationship of disorders in the transit of a single solid meal to symptom patterns. Gut, 24:405 (1983).

32. A. Molla, A. M. Molla, S. A. Sarker and M. Khatun. Wholegut transit time and its relationship to absorption of macronutrients during diarrhoea and after recovery. Scand. J. Gastroent., 18:537 (1983).

33. J. Collin, K. A. Kelly and S. F. Phillips. Increased canine jejunal absorption of water, glucose and sodium with intestinal pacing. Dig. Dis. Sci., 23:1121 (1978).

34. J. Collin, K. A. Kelly and S. F. Phillips. Absorption from the jejunum is increased by forward and backward pacing. Br. J. Surg., 66:489 (1979).

35. H. Gladen and K. A. Kelly. Enhancing absorption in the canine short bowel syndrome by intestinal pacing. Surgery, 88:281 (1980).

36. H. Gladen and K. A. Kelly. Electrical pacing for short bowel syndrome. Surg. Gynecol. Obstet., 153:697 (1981).

37. J. S. McKay, B. D. Linaker and L. A. Turnberg. The influence of opiates on ion transport across rabbit ileal mucosa. Gastroenterology, 80:279 (1981).

38. F. D. Loo, S. Sarna, K. H. Soergel, J.A. Cunningham, C. M. Wood and V. E. Cowles. Effect of morphine on human jejunal motility and flow in the fed state. Gastroenterology, 84:1233 (1983).

39. S. Sarna, R. E. Condon and V. E. Cowles. Morphine versus motilin in the initiation of the migrating motor complexes. Dig. Dis. Sci., 27:656 (1982).

40. K. A. Kelly. Motility of the stomach and gastroduodenal junction. Physiology of the Gastrointestinal Tract, L. R. Johnson (ed.), Raven Press, New York (1981).

41. J. H. Meyer. Chronic morbidity after gastric surgery. Gastrointestinal Disease, M. H. Sleisenger and J. S. Fordtran (eds.). W. B. Saunders, Philadelphia (1978).

42. A. Cortot, S. F. Phillips and J.-R. Malagelada. Different rates of fat absorption from homogenized and solid meals. GUT, 19:968 (1978).

43. M. Kelley, E. A. Gordon and J. A. DeWeese. Pressure studies of the ileocolonic junctional zone of dogs. Am. J. Physiol., 209:333 (1965).

44. S. Cohen, L. D. Harris and R. Levitan. Manometric characteristics of the human ileocecal junctional zone. Gastroenterology, 54:72 (1968).

45. E. Quigley, B. Taylor, J. Dent, K. A. Kelly and S. F. Phillips.
     Interdigestive and postprandial pressures in the ileo-cecal
     sphincter. Gastroenterology, 82:1153 (1982).
46. E. M. M. Quigley and S. F. Phillips. Interdigestive
     patterns of intraluminal pressure at the canine ileocolonic
     junction. Gastroenterology, 84:1279 (1983).
47. E. M. M. Quigley, S. F. Phillips, M. Wienbeck and R. L. Tucker.
     Fasting patterns of motility at the ileocolonic junction
     in normal man (abstract). Gastroenterology, 84:1279 (1983).
48. B. F. Hambleton. Note upon the movements of the intestinal
     villi. Am. J. Physiol., 34:446 (1914).
49. C. E. King and L. Arnold. The activities of the intestinal
     mucosal motor mechanism. Am. J. Physiol., 59:97 (19220.
50. J. T. Sessions, S. R. Viegas de Indrade and E. Kokas.
     Intestinal villi: Forward motility in relation to function.
     In Progress in Gastroenterology, G. B. J. Glass (ed.), Grune &
     Stratton, New York (1968).
50. E. Kokas, J. L. Davis and W. D. Brunson. Separation
     of villikinin-like substance from intestinal mucosal extract.
     Arch. Int. Pharmacodyn. Ther., 191:310 (1971).
52. W. L. Joyner and E. Kokas. Effect of venous gastrointestinal
     hormones and vasoactive substances on villous motility. Comp.
     Biochem. Physiol., 46A:171 (1973).
53. B. Sandstrom. A contribution to the concept of brush border
     function. Observations in intestinal epithelium in tissue
     culture. Cytobiologie, 3:293 (1971).
54. A. Bretscher and K. Weber. Localization of action and
     microfilament associated proteins in the microvilli and
     terminal web of the intestinal brush border by
     immunofluorescence microscopy. J. Cell Biol., 79:839 (1978).
55. D.R. Burgess. Reactivation of intestinal epithelial cell
     brush border motility: ATP-dependent contraction via a
     terminal web contractile ring. J. Cell Biol., 94:853 (1982).
56. T.C.S. Keller and M.S. Mooseker. Ca^{++}-calmodulin-dependent
     phosphorylation of myosin, and its role in brush border
     contraction in vitro. J. Cell Biol., 95:943 (1982).
57. J. S. Trier and J. L. Madara. Functional morphology of
     the mucosa of the small intestine. Physiology of the
     Gastrointestinal Tract, L. R. Johnson (ed.), Raven Press, New
     York (1981).
58. F. Angel, P. F. Schmalz, K. G. Morgan, V. L. W. Go and
     J. H. Szurszewski. Innervation of the mucularis mucosa
     in the canine stomach and colon. Scand. J. Gastroenterol.,
     17:71 (1982).
57. F. Angel, V. L. W. Go, P. F. Schmalz and J. H. Szurszewski.
     Vasoactive intestinal polypeptide: a putative
     neurotransmitter in the canine gastric muscularis mucosa. J.
     Physiol., in press.

60. J. M. Dietschy, V. L. Salle and F. A. Wilson. (1971). Unstirred water layers and absorption across the intestinal mucosa. Gastroenterology, 61:932 (1971).

61. J. S. Lee. Effect of stretching and stirring on water and glucose absorption by canine mucosal membrane. J. Physiol. (London), 335:335 (1983).

THE ENTERO-INSULAR AXIS

Susan M. Wood

Department of Medicine, Hammersmith Hospital
Du Cane Road, London

INTRODUCTION

Although circulating glucose is the prime regulator of insulin secretion, it is unlikely that the insulin rise occurring in response to a meal is mediated solely by a change in the glucose concentration bathing the B cell. If this were the case one would expect to observe a large rise in plasma glucose followed by a rise in insulin, such a delay in the insulin response would be unlikely to maintain glucose homeostatis. In practice plasma glucose and insulin rise in parallel, suggesting a mechanism whereby insulin requirements are anticipated by the B cell, resulting in appropriate insulin secretion to hold the postprandial glucose rise within narrow limits. The most logical site for such a regulatory mechanism would seem to be the gut. The first appreciation of gut regulation of the pancreas began as early as 1902 when Bayliss and Starling introduced the concept of 'chemical regulation'. At that time they showed that the intravenous injection of an extract of intestinal mucosa stimulated pancreatic exocrine secretion in the dog to the same extent as acid placed in the gut; and acid produced the same effect even when all neural connections between gut and pancreas were cut.[1] The chemical messenger within these extracts was of course secretin, which was not to be isolated until 1952.[2]

It was soon to be suggested that intestinal extracts also contained chemical messengers with the capacity to stimulate the endocrine pancreas. Moore, Edie and Abram hypothesised that diabetes was due to the absence of such an intestinal stimulant of the internal secretions of the pancreas. They attempted to test this by treating three diabetic patients with intestinal extracts, two showed a limited reduction of glycosuria.[3] It was much later

259

that LaBarre and others took this idea a little further and performed cross circulation experiments to demonstrate that intravenous injections of crude secretin lowered blood glucose.[4] They concluded that crude secretin contained an 'incretin' and an 'excretin' which could stimulate the endocrine and exocrine pancreas respectively.

With the advent of radioimmunoassay it became possible for McIntyre and others to show that oral glucose resulted in a much greater release of insulin than equivalent amounts of intravenous glucose.[5,6] Since then the signals mediating this enteric enhancement of insulin secretion have been vigorously investigated. In 1969 Unger and Eisentraut introduced the term 'entero-insular axis' to describe these mechanisms which were originally thought to be purely hormonal in origin.[7] It is of course now appreciated that cholinergic, adrenergic and peptidergic neural signals are likely to have equally important effects.[8,9]

I shall briefly discuss below the studies that have been carried out to attempt to define the hormonal mediators of the enter-insular axis. The role of the autonomic nervous system has proved difficult to study, most of the work has necessarily been carried out in animals, while some indirect methods of study have been used to confirm these findings in man.

HORMONAL REGULATION

Virtually all the established gut hormones have been investigated for insulin releasing activity. None fully satisfy the criteria for an 'incretin' i.e. (i) release by oral nutrients, in particular glucose, and (ii) the capacity to release insulin at the hormonal concentrations occurring postprandially.[8,10]

Regarding the first of these criteria, the only gut hormones released by glucose are glucose dependent insulinotropic peptide (GIP), gastrin and enteroglucagon where the gastrin and enteroglucagon responses are small compared to that of GIP.[11] Cholecystokinin (CCK) is released by protein, fat and acid, while secretin rises in response to only protein and acid. Since glucose absorption is a prerequisite for postprandial insulin secretion, hormones not released by oral glucose are unlikely to be major incretins, however this does not prevent their enhancement of insulin secretion in the context of a mixed meal. Of the hormones released by glucose, few fulfil the second criteria for incretin. Exogenous gastrin augments glucose induced insulin release only at concentrations reached after a protein meal[11], but its endogenous release adds little to amino acid stimulated insulin secretion.[12] An effect of enteroglucagon on insulin secretion occurs only at higher concentrations than those occurring postprandially. Glucose dependant insulinotropic peptide (GIP) has been put forward for many years as the strongest candidate for 'incretin'[8,13], in that it produces a glucose dependent secretion of insulin, and data suggests that there is feedback control of GIP release by insulin. There is however considerable evidence to suggest that GIP only has significant insulinotropic effects at high concentrations and during hyperglycaemia.[14]

The role of the hormones released by protein in the enhancement of insulin secretion during a mixed meal is still under question. The insulin response to high doses of secretin is rapid and short lived, and should be considered as a pharmacological effect. There is therefore little good evidence to implicate secretin in the control of insulin secretion.[15,16] The evidence for cholecystokinin (CCK) as an incretin is difficult to assess, in view of the problems of radioimmunoassay of this peptide, its multiple molecular forms, and the likelihood that in many situations it appears to act as a neurotransmitter. This may apply to the islet, making application of the criteria for incretin inappropriate. Its true mode of action remains to be elucidated but both CCK-4 and CCK-33 have been reported to enhance glucose stimulated insulin secretion in vitro and in vivo. [17,18]

A rather different approach to the problem has come from the use of intubation-perfusion techniques that allow manipulation regarding which segments of bowel are exposed to a meal. By this means it has been found that the bowel distal to the ligament of Treitz has the most influence on the entero-insular axis, with little effect arising from the gastroduodenal region.[19] This would confirm the evidence discussed above that gastrin, secretin and cholecystokinin are not major insulinotropic peptides.

Most interest has been concentrated on the mechanisms of the entero-insular axis involved in augmentation of the insulin response and little on how these mechanisms may also influence the secretion of other islet hormones, glucagon and pancreatic polypeptide. This is understandable with regard to glucagon where ingestion of a mixed meal leads to little change in glucagon in normal man. However it has been suggested that the abnormalities of glucagon secretion occurring in disease states such as diabetes are partly attributable to entero-insular mechanisms. [20]Certainly hormones such as GIP, cholecystokinin and secretin have been shown to have glucagonotropic effects in vivo.[18] The enteropancreatic stimulation of PP would appear to be mainly neural. Oral protein and fat are the most potent nutrient stimulants of PP secretion, while glucose has a much smaller effect. It was previously thought that the second phase of the PP response to food was mediated by cholecystokinin. However there is now considerable evidence for a vagal, cholinergic reflex.[21] It is conceivable that CCK may be involved as a neurotransmitter or neuromodulator in this pathway.[22]

As yet none of the known gastrointestinal peptides adequately fulfil the requirements for the hormonal component of the entero-insular axis, it is possible that as yet unidentified peptides are involved, or perhaps more likely several peptides act in unison.

NEURAL REGULATION

The Islets of Langerhans are richly innervated by the three divisions of the autonomic nervous system, parasympathetic, symp-athetic and peptidergic.[9,23,24] The physiological importance of the islet innervation has been until recently somewhat neglected on the basis of an early report by Minkowsky in 1893 that diabetes did not occur in animals with functional pancreatic transplants, i.e. with denervated pancreas. Although this illustrates that suffi-cient insulin secretion to prevent diabetes occurs in the den-nervated state, it can give no indication of the role of innervation under normal conditions. Siegel and his colleagues have recently shown that intraportal transplantations of isogenic islets in rats leads to abnormal oral glucose tolerance with normal intravenous glucose tolerance, supporting a neural component of the entero-insular axis.[25]

Many studies have been carried out to investigate neural control of islet hormone secretion, these have been well reviewed.[9,24,26]

PARASYMPATHETIC INFLUENCE ON ISLET SECRETION.

Early experiments to investigate the effects of vagal stimulation were limited by the inability to directly measure insulin, however a number of studies showed significant hypo-glycaemia during vagal stimulation [27,28] A variety of approaches have been used in more recent work. Vagal stimulation of the isolated perfused pancreas [29,30] demonstrated a direct stimulant effect on insulin secretion. Studies in vivo have been carried out in both the anaesthetized and conscious animal, where vagal stimulation results in a glucose dependent enhancement of insulin secretion.[31,32,33] The effects of antagonists on this response differs with the species studied suggesting that the neuro-transmitter is not always acetylcholine. Although in the rat and calf the response was shown to be blocked by atropine, it was not in the pig and cat. In a series of experiments in the pig, hexamethonium but not atropine blocked the effects of vagal stimulation,[34] atropine and not hexamethonium blocked the effect of intra-arterial acetylcholine.[35] This would suggest that the post ganglionic neurotransmitter released by vagal nerve stimulation is non-cholinergic in some species and is perhaps a peptide.[33-35] Bloom and Edwards have shown that vagal stimulation in the calf releases VIP, a response not affected by atropine; however in this species vagal stimulated insulin release was blocked by atropine.[32]

The results of studies looking at the effects of vagotomy on insulin secretion are somewhat conflicting, some impairment of insulin secretion occurs after this procedure although in some species this has been difficult to demonstrate.[9]

The importance of the parasympathetic nervous system in the regulation of glucagon secretion has been demonstrated in a number of species by infusion of acetylcholine, stimulation of the vagus nerve and the use of deoxyglucose to induce intracellular hypoglycaemia, in the presence and absence of antagonists.[32-35] Its role in man remains controversial limited by the indirect approach of the studies.[36,37]

The secretion of pancreatic polypeptide (PP) in response to food and hypoglycaemia is strongly influenced by the cholinergic nervous system. Infusion of acetylcholine and vagal nerve stimulation potently release PP.[21,32] In some species these effects are totally blocked by atropine, in others only partially. The PP response to insulin or deoxyglucose induced hypoglycaemia is much reduced by atropine and vagotomy in all species including man.[38] The post-prandial rise in PP is biphasic and seems to be under several control mechanisms, the first phase is eliminated while the second phase only significantly reduced by vagotomy.[39] Although the vagus is an important regulator of PP secretion the data suggests that other non vagal mechanisms are also involved.

The influece of the vagus nerve on somatostatin release is complicated by the multiple sources of the peptide from stomach, intestine and pancreas. The results of the studies looking at the effects of vagal nerve stimulation, acetylcholine and vagotomy are conflicting, with both stimulatory and inhibitory effects in different species, and no common pattern emerging.[40]

There is no doubt from the large amount of evidence available in animals that cholinergic mechanisms, many of these via the vagus nerve, are important in regulation of insulin, glucagon and PP secretion from the islet. The story is not quite so clear in man but this I suspect reflects the limitations resulting from indirect studies. It would seem also that the vagus contains non cholinergic fibres which have important effects on islet function.

Sympathetic nerves reach the pancreas via the splanchnic nerves, their influence on islet cell function has been investigated both in vitro and in vivo by nerve stimulation studies and by the use of specific adrenergic agonists and antagonists. The findings have been comprehensively reviewed.[9,24,26]

Stimulation of the splanchnic nerves inhibits insulin secretion in all species studied.[41,42] The use of specific receptor antagonists has shown this to be an effect on α_2 adrenergic receptors,[4,3] however when these receptors are blocked, nerve stimulation or infusion of catecholamines can stimulate release of insulin by an action on β_2 adrenergic receptors.[44] The α and β receptors regulating insulin secretion appear to be closely associated to each other on the B cell. Small changes in the concentration of the endogenous agonists, noradrenaline and adrenaline and other alterations in the environment of the receptor can profoundly influence whether the final response to sympathetic activation is stimulatory or inhibitory. At low concentrations noradrenaline stimulates β_2-receptors and insulin secretion, at physiologically higher concentrations α_2 - receptors are activated with inhibition of secretion.[9] Basal insulin secretion appears to be under some degree of sympathetic neural regulation since basal concentrations fall during β-blockade.[45] Interactions between cholinergic and adrenergic influences on the B cell are demonstrated by the finding that splanchnic nerve stimulation abolishes or reduces the increase in insulin secretion elicited by vagal stimulation.[46]

Splanchnic nerve stimulation also releases pancreatic glucagon, the effect being greater at lower glucose concentrations.[42,47] In many species this appears to be mediated by interaction with both α and β adrenergic receptors.[48] However, in the calf neither α nor β receptor antagonists influence the response to nerve stimulation, suggesting that a nonadrenergic neurotransmitter is involved.[49] Recently Bloom and Edwards have shown that splanchnic nerve stimulation releases bombesin-like immunoreactivity, this may prove to be the mediator of nerve stimulated glucagon secretion in the calf.

Combined vagal and splanchnic nerve stimulation in the pig have an additive effect in stimulating glucagon secretion, providing a mechanism for potent release of this peptide during profound hypoglycaemia when both nervous systems would be activated.[46] It has been suggested that the sympathetic nervous system mediates stress-induced glucagon secretion in animals, while the parasympathetic is involved in homeostatic glucagon release for maintenance of normoglycaemia. These differential roles are not so clear cut in man.[50]

The role of adrenergic regulation of PP secretion would seem to be minor compared to the involvement of cholinergic mechanisms. Stimulation of the splanchnic nerves release PP in the calf,[51] and in the perfused pancreas catecholamines raise PP levels, the effect being blocked by β adrenergic receptor antagonists.[52] The PP rise in man reported during exercise also may be mediated by activation of β receptors.[53]

Somatostatin release is stimulated by β adrenergic agonists, and inhibited by α agonists in the isolated canine pancreas.[48] Stimulation of the splanchnic nerve inhibits pancreatic somatostatin secretion[54], but stimulates its release from the stomach in the rat.[40] In vivo chemical sympathectomy has been shown to reduce postprandial gastric and pancreatic somatostatin release in the dog.[55] The data so far available supports the likelihood of considerable adrenergic influence on somatostatin release in the dog.[55]

PEPTIDERGIC INFLUENCE ON ISLET SECRETION

With the aid of immunocytochemical techniques a number of peptides have been demonstrated in the vagus and splanchnic nerves, as well as in the intrinsic fibres innervating the pancreas.[56,57,58] The evidence to suggest that they function as neurotransmitters and neuromodulators of the gastroenteropancreatic system will be discussed below for each peptide.

Vasoactive Intestinal Polypeptide (VIP)

Specific immunocytochemical techniques have shown VIP to be present in the nerve fibres supplying the ganglia, islets and blood vessels of the endocrine pancreas.[57,58] A number of studies have shown that VIP can stimulate islet peptide secretion from the isolated pancreas, the responses vary from species to species.[59,60] Intravenous infusions in the whole animal require large concentrations to produce any increase in insulin secretion,[61] since the physiological circulating concentration of VIP is very low, it is unlikely to be acting as a hormone but rather as a neurotransmitter. Vagal stimulation releases VIP from peptidergic nerves[32] and it is this peptide which is likely to mediate the glucose dependent, glucagon and insulin responses to vagal stimulation in the pig, which are neither blocked by atropine nor by adrenergic receptor antagonists.[33] There seems however to be species variation in the vagal neurotransmitter involved in the stimulation of insulin and glucagon secretion, since in the calf this is blocked by atropine, despite a concomitant release of VIP, suggesting that acetylcholine is the transmitter in this species.[32] Therefore despite the wealth of evidence in support of VIP as a neurotransmitter released from postganglionic parasympathetic nerve terminals in the gut, its role is not so clear cut in the islet. It is possible that in those species where the effects of vagal stimulation on islet secretions are blocked by atropine, that the VIP released is acting to enhance the binding of acetylcholine to muscarinic receptors, so potentiating acetylcholine's actions, an effect reported in cat submandibular salivary gland.[62]

Cholecystokinin and Gastrin like Peptides.

Numerous nerve fibres reacting with antisera against the COOH-terminal tetrapeptide of CCK, which is common also to the gastrins, have been found to innervate the ganglia and islets of the pancreas.[17,22] These "CCK nerves" are reported to release a small molecular form of CCK, presumed to be tetrin by Rehfeld and his colleagues[63], however there still remains some controversy over the nature of this molecular form of CCK.[64]

Studies in the perfused porcine pancreas show that CCK-39, CCK-33 and CCK-8 at concentrations between 10^{-11} to 10^{-9} M have no effect on insulin or glucagon secretion; similarly the larger gastrins G-34, G-17 and G-14 only have effects at pathological concentrations. In contrast the newly characterised free tetrapeptide amide, tetrin, is a potent stimulus of insulin and glucagon secretion at low concentrations.[65] The effects of intravenous infusions of the CCK molecular forms differ from their effects on the perfused pancreas, for instance CCK-8 and CCK-39 stimulate insulin secretion dose dependently, an effect blocked by muscarinic or β adrenergic antagonists.[66] CCK-39 but not CCK-8 has been found to potentiate glucose or carbachol stimulated insulin secretion, suggesting that this action is dependent on a part of the molecule beyond the C-terminal octapeptide.[67] These studies tend to confirm that the larger molecular forms of CCK act as circulating hormones and their effects on the B cell are probably indirect; whereas the more rapidly metabolised smaller CCK forms are more likely to be released directly on to the islet from peptidergic nerve fibres.

Bombesin-Like Peptides

A peptide, immunoreactivily similar to the amphibian tetradecapeptide bombesin has been identified in intrinsic nerves throughout the mammalian gut and pancreas.[68] It has been shown that stimulation of the splanchnic nerves in the calf results in a rise in arterial bombesin-like immunoreactivity, which is greatest when stimulation is intermittent and at high frequency. More recently a 27 amino acid peptide, gastrin releasing peptide (GRP), homologous with bombesin at the biologically active carboxy terminal end of the molecule, has been isolated from porcine gut.[69] Immunostaining using specific anti-GRP antibodies has demonstrated GRP nerve fibres within porcine intrapancreatic ganglia. It is likely that (GRP-27) is the active neuropeptide present in mammalian tissues, although a molecular form identical with amphibian bombesin GRP (14-27) is also found to be present.[70] Bombesin stimulates the secretion of insulin by a direct effect,[71] as well as indirectly through release of a number of potential insulinotropic peptides, neurotensin, cholecystokinin and gastrin, as shown by infusion studies in dog and man.[72,73] There is considerable species variation in the response of the islet peptides to bombesin and GRP, with most potent effects on PP and glucagon being found in the dog.[73] As regards the influence of the other islet peptides on GRP/bombesin it is of interest that somatostatin has been shown to inhibit bombesin-stimulated insulin secretion in the dog.[74] The presence of somatostatin and bombesin-like peptides within the islet would suggest that regulation of islet cell secretions may be maintained by a balance between the effects of these two mutually antagonistic peptides.

Neurotensin

Neurotensin, a tridecapeptide originally isolated from the hypothalamus is found in other areas of the brain, and in the gut in endocrine cells. Carraway and Leeman have also reported its presence in the rat pancreas,[76] but this has not been confirmed by other authors or in other species. Neurotensin has been found to have a dual effect on the endocrine pancreas in vitro: at low glucose concentrations it stimulates insulin, glucagon and somatostatin secretion, while at high glucose concentrations their secretion is inhibited.[77] Intravenous infusions of neurotensin result in very variable islet peptide responses, the large glucose-dependent rise in plasma insulin and PP observed in the calf is seen neither in man nor the mouse.[78,79] It would seem from these studies that neurotensin has no clearly defined effects on islet peptide secretion. However on the basis of its rise in plasma after food, and its effects in some species, it has been put forward as one of the possible hormonal components of the enteroinsular axis.

Opioid Peptides

Immunoreactive enkephalin and endorphin have been identified in pancreatic islets and ganglia in both the cat and man,[57] and have been shown to stimulate glucose dependent insulin and glucagon secretion in the isolated perfused dog pancreas. These effects may be mediated by a suppression of somatostatin secretion which occurs concomittantly.[40] The effects of met- and leu-enkephalin on insulin secretion from isolated islets have been found to be dose dependent, stimulating at low but inhibiting at high concentrations. Bolus injections of β endorphin in man results in a rapid rise in plasma insulin, glucagon, and glucose.[80] The importance of opioids in islet regulation remains speculative. An altered sensitivity to these peptides in Type II diabetes has been suggested on the basis of a reversal of the chlorpropamide alcohol facial flush, by naloxone, and by precipitation of the flush by infusion of enkephalin.[81] This data remains to be confirmed.

Large molecular weight variants of Leu and Met-enkephalin are now being characterised including Met-enkephalin Arg[6] Phe[7]. The C-terminal tetrapeptide of this compound exists in an amidated form (FMRF amide), which is of interest since it has some structural similarities to the C-terminal tetrapeptide of CCK and gastrin.[82] It therefore may prove to influence insulin secretion.

Other Neuropeptides

Two newly characterised peptides PHI and PYY have been isolated from porcine gut by a chemical method which relies on detection of a C-terminal amide.[83] PHI is a further member of the secretin family, while PYY is structurally similar to pancreatic polypeptide. PHI has been found in the brain, gut and pancreas in a number of species and shown to stimulate basal and glucose induced insulin secretion, and enhance arginine stimulated glucagon secretion in the perfused isolated rat pancreas.[84] These effects are similar to those of VIP except PHI has a more prolonged action. It is possible that PHI may act as a neurotransmitter or neuromodulator in the islet.

Substance P has been shown by radioimmunoassay and immunohisto-chemistry to be present in septal nerve fibres and ganglia of the cat pancreas.[57] Its effect on islet peptide secretion varies in different species, inhibiting insulin seretion in mice, while stimulating insulin, glucagon and somatostatin in the dog.[85]

Luteinizing hormone-releasing factor (LRF) and thyrotrophin releasing hormone (TRH) have both been found in islet cells, their role, like the many unknown peptides that no doubt remain to be localised in the islet, is currently undefined.

CONCLUSIONS

Glucose homeostasis is primarily dependent upon regulated insulin secretion from the B cell. It is therefore not surprising that many mechanisms exist to allow the B cell to respond appropriately to the changing internal and external environment. Although the exact mechanisms and mediators involved in this regulatory system are not fully known it is likely that neural and hormonal signals from the gut allow a rapid stimulation of insulin secretion prior to any change in circulating glucose. The close contact between the islet cells through gap junctions and interdigitating processes allows the necessary rapid intercellular communication. The intrapancreatic ganglia provide another site for the integration of neural signals from the central nervous system, gut and liver. In this way the large input of information received by the islet can be modified to produce an appropriate and rapidly changing insulin secretion which anticipates rather than follows peripheral insulin requirement.

REFERENCES

1. W. M. Bayliss and E. H. Starling, On the causation of the so called peripheral reflex secretion of the pancreas, Proc Roy Soc. 69:352 (1902)

2. J. E. Jorpes and V. Mutt, The preparation of secretin, Biochem J 52:328 (1952)

3. B. Moore, E. S. Edie and J. H. Abram, On the treatment of diabetes mellitis by acid extract of duodenal mucous membrane, Biochem J. 1:28 (1906)

4. J. La Barre and E. V. Still, Studies on the physiology of secretin. III. Further studies on the effects of secretin on the blood sugar, Am J Physiol. 91:649 (1930)

5. N. McIntyre, C. D. Holdsworth and D. S. Turner, A new interpretation of oral glucose tolerance, Lancet. ii:20 (1964)

6. M. J. Perley and D. M. Kipnis, Plasma insulin responses to oral and intravenous glucose: Studies in normal and diabetic subjects, J Clin Invest. 46:1954 (1967)

7. R. H. Unger and A. M. Eisentraut, Entero-insular axis, Arch Intern Med. 123:261 (1979)

8. W. Creutzfeldt, The incretin concept today, Diabetologia. 16:75 (1979)

9. R. E. Miller, Pancreatic neuroendocrinology: peripheral neural mechanisms in the regulation of the Islets of Langerhams, Endocrine Reviews 2: 471 (1981)

10. W. Creutzfeldt, R. Ebert, M. Nauck and F. Stockman, Disturbances of the entero-insular axis, Scand J Gastroenterol. 18 Supp 82:111(1983)

11. J. F. Rehfeld and F. Stadil, Effect of gastrin on basal and glucose stimulated insulin secretion in man, J Clin Invest. 52:1415 (1973)

12. J. F. Rehfeld and F. Stadil, The glucose induced gastrointestinal stimulation of insulin secretion in man: relation to age and to gastrin release, Eur J Clin Invest. 5:273 (1975)

13. D. K. Andersen, D. Elahi, J. C. Brown, J. D. Tobin and R. Andres, Oral glucose augmentation of insulin release, J Clin Invest. 62:152 (1978)

14. D. L. Sarson, S. M. Wood, D. Holder and S. R. Bloom, The effect of glucose dependent insulinotropic polypeptide infused at physiological concentrations on the release of insulin in man, Diabetologia. 22:33(1982)

15. J. Fahrenkrug, O. B. Schaffalitzky de Muckadell and C. Kuhl, Effect of secretin on basal and glucose stimulated insulin secretion in man, Diabetologia 14:229(1978)

16. J. J. Holst, S. L. Jensen, O. B. Schaffalitzky de Muckadell and J. Fahrenkrug, Secretin and vasoactive intestinal polypeptide in the control of the endocrine pancreas, Front Hormone Res. 7:119(1980)

17. J. F. Rehfeld and S. L. Jensen, The effect of gastrin and cholecystokinin on the endocrine pancreas, Front Hormone Res. 7:107(1980)

18. J. Szecowka, P. E. Lins and S. Efendic, Effects of cholecystokinin, gastric inhibitory polypeptide and secretin on insulin and glucagon secretion in rats, Endocrinology. 110:1268 (1982)

19. V. L. W. Go and L. J. Miller, The role of gastrointestinal hormones in the control of postprandial and interdigestive gastrointestinal function, Scand J Gastroenterol. 18 Supp 82:133 (1983)

20. J. Dupre, Y. Caussignac, M. Champion, M. Kobric, T. J. McDonald, N. W. Rodger, S. A. Ross, G. A. Shepherd and S. Van Vliet, Gastrointestinal hormones: the entero-insular axis and the secretion of glucagon, Front Hormone Res. 7:92 (1980)

21. T. W. Schwartz, Entero-insular axis for pancreatic polypeptide, Front Hormone Res. 7:82 (1980)

22. L. I. Larsson and J. F. Rehfeld, Localisation and molecular heterogeneity of cholecystokinin in the central and peripheral nervous system, Brain Res. 165:20 (1979)

23. E. Van Campen Hout, Contributions a l'etude de histogenese du pancreas chez quelque maminiferes les complexes sympathetic insulinaires, Archives de Biologie Liege. 37:121 (1927)

24. S. C. Woods and D. Porte, Neural control of the endocrine pancreas, Physiol Rev. 54:596 (1974)

25. E. G. Siegel, E. R. Trimble, A. E. Renold and H. R. Berthoud, Importance of preabsorptive insulin release in the oral glucose tolerance: studies in pancreatic islet transplanted rats, Gut. 21:1002 (1980)

26. P. H. Smith and D. Porte, Neuropharmacology of the pancreatic islets, Ann Rev Pharmacol Toxicol. 16:269 (1979)

27. S. W. Britton, Studies on the conditions of activity in endocrine glands (XVIII): the nervous control of insulin secretion, Am J Physiol. 74:29 (1925)

28. J. La Barre, Sur L'augmentation de la teneur en insuline du sang veineux pancreatique apres excitation du nerf vague compt, Rend Soc Biol. 96:193 (1927)

29. J. A. Findlay, J. R. Gill, J. E. Lever, P. J. Randle and J. L. B Spriggs, Increased insulin output following stimulation of the vagal supply to the perfused rabbit pancreas, J Anat. 104:580 (1969)

30 A. Orsetti and F. Passebois, The production of insulin by isolated fragments of pancreas directly stimulated by way of their vagal nerve fibres. Importance of the glucose concentration of the medium, Diabetologia. 11:367 (1975)

31. K. Uvnas Wallenstein and G. Nilsson, A quantitative study of the insulin release induced by vagal stimulation in anaesthetised cats, Acta Physiol Scand. 102:137 (1978)

32. S. R. Bloom and A. V. Edwards, Pancreatic endocrine responses to stimulation of the peripheral ends of the vagus nerve in conscious calf, J Physiol. 315:31 (1981)

33. J. J. Holst, R. Gronholt, O. B. Schaffalitzky de Muckadell and J. Fahrenkrug, Nervous control of pancreatic endocrine secretion. I. Insulin and glucagon responses to electrical stimulation of the vagus nerve, Acta Physiol Scand. 111:1 (1981)

34. J. J. Holst, R. Gronholt, O. B. Shaffalitzky de Muckadell and J. Fahrenkrug, Nervous control of pancreatic endocrine secretion in pigs. II. The effect of pharmacological blocking agents on the response of vagal stimulation. Acta Physiol Scand. 111:9 (1981)

35. J. J. Holst, O. B. Schaffalitzky de Muckadell, J. Fahrenkrug, S. Linkaer, O. V. Nilsson and T. W. Schwartz, Nervous control of pancreatic endocrine secretion in pigs. III. The effects of acetylcholine on the pancreatic secretion of insulin and glucagon, Acta Physiol Scand. 111:15 (1981)

36. S. R. Bloom, N. J. A. Vaughn and R. C. G. Russell, Vagal control of glucagon release in man, Lancet. 2:546 (1974)

37. J. Palmer, P. Werner, P. Hollander and J. Ensinck, Evaluation of the control of glucagon secretion by the parasympathetic nervous system in man, Metabolism. 28:549 (1979)

38. J. A. Hedo, M. L. Vallanueva and J. Mario, Stimulation of pancreatic polypeptide and glucagon secretion by deoxy-D-glucose in man: evidence of cholinergic mediation, J Clin Endocrinol Metab. 47:366 (1978)

39. J. C. Floyd and A. I. Vinik, Pancreatic polypeptide, in: "Gut Hormones", S. R. Bloom, and J. M. Polak, ed. Churchill Livingstone, London (1981).

40. V. Schusdziarra, Somatostatin - a regulatory modulator connecting nutrient entry and metabolism, Horm Metab Res. 12:563 (1980)

41. D. Porte, L. Girardier, J. Seydoux, Y. Kanazawa and J. Posternak, Neural regulation of insulin secretion in the dog, J Clin Invest. 52:210 (1973)

42. S. R. Bloom and A. V. Edwards, The release of pancreatic glucagon and inhibition of insulin in response to stimulation of the sympathetic innervatio, J Physiol. 253:57 (1975)

43. T. Nakadate, T. Nakaki, T. Muraki and R. Kato, Adrenergic regulation of blood glucose levels: possible involvement of post synaptic alpha-2 type adrenergic receptors regulating insulin release, J Pharmacol Exp Ther. 215:226 (1980)

44. A. Loubatieres, M. M. Mariani, G. Sorel and L. Savi, The action of β adrenergic blocking and stimulating agents on insulin secretion, characterisation of the type of β receptor, Diabetologia. 7:127 (1971)

45. C. Y. Goodner, D. J. Koerker, J. H. Werrbach, P. Toivola and C. C. Gale, Adrenergic regulation of lipolysis and insulin secretion in the fasted baboon, Am J Physiol. 224:534 (1973)

46. J. J. Holst, R. Gronholt, O. B. Schaffalitzky de Muckadell and J. Fahrenkrug, Nervous control of pancreatic endocrine secretion in pigs V. influence of the sympathetic nervous system on the pancreatic secretion of insulin and glucagon, and on the insulin and glucagon response to vagal stimulation, Acta Physiol Scand, 113:279 (1981)

47. E. B. Marliss, L. Girardier, J. Seydoux, C. B. Wolheim, Y. Kanazawa, L. Orci, A. E. Renold and D. Porte, Glucagon release induced by pancreatic nerve stimulation in the dog, J Clin Invest. 52:1246 (1973)

48. E. Samols and W. C. Weir, Adrenergic modulation of pancreatic A, B and D cells, J Clin invest. 63:230 (1979)

49. S. R. Bloom and A. V. Edwards, Certain pharmacological characteristics of the release of pancreatic glucagon in response to stimulation of the splanchnic nerves, J Physiol. 280:25 (1978)

50. P. L. Werner, J. W. Benson, J. B. Brodsky, P. M. Hollander, C. M. Asplin, D. G. Johnson and J. P. Palmer, Comparison of glucagon responses to 2-deoxy-D-glucose and hypoglycaemia in man, Am J Physiol. 239:E227 (1980)

51. S. R. Bloom and A. V. Edwards, Pancreatic endocrine responses to stimulation of the peripheral ends of the splanchnic nerves in the conscious adrenalectomised calf, J Physiol. 308:39 (1980).

52. E. Samols, G. C. Weir, Y. C. Patel, S. W. Loo and K. H. Gabbay, Autonomic control of somatostatin and pancreatic secretion by isolated perfused pancreas, Clin Res. 28:499 (1977)

53. D. Berge, J. C. Floyd, R. M. Lampmam and S. S. Fajans, The effect of adrenergic receptor blockade on the exercise induced rise in pancreatic polypeptide in man, J Clin Endocrinol Metab. 50:33 (1980)

54. M. W. Roy, M. S. Jones and R. E. Miller, Pancreatic somatostatin secretion is suppressed by pancreatic nerve stimulation, Diabetologia. 20:102 (1981)

55. V. Schusdziarra, D. Rouiller, V. Harris, R. Dey and R. H. Unger, Plasma somatostatin like immunoreactivity in chemically sympathectomised dogs, Horm Metab Res. 12:656 (1980)

56. T. Hokfelt, L. G. Elfvin, R. Elde, M. Schultz, M. Goldstein and R. Luft, Occurrences of somatostatin like immunoreactivity in some peripheral sympathetic noradrenergic neurones, Proc Natl Acad Sci USA. 74:3587 (1977)

57. L. I. Larsson, Innervation of the pancreas by substance P, enkephalin, vasoactive intestinal peptide and gastrin/CCK immunoreactive nerves, J Histochem Cytochem. 27:1283 (1979)

58. A. E. Bishop, J. M. Polak, I. C. Green, M. G. Bryant and S. R. Bloom, Location of VIP in the pancreas of man and rat, Diabetologia. 18:73 (1980)

59. M. Schebalin, S. I. Said and G. M. Maklouf, Stimulation of insulin and glucagon secretion by vasoactive intestinal peptide, Am J Physiol. 232:E197 (1977)

60. E. Ipp, R. E. Dobbs and R. H. Unger, Vasoactive intestinal peptide stimulates pancreatic somatostatin release, Febs Lett. 90:76 (1978)

61. B. Ahren and I. Lundquist, Effects of vasoactive intestinal polypeptide (VIP), secretin and gastrin on insulin secretion in the mouse, Diabetologia. 20:54 (1981)

62. J. M. Lundberg, B. Hedlund, and T. Burtfai, Vasoactive intestinal polypeptide enhances muscarinic ligand binding in cat submandibular salivary gland, Nature. 295:147 (1982)

63. J. F. Rehfeld, L. I. Larsson, N. R. Goltermann, T. W. Schwartz, J. J. Holst, S. L. Jensen and J, S, Morley, Neural regulation of pancreatic hormone secretion by the C-terminal tetrapeptide of CCK, Nature. 284,33 (1980)

64. G. J. Dockray, R. A. Gregory, J. F. Rehfeld, L. I. Larsson, N. R. Goltermann, T. W. Schwartz, S. L. Jensen and J. S. Morley, Does the C-terminal tetrapeptide of gastrin and CCK exist as an entity? Nature. 286:742 (1980)

65. J F Rehfeld and S L Jensen, The effect of gastrin and cholecystokinin on the endocrine pancreas, Front Hormone Res. 7:107 (1980)

66. R M Williams and J Champagne, Effects of cholecystokinin, secretin and pancreatic polypeptide on secretion of GIP, insulin and glucagon, Life Sci. 25:947 (1979)

67. B. Ahren and I. Lundquist, Effects of two cholecystokinin variants, CCK39 and CCK8 on basal and stimulated insulin secretion, Acta Diabet Lat. 18, 3: 347 (1981)

68. J. B. Furness and M. Costa, Types of nerves in the enteric nervous system, Neuroscience. 5:1(1980)

69. T. J. MacDonald, H. Jornvall, G. Nilsson, M. Vagne, M. Ghatei, S. R. Bloom and V. Mutt, Characterisation of a gastrin releasing peptide from porcine non-antral gastric tissue, Biochem and Biophys Res Commun. 90:227 (1979)

70. N. Yanaihara, C. Yanaihara, T. Mochizuki, K. Iwahara, T. Fujita and T. Iwanaga, Immunoreactive GRP, Peptides 2. Suppl 2: 185 (1981)

71. E. Ipp and R. H. Unger, Bombesin stimulates the release of insulin and glucagon, but not pancreatic somatostatin from the isolated perfused dog pancreas, Endocrine Res Commun. 6:37 (1979)

72. M. A. Ghatei, R. T. Jung, J. C. Stevenson, C. J. Hillyard, T. E. Adrian, Y. C. Lee, N. D. Christofides, D. L. Sarson, K. Mashiter, I. McIntyre and S. R. Bloom, Bombesin: Action on gut hormones and calcium in man, J Clin Endocrinol Metab. 54:980 (1982)

73. T J MacDonald, M A Ghatei, S R Bloom, N S Track, J Radziuk, J Dupre and V Mutt, A qualitative comparison of canine plasma gastroenteropancreatic hormone responses to bombesin and the porcine gastrin releasing peptide (GRP). Regul Pept. 2:293 (1981)

74. N. Vaysse, L. Pradayrol, J. A. Chayvialle, F. Pignal, J. O. Esteve, C. Susini, F. Descos and A. Ribet, Effect of somatostatin-14 and somatostatin-28 on bombesin stimulated release of gastrin, insulin and glucagon in the dog, Endocrinology. 108:1843 (1981)

75. R. Carraway and L. E. Leeman, The isolation of a new hypotensive peptide, neurotensin from bovine hypothalami, J Biol Chem. 248:6854 (1973)

76. R. Carraway and L. E. Leeman, Radioimmunoassay for neurotensin, a hypothalamic peptide, J Biol Chem. 251:7035 (1976)

77. J. Dolais-Kitabgi, P. Kitabgi, P. Brazeau and P. Freychet, Effect of neurotensin on insulin, glucagon and somatostatin release from isolated pancreatic islets, Endocrinology. 105:256 (1979)

78. A. M. Blackburn, D. R. Fletcher, T. E. Adrian and S. R. Bloom, Neurotensin infusions in man:Pharmacokinetics and effect on gastrointestinal and pituitary hormones, J Clin Endocrinol Metab. 51:1257 (1980)

79. I. Lundquist, F. Sundler, B. Ahren, J. Aluments and R. Hakanson, Somatostatin, pancreatic polypeptide, substance P and neurotensin: Cellular distribution and effects on stimulated insulin secretion in the mouse, Endocrinology. 104:832 (1979)

80. I. C. Green, D. Perrin, K. C. Pedley, R. D. G. Leslie and D. A. Pyke, Effect of enkephalins and morphine on insulin secretion from isolated rat islets, Diabetologia. 19:158 (2980)

81. R. D. G. Leslie, D. A. Pyke and W. A. Stubbs, Sensitivity to enkephalin as a cause of non-insulin dependent diabetes, Lancet. II:341 (1979)

82. G. J. Dockray, C. Vaillant and R. G. Williams, New vertebrate brain-gut peptide related to a mollusion neuropeptide and opioid peptide, Nature. 293:656 (1981)

83. K. Tatemoto and V. Mutt, Isolation of two novel candidate hormones using a chemical method for finding naturally occurring polypeptides, Nature. 285:417 (1980)

84. K. Szecowka, K. Tatemoto, V. Mutt and S. Efendic, Interaction of a newly isolated intestinal polypeptide (PHI) with glucose and arginine to effect the secretion of insulin and glucagon, Life Sciences. 26:435 (1980)

85. L. Hermansen, Effects on substance P and other peptides on the release of somatostatin, insulin, and glucagon in vitro, Endocrinology. 107:256 (1980)

NEURO-HORMONAL CONTROL OF EXOCRINE PANCREATIC SECRETION IN HUMANS AND ANIMALS

Manfred V Singer

Universitätsklinikum Essen
Medizinische Klinik und Poliklinik
Abt Gastroenterologie
Hufelandstr 55, D-4300 Essen 1
Federal Republic of Germany

It is generally believed and written in many current medical text books that gastrointestinal hormones play a dominant physiological role in the control of pancreatic exocrine secretion in response to a meal. Many effects of vagal cholinergic nerves on pancreatic secretion are believed to be due to indirect effects on hormone release rather than direct effects on the pancreas. However, several recent studies support an important role for direct cholinergic vagal regulation of both enzyme and bicarbonate secretion from the pancreas.

The debate whether the nervous system or the hormones are more important in the regulation of pancreatic secretion under physiological conditions originated in 1902 when Bayliss and Starling discovered the "first" hormone secretin and induced the completely new concept of blood-borne chemical messengers or hormones. Being unable to repeat Pavlov's observations on the effects of peripheral vagal stimulation, they drew the premature conclusion that "the nervous process of pancreatic secretion is superfluous and therefore improbable" (Bayliss and Starling, 1902). Until the discovery of secretin, the doctrine of "nervism" which stated that most of the body functions are regulated by the nervous system was the predominant view. During the last 70 years scientists were preoccupied with the isolation and synthesis of the many newly discovered peptide hormones of the gut. Neural influences on the secretion of the pancreas were almost completely neglected. This imbalance is now being redressed because recent studies show the outstanding importance of nerves for the regulation of gastrointestinal function. Comparisons concerning the relative importance of hormonal and nervous mechanisms have been made in the almost complete absence of knowledge of the complexity of both neuro-hormonal and hormonal-hormonal relationships, and the extent to which different regions of the gut affect the pancreas. Thus, we are just about beginning to understand these complex inter-relationships.

Neither the function nor the control mechanisms of the inter-digestive (basal) pancreatic exocrine secretion are understood. Boldyreff (1911) noted that cyclic pancreatic flow occurs in the dog coincident with periodic contractions of the upper small intestine. Only recently we have learned that also in humans that there is a close association of pancreatic interdigestive secretion into the duodenum and the different phases of duodenal motor activity. There were distinct differences in the duodenal enzyme output of the pancreas between the four phases of duodenal interdigestive motor activity; increased pancreatic enzyme output started during phase II and peaked just before the onset of phase III. Peak enzyme secretory activity associated with the migrating motor complex reached about one third of maximal secretory rates.

Possible control mechanisms of interdigestive pancreatic secretions are:

1. an inherent automaticity of the gland,
2. a continuous or phasic secretion of gastrointestinal hormones such as secretin and cholecystokinin, at very low levels,
3. release of acetylcholine and other transmitters by the extrinsic and intrinsic innervation of the gland.

The control of pancreatic exocrine secretion in response to a meal has been traditionally divided for descriptive purposes into three phases - cephalic, gastric and intestinal - according to the site at which the stimuli act. These phases, however, are not separate but overlap one another in the time sequence of digestion. The main secretory nerves of the pancreas are the vagus nerves. Pancreatic bicarbonate and enzyme responses to stimuli of the cephalic and gastric phases are, directly or indirectly, mediated by the vagus nerves. The only identified hormonal mediator of the gastric phase is gastrin. In humans and some animals, such as the dog and cat, the cephalic and gastric phases of pancreatic exocrine secretion affect pancreatic enzyme output rather than the secretion of water and bicarbonate.

The intestinal phase is quantitatively the most important for the pancreatic response to a meal. The reduced pancreatic response to a meal after vagotomy is mainly due to a decreased response to intestinal stimuli. During the intestinal phase of pancreatic response to a meal pancreatic water and bicarbonate outputs are mainly stimulated by the hormone secretin, which is released by gastric acid entering the duodenum. Another important mechanism is the potentia-

tion of secretin action by neuro-hormonal and hormonal-hormonal interactions.   There is evidence for cholinergic vagal effects of pancreatic bicarbonate secretion.   Bicarbonate response to low, but
not high, doses of secretin may be decreased after vagotomy, suggesting that acetylcholine potentiates the action of secretin.   Vagotomy or atropine decrease the intestinal response to HCl, but neither
affects immunoreactive secretin release.   This suggests that basally
released acetylcholine (and perhaps acetylcholine released by HCl
via an enteropancreatic vago-vagal reflex) and secretin released
by HCl interact at the cellular sites of pancreatic bicarbonate
secretion.

Pancreatic enzyme secretion during the intestinal phase was
generally believed to be mediated exclusively by the hormone cholecystokinin.   However, recent work has provided strong evidence for
the existence of enteropancreatic cholinergic vago-vagal reflexes,
mediating the pancreatic enzyme response to intestinal stimuli such
as amino acids, fatty acids and HCl.   Observations of the behaviour
of a transplanted pancreas, and the effects of truncal vagotomy and
atropine on the secretory response of the transplanted pancreas and
the intact in situ pancreas, have supported the hypothesis that enteropancreatic reflexes are quantitatively important mediators of
the pancreatic enzyme response to intestinal stimulants.

During the recent years, considerable evidence has been accumu-
lated demonstrating that inhibitory as well as stimulatory factors
act to regulate pancreatic exocrine secretion.   Several polypeptides, such as somatostatin, pancreatic polypeptide, glucagon and
enkephalins have been shown to inhibit pancreatic secretion when
given exogenously.   Whether these agents are of physiological importance remains to be established.   Inhibition of exocrine pancreatic secretion has also been shown to be induced by hyperglycaemia
and ileal or colonic perfusion with oleate.   The resulting inhibition of pancreatic secretion has been postulated to be due to release
of the hormone called "pancreatone" or "anticholecystokinin peptide"
(ACP).   There is also evidence for neurally mediated inhibition of
pancreatic secretion acting by way of the splanchnic nerves.

The concept of paracrine secretion has only recently emerged,
and is a hypothetical concept, not an established mechanism.   For
endocrine (hormonal) secretion, measurement of blood peptide concentrations gives an index of how much has been released from the stores
and is available for action on target cells.   For paracrine secretion, we do not have comparable methods for measuring the released
peptide available for action on target cells.   Only in the case of
somatostatin, there is a good structural basis for possible paracrine
function in the pancreas and the stomach.   Long processes extend
from antral somatostatin cells to adjacent cells, including G cells,
thus supporting the idea that this peptide may act on adjacent cells
without entering the circulation.   The discovery of the paracrine

mechanism makes the understanding of regulation of exocrine pancreatic secretion even more complex than has been believed so far.

SUGGESTED REFERENCES FOR FURTHER READING

Malagelada J.-R.:
Gastric, pancreatic, and biliary responses to a meal.
Physiology of the Gastrointestinal Tract, edited by L.R. Johnson,
Raven Press, New York 1981, 893-924.

Meyer J.H.:
Control of pancreatic exocrine secretion.
Physiology of the Gastrointestinal Tract, edited by L.R. Johnson,
Raven Press, New York 1981, 821-829.

Singer M.V., T.E. Solomon and M.I. Grossman:
Effects of atropine on secretion from intact and transplanted pancreas in the dog.
Am. J. Physiol. 238: G18-22 (1980).

Singer M.V., T.E. Solomon, J. Wood and M.I. Grossman:
Latency of pancreatic enzyme response to intraduodenal stimulants.
Am. J. Physiol. 238: G23-29 (1980).

Singer M.V., T.E. Solomon, H. Rammert, F. Caspary, W. Niebel,
H. Goebell and M.I. Grossman:
Effect of atropine on pancreatic response to HCl and secretin.
Am. J. Physiol. 240: G376-380 (1981).

Singer M.V., W. Niebel, D. Hoffmeister, J. Elsahoff and H. Goebell:
Dose response effects on pancreatic response to low doses of secretin.
Gastroenterology 82: 1182 (1982) (Abstract).

Singer M.V.:
Latency of pancreatic fluid secretory response to intestinal
stimulants in the dog.
J. Physiol. 339: 75-85 (1983).

Solomon T.E. and M.I. Grossman:
Effect of atropine and vagotomy on transplanted pancreas.
Am. J. Physiol. 236: E186-190 (1979).

Solomon T.E.:
Neuro-hormonal control of the pancreas.
In: Gut Hormones, edited by S.R. Bloom and J.M. Polak, Churchill
Livingstone, Edinburgh, London, Melbourne and New York 1981,
499-503.

ACUTE AND CHRONIC ACTIONS OF ALCOHOL ON PANCREATIC EXOCRINE

SECRETION IN HUMANS AND ANIMALS

Manfred V Singer

Universitatslkinikum Essn
Abt fur Gastroenterologie
Hufelandstr 55, 4300 Essen 1
Federal Republic of Germany

There is considerable experimental evidence that acute and
chronic administration of ethanol induces secretory modifications
of the pancreas in humans and laboratory animals.   Acute intravenous administration of ethanol inhibits the stimulation by secretin
and cholecystokinin of pancreatic water, bicarbonate and protein in
non-alcoholic humans and most species of animals tested.   In vitro
studies suggest a direct toxic action of ethanol on the pancreatic
acinar and ductal cells, but the precise mechanism has not been
identified.   Since atropine, pentolinium and truncal vagotomy diminished the ethanol-induced inhibition of pancreatic exocrine secretion in the intact animal, it was postulated that the action of
ethanol on the pancreas is at least partly mediated by inhibitory
cholinergic mechanisms (eg inhibitory fibres of the vagal nerves).
Whether the extrinsic and intrinsic peptidergic nerves and paracrine
transmitters are involved is not known.   It is also conceivable
that intravenous ethanol inhibits hormonally induced pancreatic
secretion by blocking the pancreatic response to these secretagogues
(eg by distorting their receptors).

Ethanol given intragastrically (without diversion of gastric
juice) or intraduodenally has been shown to produce either no change
or a slight and variable increase in basal (interdigestive) and hormonally induced pancreatic exocrine secretion in humans and other
animal species.   With intragastric instillation of ethanol in laboratory animals this stimulatory action is probably due to release
of gastrin by ethanol and subsequent direct (gastrin itself) and
indirect (acid secreted in response to gastrin causing secretin release) effects on the pancreas.   In humans, however, it is uncert-
tain whether the mechanism is operative.   The stimulatory action
of intraduodenal ethanol on the pancreas might be mediated either

281

by neural reflexes or the release of gastrointestinal hormones.

Little is known about the releasing action of ethanol on gastro-intestinal hormones. In humans, whisky or pure ethanol in different concentrations do not stimulate gastrin release. Beer, red and white wine, however, are potent gastrin releasers. Neither pure alcohol nor the above-mentioned alcoholic beverages release pancreatic polypeptide in humans. In dogs, only a high dose (2.7g/kg body weight) of intragastric ethanol caused a small increase in plasma levels of pancreatic polypeptide which was only 12% of the response seen after a meal. Therefore, it is unlikely that pancreatic polypeptide is the hormonal mediator of the ethanol-induced inhibition of exocrine pancreatic secretion in humans and dogs. Whether the inhibitory action of ethanol is mediated by release of other gastrointestinal hormones, eg neurotensin, has not been studied.

The results of the action of chronic alcoholism on interdigestive (basal) pancreatic secretion in humans and animals are inconclusive. There is some evidence that in chronic alcoholic humans and dogs basal secretion of pancreatic enzymes is increased whereas bicarbonate output and water putput are decreased.

Pancreatic response to intravenous ethanol is different in non-alcoholic and alcoholic dogs, and depends on the duration of chronic alcoholism. In dogs receiving ethanol 2g/kg intragastrically each day for at least 12 months, an intravenous infusion of ethanol (1.5 g/kg) no longer inhibited but increased the hormonally stimulated pancreatic bicarbonate and protein output. In alcoholic men, the reversal of the action of intravenous ethanol was not observed, but the inhibitory action of alcohol disappeared. As stated earlier, atropine prevented the ethanol-induced inhibition of pancreatic secretion in the non-alcoholic period; it also prevented the stimulatory action of intravenous ethanol on the dog pancreas after one year of chronic alcoholism.

After 12 and 24 months of alcoholism, protein output by the pancreas in response to cholecystokinin was not modified. After only 6 months of chronic ethanol feeding the maximal volume and bicarbonate responses to secretin were higher in chronic alcoholic than in control dogs. This was still the case after 12 and 24 months of ethanol feeding. Atropine did not alter the bicarbonate response in alcoholic or non-alcoholic dogs. Paradoxically secretin stimulated the protein output in alcoholic but not in non-alcoholic dogs.

As soon as 6 weeks of chronic alcohol administration, dogs secreted precipitates of protein through the pancreatic cannula. According to Sarles, these precipitates consist of proteins normally found in pancreatic juice and are believed to be due to their hyperconcentration by ethanol. Intraductal proteins form the matrix of

282

calcified pancreatic calculi.   The 3-dimensional anatomical studies
of the pancreas suggest that protein-precipitates and calculi form
the first lesion of chronic pancreatitis in man.   In alcoholics
without pancreatic disease, the concentration of protein in pancreatic juice was found to be higher than in non-alcoholic controls.

The protein-precipitates as well as the pancreatic stones can
be dissolved in vivo and in vitro by citrate and other calcium
chelators.

Recently, the group of Sarles has found a protein which they
call "pancreatic stone protein" and which constitutes a stable fraction of juice protein in controls, in alcoholics without pancreatic
lesions and in patients with acute pancreatitis amounting to 18%
of total pancreatic juice protein.   From preliminary observations
it would appear that the concentration of this protein is low in congenital and in alcoholic calcified pancreatitis.   The authors specu-
lated that this reduced concentration of pancreatic stone protein
could explain the spontaneous development of hereditary pancreatitis
and the individual risk of developing alcoholic pancreatitis.

Little is known about the basal and stimulated plasma concentrations of gastrointestinal hormones in chronic alcoholic humans
and animals.   Normal, decreased or increased basal levels of gastrin have been found in chronic alcoholic humans.   The same is
true for basal and stimulated gastric acid secretion in patients
with chronic alcoholic pancreatitis.   In one study, plasma gastrin
levels in response to a meal were higher in patients with chronic
alcoholic pancreatitis or in "normal" alcoholics than in non-alcoholic controls.   In chronic alcoholic dogs lower plasma levels of
secretin in response to intraduodenal HCl have been found than in
non-alcoholic control dogs.   Whether the release of other gastrointestinal hormones such as cholecystokinin, VIP, somatostatin and
pancreatic polypeptide is altered by chronic alcoholism has not been
studied systematically.

In chronic alcoholism the dietary regimen associated with alcohol feeding seems to be important for the action of alcohol on the
pancreas.   In rats, ethanol feeding together with a diet rich in
protein and fat resulted in an increased pancreatic enzyme secretion,
whereas the opposite action was seen with a diet low in fat and protein.   Contrary to the results in dog, studies on the long-term
effect of ethanol feeding on the pancreas of rats have given con-
tradictory results and are therefore inconclusive.   In humans, it
has been shown that the risk of developing chronic pancreatitis
increases logarithmically with rising alcohol consumption.   High
protein intake, and both high and low fat intake, clearly increase
the risk.   There is a logarithmic increase in the risk with high
protein intake, but the effect of protein is much less than that of

alcohol.   In the case of fat intake, the lowest risk was observed
with an average diet (containing 80-110g per day), the highest with
a high fat diet, and an intermediate risk with a low fat diet.   The
effect of alcohol, protein and fat was additive.   While in Europe
chronic alcoholic pancreatitis is often associated with a high alcohol, high fat, high protein diet, a recent North American study found
that the disease occurred with low fat and protein intakes but an
alcohol consumption which was much higher than in European series.

In conclusion, despite the many animal and the few human studies
the mechanisms by which chronic oral ingestion of alcohol influence
the pancreas are still not defined.   Whether ethanol-induced changes
in the release of gastrointestinal hormones and/or alterations of
the neural tone of the pancreas are responsible for the effects of
chronic alcoholism on the pancreas is still speculative.   In addition, there is still a lot of descriptive work to do.   Thus, under
well-controlled conditions dose-response curves of basal and hormonally stimulated pancreatic response to increasing doses of ethanol
given by different routes need to be done.   There are also no studies on the action of different doses of ethanol on pancreatic dose-
response curves to intestinal stimulants such as HCl, amino acids
and fatty acids.   The action of acute and chronic ethanol administered on the different phases of basal pancreatic secretion needs
to be clarified, as do the close inter-relationships between the
interdigestive motor complex and pancreatic exocrine secretion.
Since in the animal species studied so far, pancreatic lesions
similar to chronic alcoholic human pancreatitis could not be produced
we should search for a more suitable model to elucidate the action
of chronic alcohol feeding.

The acute action of alcoholic beverages on exocrine pancreatic
secretion in humans is completely unknown.   Since humans rarely
ingest pure ethanol and since other constituents of alcoholic beverages such as beer, wine, liquor, cognac, vodka and whisky should
be tested.

REFERENCES

Sarles H.:
Chronic calcifying pancreatitis - chronic alcoholic pancreatitis.
Gastroenterology 66: 604 (1974).

Sarles H., R.C. Cros and J.M. Bidart and the International Group
for the Study of Pancreatic Diseases:
A multi-center inquiry into the etiology of pancreatic diseases.
Digestion 19: 110 (1979).

Sarles H., O. Tiscornia and G. Palasciano:
Chronic alcoholism and canine exocrine pancreas secretion: A long

term follow-up study.
Gastroenterology 72: 238 (1977).

Sarles H., J. Sahel, G. Palasciano, Y. Capitaine and J. Meullenet:
Alcohol consumption and the human pancreas.
1. Alcohol induced modifications of exocrine function.
INSERM 95: 289 (1980).

Sarles H., F. Clemente, E. Colomb and A. De Caro:
Alcohol consumption and the human pancreas.
2. Alcohol induced chemical and physical modifications of pancreatic juice.   Formation of the lesions.
INSERM 95: 315 (1980).

Schmidt D.:
Studies on neurohormonal control of exocrine pancreas in dogs.
Effects of chronic ethanol feeding.
Thesis, Stockholm, Sweden 1983.

Schmidt D.N., H. Sarles and M.-A. Devaux:
Early increased pancreatic secretory capacity during alcohol adap-
tation in the dog.
Scand. J. Gastroent. 17: 49 (1982).

Schmidt D.N., M.-A. Devaux, T.M. Biedzinski and H. Sarles:
Disappearance of an inhibitory factor of exocrine pancreas secre-
tion in chronic alcoholic dogs.
Scand. J. Gastroent. 17: 761 (1982).

Singer M.V.:
Acute and chronic effects of ethanol on exocrine function in
animals.
Symposium International sur l'alcool et le tractus digestif
Bischenberg-Strasbourg (France), 6-8 Mars, 1980
INSERM 95: 339 (1980).

Singer M.V., V. Eysselein and H. Goebell:
Pancreatic polypeptide response to intragastric ethanol in humans
and dogs.
Reg. Pept. 6: 13 (1983).

Singer M.V., V. Eysselein and H. Goebell:
Beer and wine but not whisky and pure ethanol do stimulate release
of gastrin in humans.
Digestion 26: 73 (1983).

Singer M.V., H. Calden, V. Eysselein and H. Goebell:
Bier stimuliert stark, seine Inhaltsstoffe Äthanol und Aminosäuren
hingegen nur schwach die Magensäuresekretion des Menschen.

38. Tagung der Deutschen Gesellschaft für Verdauungsund Stoff-
wechselkrankheiten, 8.-10.9. 1983 in München Z. Gastroenterologie
21: 420 (1983).

DOPAMINE ANTAGONISTS AS ANTI-EMETICS AND AS STIMULANTS OF GASTRIC MOTILITY

Brian McRitchie, Christine M. McClelland, Stephen M. Cooper, David H. Turner and Gareth J. Sanger

Beecham Pharmaceuticals, Medicinal Research Centre
Coldharbour Road, The Pinnacles, Harlow, Essex. U.K.

Dopamine antagonists are commonly used to treat the symptoms of psychosis, where abnormal dopaminergic neuro-transmission in the brain is thought to be the primary cause of the illness[1,2]. Some dopamine antagonists however are not "anti-psychotic", because they do not easily cross the blood-brain barrier or they only weakly antagonise the dopamine receptors involved in psychosis[3]. Among this latter group of antagonists are drugs which are used clinically to inhibit nausea and vomiting caused by a large number of different stimuli. Examples of such drugs include the substituted benzamides metoclopramide and clebopride, and the butyrophenone derivative, domperidone (Fig. 1).

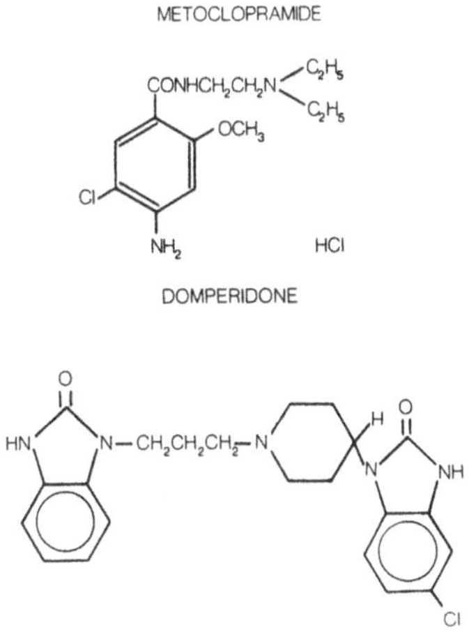

Fig. 1.

Dopamine antagonists prevent nausea and vomiting because they block the effects of dopamine in the emetic chemoreceptor trigger zone[4]. The trigger zone is located in the area postrema on the floor of the fourth ventricle, a region of the brain which is only poorly protected by the blood-brain barrier and so is responsive to many types of chemical stimuli carried in the blood and cerebrospinal fluid[5]. A dopaminergic-dependent mechanism mediates the chemorecptor response and this is then relayed to the vomiting centre in the medulla oblongata, which is responsible for co-ordinating the emetic reflex[6,7].

Emesis is not always caused by chemical stimuli acting on the chemoreceptor trigger zone and there are examples of emesis which tend to be resistant to dopamine antagonists. However, metoclopramide and domperidone have been shown to be effective antagonists of post-operative nausea and vomiting, a variety of drug-induced emesis (including emesis caused by certain analgesics or cytotoxic drugs used in cancer chemotherapy), radiation sickness and nausea and vomiting associated with a wide variety of conditions such as recurrent gastritis, migraine and dysmenorrhoea[8,9,10].

In addition to preventing dopamine-mediated emesis, certain dopamine antagonists also stimulate gastrointestinal motility. This unique action occurs mostly in the stomach and upper small intestine. Secretion of gastric acid is not affected (for metoclopramide and domperidone see[9,10]). Metoclopramide is therefore widely used to treat disorders of gut function, such as dyspepsia, reflux oesophagitis and gastric stasis associated with a variety of clinical conditions. In addition, the increased gastrointestinal motility caused by metoclopramide is used to achieve a more rapid passage of barium meals and to aid gastrological intubation procedures[8,11,10].

The following experiments briefly illustrate some of the properties of dopamine antagonists by comparing the effects of metoclopramide and domperidone on various animal models. The pharmacology of clebopride is described elsewhere[12].

INHIBITION OF APOMORPHINE-INDUCED EMESIS

The anti-emetic efficacy of metoclopramide and domperidone were assessed in groups of 8 beagle dogs of either sex (12-18kg weight), by measuring their ability to inhibit apomorphine-induced emesis. Drugs were injected subcutaneously (s.c.) 30 min prior to the apomorphine (0.1mg/kg s.c.) challenge. Metoclopramide and domperidone dose-dependently antagonised the emetic action of apomorphine. For each antagonist, the doses required to give complete protection from emesis in 50% of animals (ED_{50} values) were respectively 0.1 and 0.01mg/kg. These results are broadly in agreement with other studies in dogs[13].

Despite the relatively high potency of domperidone in the dog, similar doses of metoclopramide and domperidone are normally recommended for use in adult humans (10mg 3 or 4 times a day) and there is little clinical data to suggest any marked difference in the anti-emetic efficacy of these doses of metoclopramide and domperidone[9]. However, one noteable advantage of metoclopramide is that high intravenous doses give effective protection against vomiting caused by strongly emetic drugs used in cancer chemotherapy[14]. This contrasts with the poor protection given by the normally recommended doses of metoclopramide (see [14]), prochlorperazine[14] and high intravenous doses of domperidone[15]. Further studies are necessary to establish the precise mechanism of action of high-dose metoclopramide, as well as the optimum regimen for dosing in patients receiving cancer chemotherapy.

STIMULATION OF GASTRIC MOTILITY AND FACILITATION OF GASTRIC EMPTYING

Gastric motility is a term which comprises a number of different, complex patterns of stomach activity occurring during both 'fasting' and 'fed' conditions. In many fasting animals, including man, a relatively quiescent gastric motility is interrupted approximately every 90 min by a burst of contractile activity which is propagated the entire length of the gut, propelling undigested stomach contents in an aboral direction (known as the interdigestive "housekeeper" or migrating motor complex[16,17]). After feeding, the pattern of motility is replaced by a continuous gastric activity responsible for the efficient mixing and gradual emptying of the stomach contents. The duration of this type of gastric motility depends on the physical and chemical composition of the ingested food[18]. Finally, all gastric motility is subject to modulation by humoral and nervous systems, particularly those originating in the gut and the central nervous system[18].

We now describe the effects of metoclopramide and domperidone on two simple models of gastric motility. Firstly we investigated the effects of the drugs on the resting, spontaneous gastric activity in conscious rats. Secondly we looked for an action on the ability of the rat stomach to empty a liquid test meal. For both experiments, conscious male Wistar rats (200-500g weight) were used, which had been previously implanted with a chronic gastric fistula[19]. The rats were fasted overnight and then individually restrained in Bollman cages prior to each experiment.

Resting gastric activity was assessed from the amplitude of the pressure waves recorded via the gastric fistula over a 40 min period, before and after drug administration. Rats with a low level of gastric activity (mean amplitude <4mm Hg) were pre-selected for use, aiding the detection of drug-induced stimulation of activity. Metoclopramide increased the amplitude of pressure waves (Fig. 2).

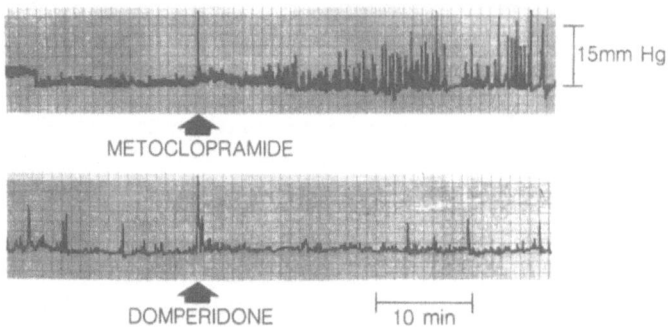

Fig. 2. Effects of metoclopramide and domperidone 5mg/kg s.c. on
the intragastric pressure changes in the chronic gastric
fistula rat. The upper trace shows the effects of administration of metoclopramide. The lower trace is from an
experiment using domperidone in a different rat.

Stimulation in each animal was of an "all or none" nature, and the
number of animals responding to metoclopramide increased with dose
over the range 0.25 to 10mg/kg administered s.c. or intragastrically
(see Fig. 3 for s.c. results). The mean ± sem increase in amplitude
in responding animals was 95 ± 16%. There were no consistent effects
of metoclopramide on either the frequency of contractions or the
baseline pressure of the stomach. Domperidone 0.25-10mg/kg did not
increase gastric activity at any dose tested, when injected s.c.
(Fig. 3) or by the intragastric route (not shown).

    The effects of metoclopramide and domperidone on gastric
emptying was assessed by measuring the recovery of a 5ml liquid test
meal of 33mM citric acid, containing phenol red 100µg/ml as a non-
absorbable marker. This test meal was chosen as it would empty from
the stomach slower than an equivalent water or saline meal[20], thereby
facilitating the detection of responses to drugs which stimulate the
rate of gastric emptying. The test meal was recovered 10 min after
instillation into the stomach via the gastric fistula. Metoclopramide
significantly increased the gastric emptying when injected s.c. 15
min prior to administration of the test meal (Table 1). Domperidone
10 or 25mg/kg s.c. had no significant effects on gastric emptying
(Table 1).

290

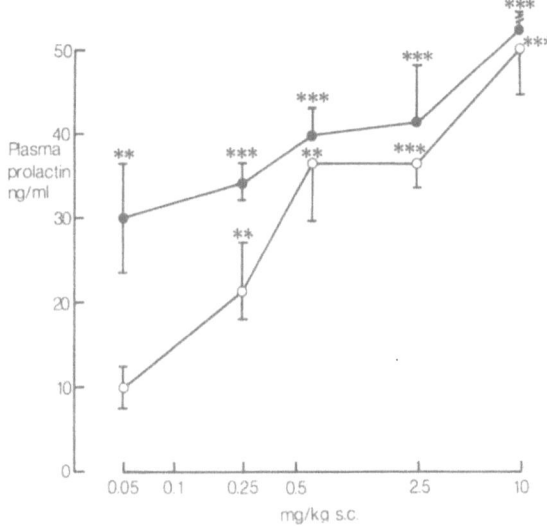

Fig. 3. Effects of metoclopramide and domperidone on the intragastric
pressure in the conscious rat. The columns represent the
number of animals which responded with a significant increase
in intragastric pressure after s.c. injection of metoclopramide (left-hand columns) or domperidone (right-hand
columns); n=10 each. The increase in the number of animals
responding with metoclopramide was dose-dependent, whereas
domperidone had no excitatory effects. For both drugs, doses
of 50mg/kg s.c. reduced intragastric pressure activity in
all animals.

Thus, the results show that metoclopramide increases gastric
motility and stomach emptying in the rat. Similar effects of
metoclopramide have been described in man, on motility recorded during
fasting and for gastric emptying of both liquids and solids[10]. In
contrast, domperidone did not stimulate rat gastric resting activity
or the emptying of the liquid test meal. In man, domperidone can
increase the motility of the gastrointestinal tract, but this is not
always a consistent action and domperidone is of doubtful benefit in
reflux oesophagitis[9], a condition which is usually successfully
treated by metoclopramide[8,10]. This reduced effectiveness of
domperidone may reflect differences in the mechanisms by which
metoclopramide and domperidone stimulate gastric motility. Unlike
metoclopramide, domperidone does not increase cholinergic-mediated
contractions in isolated muscle strips from rat[21] or human stomach
(unpublished). However, domperidone potently antagonises dopamine
and α_1-adrenoceptor-mediated inhibition of gastric motility[9]. It may
therefore be possible to detect an action of domperidone in situations
where gastric motility is reduced by an action of catecholamines.

291

Table 1: Effects of metoclopramide and domperidone on the gastric emptying of a citric acid liquid test meal in the chronic gastric fistula rat.

Drug	Dose mg/kg s.c.	% test meal emptied in 10 min. mean ± s.e.m. (n)		% Increase in emptying
		Vehicle	Drug	
METOCLOPRAMIDE	10	42.5 ± 1.5 (6)	57.3 ± 3.1 (6)	35*
DOMPERIDONE	10	66.2 ± 4.9 (6)	69.8 ± 4.7 (6)	5
	25	47.2 ± 3.1 (5)	52.0 ± 5.6 (5)	10

Comparisons were made between the vehicle and drug-treated groups of rats using a Student's 't' test ($*P < 0.05$)

Noradrenaline and adrenaline are involved in the inhibition of gastrointestinal motility caused by stress or by various inhibitory
reflexes[22,23], but the importance of a dopamine-mediated control of
gastric motility is uncertain. Dopamine may be detected in the
mucosal enterochromaffin cells, but it seems unlikely that the amine
acts as a neurotransmitter intrinsic to the gut[24]. In addition,
experiments with several different isolated gastrointestinal tissues
show that it is difficult to detect an action of dopamine on the
smooth muscle membrane or on the cholinergic nerves which is not
blocked by antagonists of α- and/or β-adrenoceptor-mediated responses
[25,26,27,28]. Nevertheless, despite the uncertainty concerning the
physiological significance of a dopamine in controlling gastric
motility, we have tested the ability of metoclopramide and domperidone
to antagonise the reduction of gastric emptying caused by a rigid
analogue of dopamine. We used 6,7-dihydroxyaminotetralin (6,7-ADTN),
which only poorly penetrates the blood-brain barrier and therefore
behaves as a peripheral dopamine agonist[29].

6,7-ADTN was injected subcutaneously into chronic gastric fistula
rats, 15 min before instillation into the stomach of a 5ml liquid
test meal containing phenol red 100µg/ml in tris buffer pH 9.0.
After 10 min the remainder of the meal was withdrawn and the effects
of 6,7-ADTN on the gastric emptying were calculated. 15 min pretreatment with 6,7-ADTN 0.04 to 50mg/kg s.c. caused a dose-dependent
inhibition of gastric emptying. In the following experiments with
metoclopramide and domperidone, a dose of 1mg/kg s.c. 6,7-ADTN was
used, slowing gastric emptying by approximately 50% of the maximum
reduction obtained with 6,7-ADTN. The mean ± sem percentage of
test meal emptied from the stomach in the 10 min period after this
dose of 6,7-ADTN was 53 ± 3.6% compared with 79 ± 2.0% in the vehicle
control group (P<0.001, n=18 each group). Injection of metoclopramide
1 to 10mg/kg s.c. or domperidone 1 to 5mg/kg s.c. 5 min after injection of 6,7-ADTN significantly increased the gastric emptying (Table
2). In similar experiments, the inhibitory effects of 6,7-ADTN were
not antagonised by the adrenoceptor antagonists prazosin 0.02-0.1
mg/kg, yohimbine 5mg/kg, phentolamine 0.2-1mg/kg or propranolol
5mg/kg, but was reversed by the dopamine antagonist haloperidol
0.1mg/kg. 6,7-ADTN may therefore act at dopamine receptors which are
different from α- or β-adrenoceptors. However, these experiments
do not tell us where the dopamine receptors may be situated. Since
experiments with various isolated gastrointestinal tissues (including
rat stomach[27]) show that most responses to dopamine on the smooth
muscle or on the cholinergic nerve are blocked by antagonists of
α- and/or β-adrenoceptors it is possible that 6,7-ADTN inhibits rat
gastric emptying by acting on dopamine receptors at other gastrointestinal sites (e.g. to modulate local hormone or peptide
release[30]), or at non-gastrointestinal sites which modulate gut
motility (e.g. the peripheral ganglia).

Table 2: Effects of metoclopramide and domperidone on rat gastric emptying after injection of 6,7-ADTN 1mg/kg s.c.

Drug	Dose mg/kg s.c.	% Test meal emptied in 10 min. mean ± s.e.m. (n)		% Increase in emptying
		Vehicle	Drug	
METOCLOPRAMIDE	0.2	65.7 ± 3.5 (6)	70.8 ± 5.0 (6)	8
	1	42.5 ± 4.2 (11)	61.9 ± 5.8 (11)	46*
	5	45.8 ± 2.5 (11)	68.7 ± 3.0 (10)	50***
	10	54.3 ± 4.8 (6)	80.8 ± 4.6 (6)	49**
DOMPERIDONE	0.2	65.7 ± 3.5 (6)	68.2 ± 5.4 (6)	4
	1	29.3 ± 3.5 (7)	49.9 ± 6.2 (7)	70*
	5	31.7 ± 4.8 (6)	67.2 ± 2.9 (6)	112***

All groups received 6,7-ADTN 5 min prior to administration of metoclopramide, domperidone or vehicle. The asterisks denote significant differences (Student's 't' test) between drug and vehicle groups (*P<0.05, **P<0.005, ***P<0.001)

Nevertheless, domperidone may increase rat gastric motility by antagonising the inhibitory effect of a dopamine agonist. In this test metoclopramide has a potency which is similar to domperidone but is uncertain to what extent this effect of metoclopramide is due to dopamine antagonism or to the more direct stimulation of gastric activity.

SIDE EFFECTS

In patients metoclopramide may occasionally cause dyskinesias, resembling tetanic spasms of the neck, back and facial muscles[31]. This action probably reflects the antagonism by metoclopramide of brain dopamine receptors involved in motor function[32]. Thus, to test for this type of dopamine antagonism we looked for the ability of drugs to inhibit apomorphine-induced climbing behaviour in the mouse, a standard pharmacological screening test for central dopamine antagonism[33].

Metoclopramide and domperidone each antagonised apomorphine-induced climbing; metoclopramide was more potent than domperidone (Table 3). The weaker effect of domperidone compared to metoclopramide is probably a reflection of the relatively poor penetration by domperidone into the central nervous system[13,9]. However, despite this poor penetration, extrapyramidal reactions do very occasionally occur with domperidone[35,36], perhaps as a consequence of an impaired blood brain barrier in these patients.

An additional side effect of dopamine antagonists is increased blood prolactin concentrations, due to antagonism of a tonic dopaminergic-mediated inhibitory control of prolactin release[37]. The site of action of dopamine in regulating prolactin release is in the anterior pituitary gland, which is outside the blood-brain barrier. Therefore, even domperidone has an ability to raise concentrations of blood prolactin, which may lead to galactorrhoea with chronic administration[38]. We have now compared the ability of metoclopramide and domperidone to increase prolactin release in rats subjected to minimal stress.

Hacking and Churchill CFY male rats (200-250g weight) were housed in groups of five with food and water ad libitum. Plasma samples were obtained by collection of body blood after decapitation, 1 hour after s.c. injection of the drugs. Prolactin concentrations were determined by double antibody radioimmunoassay (NIADDK kit). Metoclopramide caused a significant elevation in the mean blood plasma immunoreactive prolactin concentration over the dose range which also caused stimulation of rat gastric motility. Similar concentrations of domperidone also increased the blood plasma prolactin concentration (Fig. 4).

Table 3: Inhibition of apomorphine-induced climbing behaviour in the mouse.

Drug	ED_{50} mg/kg s.c. (95% confidence limits)
METOCLOPRAMIDE	0.8 (0.6-0.9)
DOMPERIDONE	2.5 (1.8-3.5)

The doses of metoclopramide or domperidone which caused a 50% reduction in the mouse climbing behaviour evoked by apomorphine 1mg/kg s.c. are expressed as ED_{50} values (method of Protais et al,[33]). Confidence limits were calculated by the method of Litchfield & Wilcoxon[34].

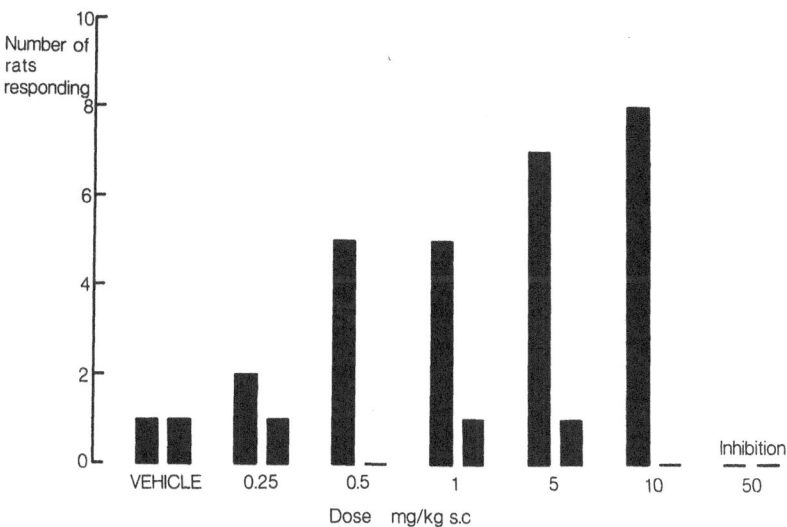

Fig. 4. Metoclopramide and domperidone dose-dependently increased
the blood plasma prolactin concentration in rats subjected
to minimal stress. The results are calculated as ng
immunoreactive prolactin/ml plasma, measured 1h after s.c.
injection of the drug. The points and the vertical bars
represent the means ± sem of 6 experiments with metoclopramide (o—o) and 5 with domperidone (●—●). Statistical
analysis was applied by comparing the results obtained for
each drug concentration with the results obtained for the
drug vehicle (Student's 't' test; *P<0.05, **P<0.01,
***P<0.001).

SUMMARY AND CONCLUSIONS

Metoclopramide and domperidone antagonise dopamine-mediated
responses in the emetic chemoreceptor trigger zone to inhibit nausea
and vomiting. However, additional factors may also be involved,
since unlike other dopamine antagonists, high-dose intravenous
metoclopramide successfully prevents emesis caused by strongly emetic
cancer chemotherapeutic agents.

Domperidone increased rat stomach activity only after gastric
emptying was reduced by a dopamine receptor stimulant, whereas
metoclopramide readily stimulated resting gastric motility and
increased low or reduced gastric emptying. This ability of metoclopramide to stimulate gastric motility appears to be unrelated to
antagonism of dopamine-induced responses in the gastrointestinal
tract[28] and could play a major role in its ability to reverse several
clinical hypomotility disorders of the upper gastrointestinal tract.

We have recently described a novel substituted benzamide, BRL 20627, which acts like metoclopramide and stimulates rat gastric motility[39,40]. However, BRL 20627 is unique because it has little or no ability to antagonise responses to dopamine in the central nervous system and anterior pituitary gland[39]. Side-effects associated with dopamine antagonists (increased blood prolactin concentrations or dyskinesias) are therefore unlikely to occur with this drug. Thus, BRL 20627 may be suitable not only for treatment of the hypomotility disorders of the upper gastrointestinal tract which are already successfully managed with metoclopramide, but also for the treatment of patients who are highly susceptable to the side-effects of dopamine antagonists (e.g. children[41] and patients with gut disorders requiring chronic treatment[38]).

The results therefore suggest that there are two distinctive actions of drugs used in the treatment of upper gut disorders.

1. Antagonism of dopamine-induced responses. This action can prevent nausea and vomiting caused by stimulation of the emetic chemoreceptor trigger zone. Antagonism of responses to dopamine may also enable a drug to increase gastric motility on occasions when it is partially suppressed by mechanisms involving catecholamines. This is the category in which domperidone would appear to belong and is also a property of metoclopramide.

2. Stimulation of gastric motility by mechanisms which may not depend on antagonism of responses to dopamine. This is a property of metoclopramide and BRL 20627, but not of domperidone.

REFERENCES

1. L. L. Iversen, Dopamine receptors in the brain, Science. 188:1084 (1975).
2. P. Seeman, Brain dopamine receptors, Pharmacol. Rev. 32:229 (1981).
3. M. Stanley, A. Lautin, J. Rotrosen, and S. Gershon, Antipsychotic efficacy of metoclopramide: Do DA/neuroleptic receptors mediate the action of anti-psychotic drugs? IRCS/Med. Sci. 7:322 (1979).
4. J. Perrot, G. Nahas, C. Laville, and A. Debay, Substituted benzamides as antiemetics, in: "Treatment of cancer chemotherapy-induced nausea and vomiting", D. S. Poster, J. S. Penta and S. Bruno, ed., Masson Publishing USA, Inc. (1982).
5. H. L. Borison, Area postrema? Chemoreceptor trigger zone for vomiting - Is that all? Life Sci. 14:1807 (1974).
6. H. L. Borison and S. C. Wang, Physiology and pharmacology of vomiting, Pharmacol. Rev. 5:193 (1953).

298

7. H. L. Borison and L. E. McCarthy, Physiologic basis of nausea and vomiting, in: "Treatment of cancer chemotherapy-induced nausea and vomiting", D. S. Poster, J. S. Penta and S. Bruno, ed., Masson Publishing USA, Inc. (1982).

8. R. M. Pinder, R. N. Brogden, P. R. Sawyer, T. M. Speight, and G. S. Avery, Metoclopramide: A review of its pharmacological properties and clinical use, Drugs, 12:81 (1976).

9. R. N. Brogden, A. A. Carmine, R. C. Heel, T. M. Speight, and G. S. Avery, Domperidone: A review of its pharmacological activity, pharmacokinetics and therapeutic efficacy in the symptomatic treatment of chronic dyspepsia and as an anti-emetic, Drugs, 24:360 (1982).

10. R. A. Harrington, C. W. Hamilton, R. N. Brogden, J. A. Linkewich, J. A. Romankiewicz, and R. C. Heel, Metoclopramide: An updated review of its pharmacological properties and clinical use, Drugs, 25:451 (1983).

11. K. Schulze-Delrieu, Metoclopramide, Gastroenterol. 77:768 (1979).

12. D. J. Roberts, The pharmacological basis of the therapeutic activity of clebopride and related substituted benzamides, Curr. Ther. Res. 31 (Suppl.):1 (1982).

13. A. Wauquier, C. J. E. Niemegeers, and P. A. J. Janssen, Neuro-pharmacological comparison between domperidone and metoclo-pramide, Jap. J. Pharmac. 31:305 (1981).

14. R. J. Gralla, L. M. Itri, S. E. Pisko, A. E. Squillante, D. P. Kelson, D. W. Braun, L. A. Bordin, T. J. Braun, and C. W. Young, Antiemetic efficacy of high-dose metoclopramide: Randomized trials with placebo and prochlorperazine in patients with chemotherapy-induced nausea and vomiting, New Eng. J. Med. 305:905 (1981).

15. R. A. Joss, A. Goldhirsch, K. W. Brunner, and R. L. Galeazzi, Sudden death in cancer patient on high-dose domperidone, Lancet. 1:1019 (1982).

16. J. H. Szurszewski and C. F. Code, Activity fronts of the canine small intestine, Gastroenterol. 54:1304 (1968).

17. C. F. Code and J. F. Schlegel, The gastrointestinal interdiges-tive housekeeper, Proc. 4th Int. Sym. Gastrointestinal Moti-lity. Mitchell, Vancouver, pp 631-634 (1974).

18. A. R. Cooke, Control of gastric emptying and motility, Gastroenterol. 68:804 (1975).

19. A. Lane, A. C. Ivy, and E. K. Ivy, Response of the chronic gastric fistula rat to histamine, Am. J. Physiol. 190:221 (1957).

20. J. N. Hunt and M. T. Knox, The regulation of gastric emptying of meals containing citric acid and salts of citric acid, J. Physiol. 163:34 (1962).

21. C. M. McClelland and G. J. Sanger, Effects of metoclopramide and domperidone on cholinergic responses in rat isolated stomach, Br. J. Pharmac. 77, Proc. Suppl: 539P (1982).

22. J. B. Furness and M. Costa, The adrenergic innervation of the gastrointestinal tract, Ergeb. Physiol. 69:1 (1974).

23. P. L. R. Andrews, D. Grundy, and I. N. C. Lawes, The role of the vagus and splanchnic nerves in the regulation of intragastric pressure in the ferret, J. Physiol. 307:401 (1980).

24. J. B. Furness and M. Costa, Indentification of gastrointestinal neurotransmitters, in: "Handb. Exp. Pharmacol, 59, Mediators and Drugs in Gastrointestinal Motility. I.", G. Bertaccini, ed., Springer-Verlag, Berlin, Heidelberg, New York (1982).

25. J. M. Van Neuten, Is dopamine an inhibitory modulator of gastric motility? Trends in Pharmacological Sciences. May:233 (1980).

26. H. A. Sahyoun, B. Costall, and R. J. Naylor, Catecholamine-induced relaxation and contraction of the lower oesophageal and pyloric sphincters of guinea-pig stomach: Modification by domperidone, J. Pharm. Pharmacol. 34:318 (1982).

27. R. A. Lefebvre, J. P. Blancquaert, J. L. Willems, and M. G. Bogaert, In vitro study of the inhibitory effects of dopamine on the rat gastric fundus, Naunyn-Schmiedeberg's Arch. Pharmacol. 322:228 (1983).

28. G. J. Sanger, Mechanisms by which metoclopramide can increase gastrointestinal motility, in: "This book".

29. G. N. Woodruff, A. O. Eikhawad, and R. M. Pinder, Long lasting stimulation of locomotor activity produced by the intra-ventricular injection of a cyclic analogue of dopamine into conscious mice, Eur. J. Pharmacol. 25:80 (1974).

30. K. Uvnäs-Wallensten and M. Goiny, Dopaminergic control of gastro-intestinal hormones, in: "Apomorphine and other dopamino-mimetics, Vol. 1: Basic Pharmacology", G. L. Gessa and G. U. Corsini, ed., Raven Press, New York (1981).

31. D. L. Cochlin, Dystonic reactions due to metoclopramide and phenothiazines resembling tetanus, Br. J. Clin. Pract. 28:201 (1974).

32. D. Tarsy, J. D. Parkes, and C. D. Marsden, Metoclopramide and pimozide in Parkinson's disease and levodopa-induced dyskin-easias, J. Neurol. Neurosurg. and Psychiatry. 38:331 (1975).

33. P. Protais, J. Costentin, and J. C. Schwartz, Climbing behaviour induced by apomorphine in mice: A simple test for the study of dopamine receptors in striatum, Psychopharmacol. 50:1 (1976).

34. M. T. Litchfield and F. Wilcoxon, A simplified method of eval-uating dose-effect experiments, J. Pharmac. 96:99 (1949).

35. P. Sol, B. Pelet, and J-P. Guignard, Extrapyramidal reactions to domperidone, Lancet. 2(8198):802 (1980).

36. M. Gance, J. Bury, L. Burton, and P. J. Delwaide, Syndrome neurodysleptique induit par le dompéridone, La Nouvelle Presse Médicale. 11:2298 (1982).

37. R. M. Macleod, Regulation of prolactin secretion, in: "Frontiers in Neuroendocrinology, IV"., L. Martini and W. F. Ganong, ed., Raven Press, New York (1976).

38. P. A. Cann, N. W. Read, and C. D. Holdsworth, Galactorrhoea as side effect of domperidone, Br. Med. J. 286:1395 (1983).

39. C. M. McClelland, B. McRitchie, and D. H. Turner, BRL 20627: A non-dopaminergic blocking stimulant of gastric motility, Br. J. Pharmac. 80, Proc. Suppl:569P (1983).

40. C. M. McClelland and G. J. Sanger, Increased cholinergic responses with BRL 20627 in rat isolated stomach: Comparison with metoclopramide, Br. J. Pharmac. 80, Proc. Suppl:568P (1983).

41. G. J. Reynolds, Metoclopramide in young children, Br. Med. J. 2 (6153):1713 (1978).

MECHANISMS BY WHICH METOCLOPRAMIDE CAN INCREASE GASTROINTESTINAL

MOTILITY

Gareth J. Sanger

Beecham Pharmaceuticals, Medicinal Research Centre

Coldharbour Road, The Pinnacles, Harlow, Essex. U.K.

Metoclopramide is a dopamine antagonist which has been used for many years in the clinic as an anti-emetic and to increase the motility of the stomach and upper small intestine[1,2]. However, the mechanisms by which metoclopramide increases gastrointestinal motility are not clearly understood, and may even be unrelated to dopamine antagonism. Studying the actions of metoclopramide is therefore important not only to elucidate the mechanisms, but also to further our understanding of the ways in which gut motility can be controlled. This article describes the different ways in which metoclopramide may increase gastrointestinal motility.

EFFECTS OF METOCLOPRAMIDE IN THE CENTRAL NERVOUS SYSTEM

Metoclopramide is usually considered to increase gastro-intestinal motility by a direct action on the gut itself[1,3]. Nevertheless, there may be an additional, central nervous action of metoclopramide which facilitates gut motility. In recent experiments with the guinea-pig[4], intracerebroventricular (icv) injection of metoclopramide increased the normal rate of gastric emptying, but intraperitoneal injection of metoclopramide over a wide range of concentrations increased only the gastric emptying which had been slowed by the actions of drugs such as apomorphine. Similarly in man, a therapeutic dose of metoclopramide (intravenous or oral administration) may only increase gastric emptying which is less than maximal[5]. The unusual results obtained with icv injection of metoclopramide in the guinea-pig may therefore reflect the abnormal route of administration. Further studies are required to determine if the results obtained with icv injection of metoclopramide have any significance in the clinical efficacy of the drug.

EFFECTS OF METOCLOPRAMIDE ON CHOLINERGIC-MEDIATED CONTRACTIONS IN THE GASTROINTESTINAL TRACT

Experiments with isolated whole stomach and small intestinal preparations show that the actions of metoclopramide on the gastro-intestinal tract in vivo may be detected in vitro. For example, metoclopramide increased resting myoelectrical and mechanical activity in the antrum and duodenum of the dog isolated stomach[6] and facil-itated a submaximal peristaltic response in guinea-pig isolated ileum[7,8,9]. Metoclopramide may therefore increase gastrointestinal motility at least partly by mechanisms which are independent of the central nervous system.

We have been studying the ways in which metoclopramide might increase gut motility in vitro. In man, metoclopramide mostly stimulates the motility of the upper gastrointestinal tract[5]. In addition, a number of earlier studies suggested that cholinergic mechanisms are involved in the response to metoclopramide[10,11,12,8,13,14,15,16,17,18]. We therefore looked for ways in which metoclo-pramide may affect nerve-mediated responses in different regions of the rat isolated stomach[19,20,21,22]. The results are described below and are compared with the actions of metoclopramide on rat gastric motility in vivo[23,24] and with the results obtained by ourselves and by others using different gut preparations, including human isolated stomach.

1. Rat Stomach

Effects of metoclopramide on nerve-mediated responses: Strips of rat stomach approximately 2-4mm wide and 15-20mm long were cut parallel to the longitudinal and circular muscle fibres of the fore-stomach and corpus (Fig. 1). These were suspended under a 1g load in 10ml tissue baths containing Krebs solution (NaCl 7.1; $CaCl_2$ $6H_2O$ 0.55; KH_2PO_4 0.16; KCl 0.35; $MgSO_4$ $7H_2O$ 0.29; $NaHCO_3$ 2.1; dextrose 1.0 g/l) maintained at 37°C and bubbled with 5% CO_2 in O_2. Nerve-mediated responses were evoked using electrical field stimulation (EFS) applied across two platinum wire electrodes 2.5cm long and 0.5cm apart, insulated on entry to the bathing solution and fixed either side of the stomach strip. EFS was given as bipolar rectang-ular pulses, passed in parallel through 4 pairs of electrodes in separate tissue baths. Maximum stimulator current delivered to each pair of electrodes a peak-to-peak voltage of 60-80V/cm (current was 0.48-0.58A to each electrode) at a total pulse duration of 0.5ms. Frequency-response curves were constructed using 0.5, 1, 5 and 10Hz frequencies; higher frequencies caused rapid nerve fatigue and were not used. Periods of stimulation lasted for 30s, separated by 4 min intervals. Isotonic muscle responses were magnified 4-18x and detected using transducers and pen recorders. Results are expressed as medians with ranges or semiquartile ranges in parenthesis, and

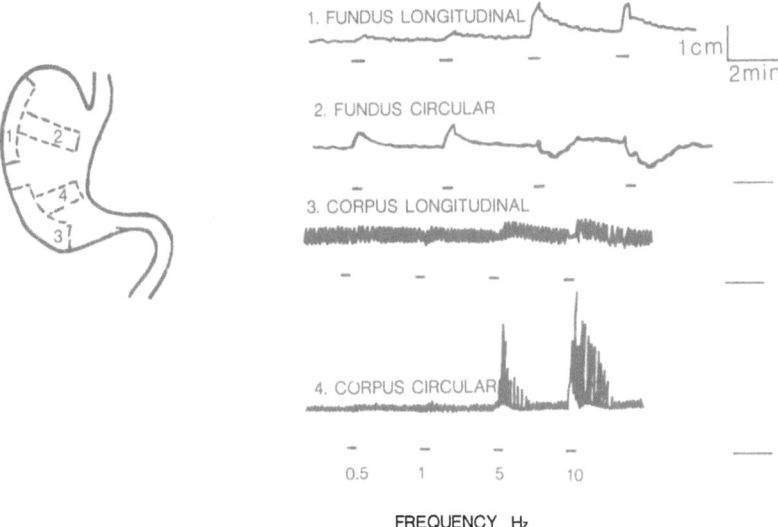

Fig. 1. Diagram showing the location of the muscle strips cut from
the rat stomach and typical records of responses obtained
with electrical stimulation (30s of bipolar 0.5ms rectangular
pulses; 60-80V/cm). The horizontal bars below the traces
indicate the period of stimulation at the frequencies shown.

analysed using the Wilcoxon matched-pairs test or the Mann-Whitney
U-test.

Each type of stomach strip responded differently to EFS (Fig. 1),
and all responses could be prevented by tetrodotoxin 0.2µg/ml.
Preliminary experiments suggested that the muscle contractions which
were evoked or increased during EFS may be due predominantly to submaximal activation of post-ganglionic cholinergic neurones. The EFS-
induced relaxations may be due to activation of non-adrenergic, non-
cholinergic inhibitory neurones, since they were not reduced by
atropine or by phentolamine and propranolol. These experiments confirmed those previously reported for the rat stomach[25,17,26,27,28].
The mechanisms of the gastrointestinal rebound or after-contractions
were not investigated.

In the forestomach longitudinal muscle, metoclopramide 1 and
10µg/ml increased the contractions to EFS, particularly at the
frequencies of 5 and 10Hz. Metoclopramide 0.1µg/ml tended to
increase the contractions to EFS, but this was not statistically
significant. Contractions to all frequencies of stimulation were
reduced by metoclopramide 100µg/ml (Fig. 2). In the presence of
atropine 1µg/ml and $BaCl_2$ 100µg/ml (which prevented contractions to
EFS and facilitated the detection of muscle relaxations by raising
the tone), metoclopramide 10µg/ml had no significant effect on the

305

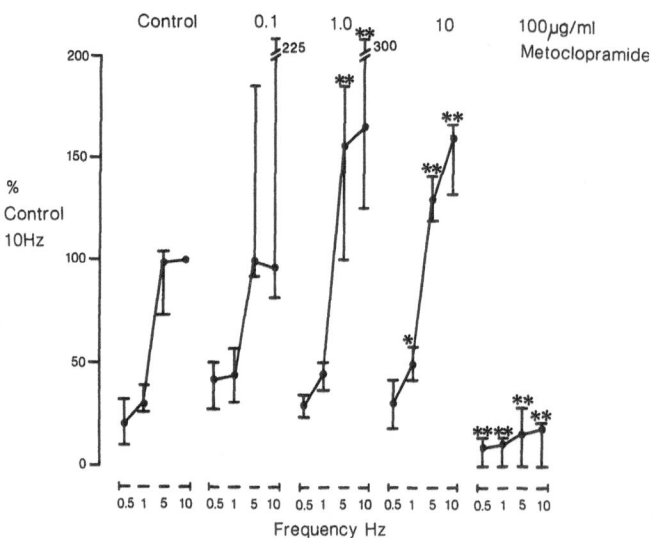

Fig. 2. Effects of metoclopramide on the contractions to electrical
stimulation in the longitudinal muscle preparation of rat
forestomach. Frequency-response curves were compared before
and after 10 min incubation of the tissue with metoclopramide; 2 increasing concentrations of metoclopramide were
tested in each tissue. Results were calculated as a percentage of the control contractions to stimulation at 10Hz. The
points represent the median values and the bars represent
the semiquartile ranges. The experiments with metoclopramide
are compared with the controls at each frequency, *P<0.1;
**P<0.05; ***P<0.01; n=12 controls or 6 with each metoclopramide concentration. In similar experiments, metoclopramide vehicle (Krebs solution) had no effects on 2 successive
frequency response curves (n=6; P>0.05 for each frequency).

relaxations caused by electrical stimulation of the inhibitory
nerves (P>0.05; n=6 for each frequency).

Metoclopramide similarly increased cholinergic-mediated contractions in the forestomach circular muscle. However, in this preparation different frequencies of EFS evoked contractions and/or relaxations (Fig. 1 and 3). Whereas EFS-induced relaxations were unaffected by metoclopramide 10µg/ml in the presence of atropine 1µg/ml, they
were reduced or prevented by metoclopramide 1 or 10µg/ml in the
absence of atropine (Fig. 3 for 10µg/ml metoclopramide). Relaxations
caused by stimulation of non-adrenergic, non-cholinergic inhibitory
nerves may therefore be indirectly reduced if the metoclopramide-
induced increase in the cholinergic response is sufficiently large
to overcome the previously dominant inhibitory nerve response to EFS.

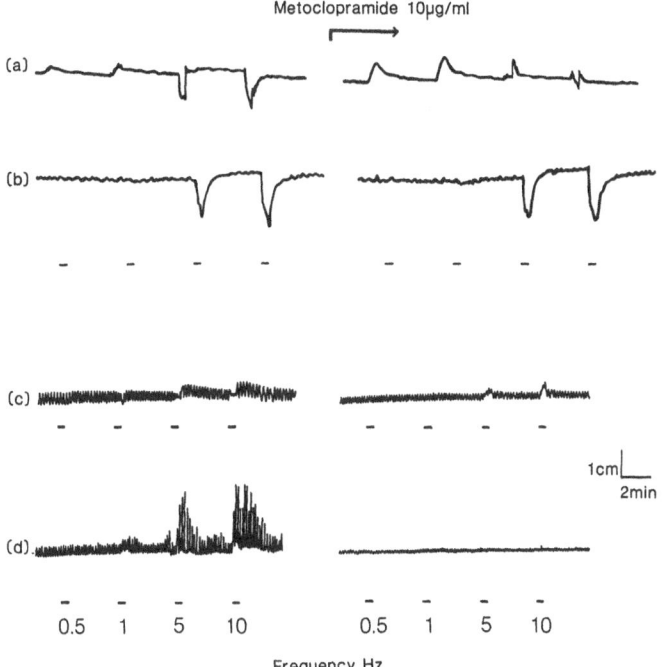

Metoclopramide 10μg/ml

(a)

(b)

(c)

1cm

2min

(d)

0.5 1 5 10   0.5 1 5 10

Frequency Hz

Fig. 3. Effects of metoclopramide 10μg/ml on the responses to electrical stimulation (30s of bipolar 0.5ms rectangular pulses;
60-80V/cm) in (a) rat forestomach circular muscle, (b) rat
forestomach circular muscle cut from the same animal but
incubated with atropine 1μg/ml, (c) rat corpus longitudinal
muscle and (d) rat corpus circular muscle. Traces were
obtained before (left hand traces) and after 10 min incubation with metoclopramide (right hand traces). The horizontal bars below the traces indicate the period of stimulation
at the frequencies shown.

     In the corpus longitudinal muscle, EFS reduced the spontaneous
muscle contractions and/or muscle tone. However, in the presence of
metoclopramide 1 or 10μg/ml, EFS at 5 and 10Hz evoked a contraction
or increased the amplitude of spontaneous contractions; rebound
contractions were not greatly affected by metoclopramide 1μg/ml but
were reduced or prevented with 10μg/ml metoclopramide (n=4 each;
Fig. 3 for 10μg/ml metoclopramide). Responses to stimulation at
0.1 and 1Hz were weak and unaffected by metoclopramide 1 or 10μg/ml.
After addition of atropine 1μg/ml to the bathing solution, inhibitory
responses to EFS were detected both before and during the presence
of metoclopramide (n=4).

     The effects of metoclopramide on nerve-mediated responses in the
corpus longitudinal muscle are therefore similar to those in the
forestomach. However, a different response to metoclopramide was

307

detected in the corpus circular muscle. In this preparation, metoclopramide 1 and 10μg/ml reduced or prevented all responses evoked by EFS (n=4 each; Fig. 3 for 10μg/ml metoclopramide). Since, in vivo, the overall effect of metoclopramide is to increase rat gastric motility[23] the importance of an inhibitory action of metoclopramide in the corpus circular muscle is not clear.

Effects of metoclopramide on acetylcholine and carbachol-induced contractions: After obtaining consistent, submaximal (approx. 50% maximum) contractions to acetylcholine (ACh; 30s contact; 10 min stimulation cycle), an increasing concentration of metoclopramide was added every 10 min immediately after washout of the preceding dose of ACh. Metoclopramide 0.001 to 10μg/ml did not increase the ACh-induced contractions in either muscle layer of the forestomach (P>0.05, n=8 for longitudinal, n=6 for circular muscle); metoclopramide 100μg/ml reduced the contractions to ACh but this was statistically significant (P<0.05) only for the longitudinal muscle. In contrast, the contractions to ACh in the corpus longitudinal muscle were increased by metoclopramide 10 and 100μg/ml; lower concentrations had no effects (n=8; Fig. 4). Similar results were obtained in corpus circular muscle except that only 100μg/ml metoclopramide significantly (P=0.05) increased the contractions to ACh (n=6).

Further experiments with the corpus longitudinal muscle showed that the metoclopramide-induced increase in the contractions to ACh were not affected by tetrodotoxin 0.2μg/ml (Fig. 4). However, when carbachol was used instead of ACh, metoclopramide did not increase the contractions. Instead, the higher concentrations of metoclopramide (10 and 100μg/ml) reduced the contractions to carbachol (Fig. 4). Since contractions to both carbachol and ACh were abolished by atropine 1μg/ml (n=6) but not affected by hexamethonium 10μg/ml (P>0.05; n=6), they may each similarly activate cholinergic muscarinic receptors. In contrast to carbachol, ACh is easily hydrolysed by cholinesterase, so metoclopramide could therefore increase contractions to ACh in the rat gastric corpus by inhibiting cholinesterase activity. This action of metoclopramide occurred in both muscle layers at the concentration of 100μg/ml (which also inhibited all neurally-mediated responses evoked by EFS), but only in the longitudinal muscle with 10μg/ml metoclopramide. Cholinesterase inhibition by metoclopramide may therefore be a relevant stimulatory mechanism of action in vivo only at the highest effective concentrations and perhaps only in certain areas of the rat stomach. Lower concentrations of metoclopramide increased cholinergic-mediated, EFS-induced responses both in the corpus longitudinal muscle and in the forestomach (where contractions to exogenous ACh were not increased by any concentration of metoclopramide). Thus, in addition to its effects on contractions to exogenous ACh, metoclopramide may increase cholinergic-mediated contractions by a pre-junctional stimulation of neural ACh release.

308

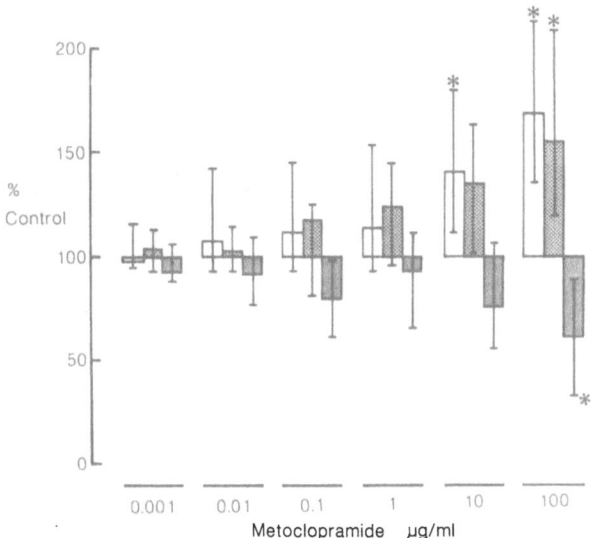

Fig. 4. Effects of increasing concentrations of metoclopramide on
submaximal contractions of rat corpus longitudinal muscle
to ACh (open columns), ACh in the presence of tetrodotoxin
0.2μg/ml (stipled columns) or to carbachol (hatched
columns). The results are expressed as a percentage of the
pre-metoclopramide control contractions and are given as
medians (columns) with semi-quartile ranges (vertical bars);
*P<0.05 compared with controls, n=8 each. Compared with the
results using just ACh, addition of tetrodotoxin had no
significant effect on the responses to metoclopramide (P>0.05
for each concentration).

Comparison of in vitro and in vivo effects of metoclopramide:
It is essential to try and relate the drug concentrations and results
obtained in vitro with drug effects obtained in vivo. For compounds
such as metoclopramide where more than one type of action may occur,
the effects which are likely to be of most importance clinically
might be expected to be those which occur at the relatively low concentrations. In the present experiments with metoclopramide, 10 or
100μg/ml increased the contractions to exogenous ACh in the rat
corpus, but 1 and 10μg/ml increased the cholinergic-mediated, EFS-
induced contractions in the rat corpus longitudinal muscle and in
the forestomach preparations. However, since small effects of drugs
may be difficult to detect by comparing frequency or dose-response
curves, the lowest effective concentration of metoclopramide for the
EFS-induced contractions could be less than 1μg/ml. We therefore
re-tested the effects of metoclopramide against consistent contractions evoked by EFS at a single frequency, using the rat forestomach
longitudinal muscle preparation.

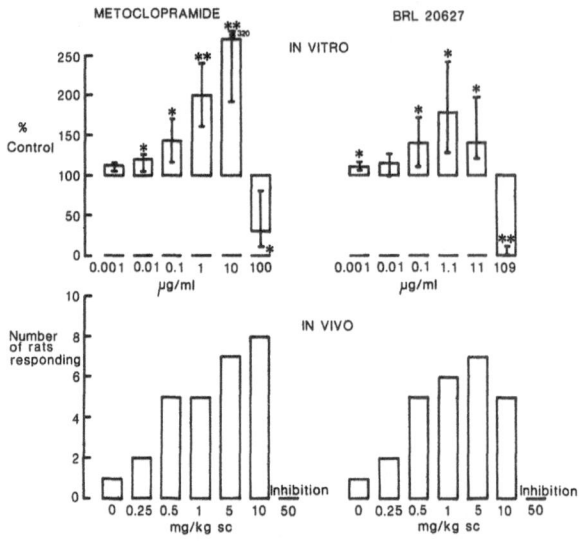

Fig. 5. Comparison between the effects of metoclopramide and BRL
20627 on (a) electrically-induced, cholinergic-mediated
contractions in rat forestomach longitudinal muscle and
(b) on the intragastric pressure changes recorded in the
conscious rat. Note the different scales of drug concentrations for the two types of experiment. In the in vitro
experiments the results were calculated as a percentage of
the pre-drug control contractions and are given as medians
(column) and semiquartile ranges (vertical bars); *P<0.05,
**P<0.01 compared with controls, n=8 each. There were no
significant differences (P>0.05) between the effects of
metoclopramide 0.001-1µg/ml and BRL 20627 0.001-1.1µg/ml
(equimolar drug concentrations). In the in vivo experiments,
the results are given as the number of animals which responded to subcutaneous injection of metoclopramide or BRL 20627
(group size = 10 each). There were no significant differences (P>0.05) between the effects of 0.25-5mg/kg s.c.
metoclopramide or BRL 20627 (base weights of compounds).

Contractions to EFS were obtained every 10 min, followed by washout of the bathing solution. Bipolar rectangular pulses of 0.5ms
width were given for 20s at the frequency of 5Hz and with the minimum
voltage required to elicit a maximum contraction. After obtaining
constant contractions to EFS, an increasing concentration of metoclopramide was added every 10 min, immediately after washout of the
bathing solution. Metoclopramide 0.01, 0.1, 1 and 10µg/ml dose-
dependently increased the contractions to EFS, whereas 100µg/ml
metoclopramide reduced the contractions (Fig. 5). Thus, in the rat
gastric forestomach preparation, very low concentrations of

metoclopramide may increase neural ACh release. These concentrations are substantially less than the concentrations which may inhibit cholinesterase activity in the rat corpus or even in extracted preparations of cholinesterase[30] which might be expected to be less affected by problems of drug access to the enzyme.

We subsequently compared the ability of metoclopramide and other substituted benzamides to increase EFS-induced cholinergic contractions in the rat isolated forestomach preparation and to stimulate rat gastric activity in vivo (see [24] for details of in vivo experiments). In particular, we compared the effects of metoclopramide and BRL 20627, a novel substituted benzamide which increases rat gastric motility but without the predicted side effects which occur with drugs which antagonise responses to dopamine in the central nervous system[23]. The dose-response curves for metoclopramide and BRL 20627 were similar for both the in vitro and the in vivo experiments; in both test systems, metoclopramide and BRL 20627 were equipotent in low concentrations, whereas at higher concentrations the differences in their actions were the same in vitro and in vivo (Fig. 5). These results therefore give added support to the suggestion that metoclopramide and BRL 20627 may increase rat gastric motility by stimulating intrinsic cholinergic activity, mostly by facilitating neuronal ACh release (see ref. [21] for details of the experiments with BRL 20627 in rat isolated stomach).

2.   Human Stomach

Specimens of human stomach were obtained at operation for benign or malignant disease, and a sample was cut away at least 6cm from any macroscopic lesion. After removal of the mucosal layers, strips of muscle approximately 4-5mm wide and 20-30mm long were cut parallel to the longitudinal muscle fibres. Each strip was suspended in tissue baths, as previously described for the rat stomach. Electrical field stimulation (EFS) was given every 10 min followed by washout of the bathing solution. Bipolar rectangular pulses of 1ms total width were given for 30s at 5Hz frequency. Maximum stimulator current was used to deliver to each pair of electrodes a peak-to-peak voltage of 80-120V/cm.

EFS caused contraction of all stomach specimens. Antagonism by tetrodotoxin 0.2μg/ml (n=3) or atropine 1μg/ml (n=6) suggested that these contractions were predominantly cholinergic-mediated, supporting the earlier results of Bennett & Stockley[29]. Nevertheless, in the presence of atropine 1μg/ml and $BaCl_2$ 100μg/ml (to raise the muscle tone), EFS caused muscle relaxations which were not prevented by a mixture of phentolamine 0.5μg/ml and propranolol 0.4μg/ml (shown to reduce noradrenaline (10-50μg/ml)-induced muscle relaxations by 90-100%; n=3), and were antagonised by tetrodotoxin 1 and 2μg/ml (n=2); tetrodotoxin 0.2μg/ml reduced the relaxations by only 48-50% (n=3).

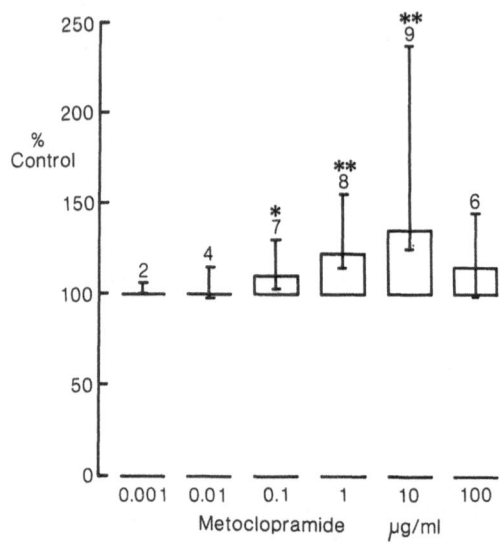

Fig. 6. Effects of increasing concentrations of metoclopramide on the contractions evoked by electrical stimulation (30s bipolar rectangular pulses, 80-120V/cm) in human isolated stomach longitudinal muscle. The results are calculated as a percentage of the pre-metoclopramide control contractions and are given as medians (columns) with semiquartile ranges (vertical bars); *P<0.05, **P<0.01 compared with controls, n=9. Numbers in parenthesis represent the number of preparations in which the contractions to electrical stimulation were increased after incubation of the tissue with metoclopramide.

Thus, in these experiments EFS-induced relaxations may be due predominantly to activation of non-adrenergic, non-cholinergic inhibitory neurones.

After obtaining consistant contractions to EFS, an increasing concentration of metoclopramide was added every 10 min. Metoclopramide 0.1, 1 and 10μg/ml significantly increased the contractions caused by EFS, whereas lower concentrations of metoclopramide had no effect (Fig. 6); there were no obvious differences between the effects of metoclopramide on muscle strips from different regions of the stomach, but the number of experiments are too small to be conclusive. In 3 further experiments, EFS-induced muscle relaxations obtained in the presence of atropine and BaCl$_2$ were both unaffected by 10 min incubation of the tissue with 10μg/ml metoclopramide.

The effects of metoclopramide on cholinergic-induced contractions in human isolated stomach were therefore similar to those found in rat stomach experiments. However, in the human stomach, metoclopramide

1 and 10μg/ml may also increase submaximal contractions to exogenous ACh. This was first shown by Eisner[10], in which these concentrations of metoclopramide increased contractions to ACh in 21 of 26 stomach specimens studied (the muscle layer was not defined). Similarly, in 3 of 4 longitudinal muscle specimens tested in our laboratory, metoclopramide 1, 10 and 100μg/ml increased submaximal ACh-induced contractions (approximately 50% maximum; 30s contact times; 10 min stimulation cycle); lower concentrations of metoclopramide had no effect.

In summary, metoclopramide 0.1-10μg/ml increased cholinergic-induced contractions in human isolated stomach. At least part of this response may be due to a pre-junctional effect of metoclopramide on ACh release, but an increase in sensitivity to the effects of ACh may be important at higher concentrations.

3. Summary of the Effects of Metoclopramide on the Cholinergic System of the Gastrointestinal Tract

The effects of metoclopramide on the gut cholinergic system of rat, guinea-pig and man are summarised in Table 1. Low concentrations of metoclopramide increased contractions caused by electrical- or nicotine-induced stimulation of cholinergic neurones in all tissues except the rat corpus circular muscle. Contractions to exogenous ACh were also increased in some tissues, usually with higher concentrations of metoclopramide. However, in guinea-pig stomach and ileum the effects on the contractions to exogenous ACh were prevented by tetrodotoxin, suggesting an involvement of nerve activity in the response to metoclopramide. In the human gut, the mechanisms by which metoclopramide may increase ACh-induced contractions have not been studied.

The relevance of the experiments with isolated colon or distal ileum may be questioned[34] on the grounds that unlike the stomach and upper small intestine, these areas of the gastrointestinal tract are not major sites of metoclopramide actions in vivo. For example, the motility of the human colon in vivo is either not affected by metoclo-pramide or only slightly increased (depending on the investigator; see Ref. [1]). However, the absence of consistant effects of metoclo-pramide in the lower gastrointestinal tract may reflect a lack of understanding of the ways in which the motility of the lower intestine is controlled (e.g. other factors may prevent or reduce the effects of metoclopramide), and/or difficulties of access for precise measurements in this area of the gut.

In most of the studies, changes in the release of neural ACh was studied by comparing the effects of metoclopramide on contractions evoked by the electrical stimulation and by exogenous ACh. For these indirect experiments it is therefore not possible to be certain that

Table 1: Effects of Metoclopramide on Contractions of Isolated Gastrointestinal Muscle Preparations Evoked by Cholinergic Stimulation or by Exogenous ACh Cholinergic-mediated contractions were evoked by electrical stimulation or by nicotine. Metoclopramide concentrations are given in parenthesis (μg/ml)

SPECIES	GUT AREA AND MUSCLE LAYER	EFFECTS ON CHOLINERGIC-MEDIATED CONTRACTIONS	EFFECTS ON CONTRACTIONS TO EXOGENOUS ACh	REFERENCES
HUMAN	STOMACH all areas, longitudinal	Increased (0.1-10)	Increased (1-100)	10, 22
	COLON longitudinal	Not tested	Increased (0.1-10)	10
RAT	STOMACH forestomach longitudinal	Increased (0.01-10), decreased (100)	No effects (<10), decreased (100)	17, 19
	forestomach circular	Increased (1 & 10; <1 not tested), decreased (100)	No effects (<100)	22
	corpus longitudinal	Increased (1 & 10; <1 or >10 not tested)	No effects (<1), increased (10 & 100; not blocked by tetrodotoxin)	22
	corpus circular	Decreased (1 & 10; <1 or >10 not tested)	No effects (<10), increased (100)	22
GUINEA-PIG	STOMACH antrum longitudinal	Increased (5; <5 not tested)	Increased (5 & 20; blocked by tetrodotoxin or hexamethonium; <5 not tested)	13
	all areas, circular	Increased (approx. 0.004-0.4; >0.4 not tested)	No effects (concentrations not given)	31
	ILEUM longitudinal	Increased (approx. 0.04-400)	Increased (approx. 0.1-10; blocked by tetrodotoxin; decreased (100)	16, 32, 33
	COLON longitudinal	Increased (0.5-10), decreased (30)	Increased (3, not blocked by tetrodotoxin; <3 not tested)	14, 15

ACh release was increased by metoclopramide. However, Kilbinger et al[32] found that metoclopramide increased ACh overflow from guinea-pig ileum, as measured by gas chromatography. It therefore seems reasonable to conclude that metoclopramide may increase neural ACh release.

4. Mechanisms by Which Metoclopramide may Increase Neural Acetylcholine Release

Metoclopramide is a dopamine antagonist in some vascular and brain tissues[35], and in the gastrointestinal tract metoclopramide may antagonise dopamine-induced stimulation of α_2-adrenoceptors which inhibit neuronal ACh release (see later). However, there is no evidence that antagonism of dopamine-induced responses plays a part in the mechanisms by which metoclopramide increases cholinergic-mediated, electrically-induced contractions in vitro[36,32,33,31].

The ability of metoclopramide to antagonise 5-hydroxytryptamine (5HT)-induced nerve-mediated responses in the gut led to the suggestion that the drug may have an action on endogenous tryptamine-like mechanisms which modulate the cholinergic response[15,7,14,16]. However, this idea is difficult to prove and there is conflicting evidence. For example, Fontaine & Reuse[37,38] described other substituted benzamides structurally related to metoclopramide, which increased cholinergic-induced contractions but did not antagonise nerve-mediated contractions to 5HT in guinea-pig ileum. More recently, Kilbinger et al[32] reported that metoclopramide increased both resting and electrically-evoked ACh release from guinea-pig ileum, but 5HT tachyphylaxis prevented only the effects of metoclopramide on resting ACh release. Nevertheless, as suggested by Kilbinger et al[32], not all 5HT-induced responses are subject to tachyphylaxis (particularly in non-gastrointestinal tissues[39]) and it remained possible that tachyphylaxis-resistant 5HT receptors are affected by metoclopramide in the gut. In another study 5HT 0.1-10 ng/ml increased submaximal electrically-induced, cholinergic-mediated contractions in guinea-pig isolated ileum, and this response was maintained for up to 15 min in the presence of 5HT[22].

A further suggestion that metoclopramide may increase neural ACh release by antagonising pre-junctional muscarinic receptors which modulate ACh release[40] has not been substantiated[32].

In our laboratory we have tried to elucidate the mechanism(s) by which metoclopramide may increase neural ACh release by studying the effects of various drug antagonists[22]. The increase caused by metoclopramide 1µg/ml in the electrically-induced cholinergic-mediated contractions of the rat forestomach longitudinal muscle was not antagonised by hexamethonium 10µg/ml, indomethacin 1µg/ml, naloxone 1µg/ml, mepyramine 0.1µg/ml or by a mixture of phentolamine

0.5μg/ml and propranolol 0.4μg/ml (Table 2). In the same experiments or in literature examples these drugs respectively reduced contractions to nicotine 100μg/ml by 100 (95-100)%, inhibited prostaglandin synthesis[51], reduced by 93 (80-100)% the inhibition of contractions to EFS caused by morphine 0.1μg/ml (median inhibition was 65%), prevented contractions to histamine 10μg/ml and reduced by 94 (75-100)% the inhibition of contractions to EFS caused by noradrenaline 10ng/ml (median inhibition was 98%) or by dopamine[42]. Similarly, in a different type of preparation of rat forestomach muscle, phentolamine or bethanidine did not antagonise the metoclopramide-induced increase in the contractions to EFS[17]. In addition tachyphylaxis to Substance P did not prevent the effects of metoclopramide (Table 2).

Tachyphylaxis of 5HT-induced muscle contractions increased the cholinergic-mediated contractions caused by EFS in 5 of the 6 experiments, and prevented a further increase with metoclopramide (Table 2). The 5HT antagonist, methysergide 10μg/ml had no effects on the contractions to EFS but reduced the response to metoclopramide; 1μg/ml methysergide had no effects on either measurement. Similarly, phenylbiguanide 10μg/ml had no significant effects, whereas 100μg/ml phenylbiguanide reduced the contractions to EFS and also the response to metoclopramide (Table 2).

There are no generally selective antagonists of nerve-mediated 5HT responses in the gastrointestinal tract, and these high concentrations of methysergide and phenylbiguanide are particularly unlikely to have a selective action against neural 5HT receptors (see ref. [43,39]). Nevertheless, methysergide 10μg/ml reduced the response to metoclopramide without affecting the contractions to EFS. Moreover, an action of metoclopramide at several other receptor sites which could be antagonised by methysergide, may be excluded by the inability of other drug antagonists to reduce the response to metoclopramide. However, it still remains a possibility that a receptor combination or receptors not considered in the present work are similarly affected by metoclopramide, methysergide and phenylbiguanide.

The experiments with rat stomach therefore do not fully explain the mechanism by which metoclopramide may increase neuronal ACh release. Others have suggested that 5HT is involved and the present work is, at best, only supportive of this possibility. The tantilising possibility that metoclopramide may affect 5HT systems which modulate neuronal ACh release must await a better understanding of the pharmacology of 5HT in the gut and the development of antagonists selective for 5HT receptors located on gastrointestinal nerves.

Table 2: Effects of Drug Antagonists and Tachyphylaxis on the Metoclopramide-induced Increase in Contractions Evoked by EFS in the Rat Forestomach. Metoclopramide 1μg/ml increased the submaximal contractions to EFS by 37 (21-73)% (n=67). After recovery and at least 1h incubation with an antagonist or after tachyphylaxis to Substance P or 5HT, the effects of metoclopramide were retested. The results are expressed as the ratio of the percentage increase with metoclopramide + antagonist/metoclopramide control. The effects of the antagonists on the contractions to EFS in the absence of meotclopramide were calculated as a percentage of the pre-antagonist control contractions. The results are given as medians; where n>6 semiquartile ranges are in parenthesis and a statistical analysis applied. *P<0.05

Antagonist	EFFECTS OF ANTAGONISTS ON:			N
	Resting muscle tone	Contractions to EFS	Response to metoclopramide	
Indomethacin 1μg/ml	Reduced	44 (28-151)	1.6 (0.4-1.0)	6
Naloxone 1μg/ml	None	101 (84-110)	1.0 (0.4-1.2)	6
Hexamethonium 10μg/ml	None	68 (55-92)	1.0 (0.7-1.7)	6
Mepyramine 0.1μg/ml	None	64 (60-68)*	0.8 (0.5-1.2)	6
Phentolamine 0.5μg/ml & Propranolol 0.4μg/ml	None	79 (48-91)	0.8 (0.2-1.3)	8
Substance P tachyphylaxis (50μg/ml)	Increased (Initial contraction to Substance P fell by 23-28%. Constant after 70-80 min).	22	3.2	2
5HT tachyphylaxis (100μg/ml)	None (Initial contraction to 5HT fell by 100 (91-103)%. Constant after 70-80 min).	139 (121-146)	0.1 (0-0.2)*	6
Methysergide 1μg/ml	Slight reduction	83 (73-115)	0.6 (0.2-1.0)	6
Methysergide 10μg/ml	None	91 (68-109)	0.4 (0.3-0.4)*	6
Phenylbiguanide 10μg/ml	Reduced	105 (96-117)	0.8 (0.6-1.3)	8
Phenylbiguanide 100μg/ml	Increased	59 (39-71)*	0.3 (0.2-0.6)*	8

ANTAGONISM BY METOCLOPRAMIDE OF DOPAMINE OR α_2-ADRENOCEPTOR-MEDIATED
INHIBITION OF GASTROINTESTINAL MOTILITY

Metoclopramide can antagonise certain dopamine-mediated
responses in isolated gut preparations, but the significance of these
results depends on the importance of dopamine as a modulator of
gastrointestinal motility.

It is unlikely that dopamine functions as a neurotransmitter in
the gut, although the amine has been detected in the enterochromaffin
cells of the mucosa[44]. Specific dopamine receptors may occur in the
opossum isolated lower oesophageal sphincter muscle, since relaxations
to dopamine were prevented by the dopamine antagonist haloperidol, but
were unaffected by tetrodotoxin or by α- and β-adrenoceptor antagonists[45]. It has also been proposed that specific dopamine receptors
exist in guinea-pig isolated stomach and ileum[46]. However, by
studying the effects of dopamine on resting muscle tone or against
cholinergic-mediated contractions, others have found no evidence for
specific dopamine receptors in guinea-pig isolated oesophagus[47],
gastro-oesophageal junction[48], stomach[49] and ileum[50,51], or in stomach
muscle strips from rat[42] and human[52]. Instead dopamine may act on α-
and β-adrenoceptors. Gastrointestinal dopamine receptors which have
been proposed on the basis of studying the effects of dopamine in vivo
must therefore be treated with caution until it can be established
that these effects of dopamine are localised to the gut (perhaps to
modulate local hormone or peptide release[52,53]) and not to other sites
which affect gut motility, such as the hypothalamus or the peripheral
ganglia.

In experiments with metoclopramide, concentrations of approximately 3 to 35µg/ml antagonised dopamine-induced inhibition of
cholinergic-mediated contractions in guinea-pig isolated ileum[36,51]
and in the rat isolated forestomach[42]. For both of these tissues
dopamine acted on those α-adrenoceptors which modulate neuronal
acetylcholine release (α_2-adrenoceptors); noradrenaline and clonidine
may act on similar receptors and their inhibitory effects were also
antagonised by metoclopramide[36,51,20,42]. Metoclopramide had no
effects on responses mediated by α- or β-adrenoceptors located on the
smooth muscle membrane of guinea-pig or rat stomach[54,20].

The lowest concentrations of metoclopramide which antagonised
α_2-adrenoceptor-mediated inhibition of cholinergic contractions are
considerably higher than the minimum concentrations of metoclopramide
which had a more direct effect on cholinergic-mediated contractions
(0.04µg/ml for guinea-pig ileum; 0.01µg/ml for rat stomach; table 2).
The effects of metoclopramide on α_2-adrenoceptors may therefore be of
relatively small importance in vivo.

EFFECTS OF METOCLOPRAMIDE ON THE RELEASE OF GASTROINTESTINAL HORMONES
AND PEPTIDES

Metoclopramide may affect blood plasma concentrations of some
gastrointestinal peptides, but in most cases it is not clear whether
metoclopramide affected the release of peptides by a direct action or
as a consequence of increased gut motility. In addition, we do not
know whether the change in peptide release was sufficient to affect
gastrointestinal motility.

In healthy volunteers, metoclopramide 10mg 3 x day for 7 days
reduced the release of gastrin in response to a meal[55]. This action
of metoclopramide may be mediated by antagonism of an action of
dopamine in the central nervous system (affecting nervous or hormonal
mechanisms which inhibit gastrin release), but the evidence was not
conclusive.

Metoclopramide improved the diarrhoea and hypokalaemia and
reduced the plasma concentrations of vasoactive intestinal polypeptide
in a patient with a pancreatic tumour[56]. In healthy volunteers,
metoclopramide 2.5 or 10mg i.v. increased serum motilin concentrations[57]. Metoclopramide 100µg/ml had no effects on the release of
motilin from human isolated mucosa[58], but this concentration of
metoclopramide is excessively high and perhaps an intact gut
cholinergic innervation may be necessary for metoclopramide to
increase the release of certain gut hormones. For example metoclopramide stimulated pancreatic polypeptide release from the human
pancreas[59]. The response to metoclopramide was prevented by atropine
but it was not established whether the peptide release was increased
as a consequence of metoclopramide stimulating gut motility (by
cholinergic-dependent mechanisms) or by an action of metoclopramide
on a cholinergic mediated control of the peptide release.

MISCELLANEOUS ACTIONS OF METOCLOPRAMIDE IN THE GASTROINTESTINAL
TRACT

In guinea-pig ileum metoclopramide may increase submaximal
contractions to acetylcholine, histamine, Substance P and barium
chloride. This effect of metoclopramide was prevented by tetrodotoxin and only partly reduced by atropine[16,9], suggesting an
involvement of non-cholinergic neurones. However, an increase in
contractions to histamine has not been confirmed by others using
similar concentrations of metoclopramide[11,38,8,33]. In addition,
metoclopramide did not increase contractions to histamine in
guinea-pig isolated colon[14]. There have been no similar studies
using human gastrointestinal preparations.

Finally, metoclopramide (approximately 1-100µg/ml) increased the tone of opossum lower oesophageal sphincter muscle. The response was not antagonised by atropine, hyosine, hexamethonium, tetrodotoxin, phentolamine, diphenhydramine or propranolol[60].

CONCLUSIONS AND FUTURE RESEARCH

The complex actions of metoclopramide on gastrointestinal motility are only just beginning to be understood. It seems probable that an important effect of metoclopramide is to increase cholinergic-mediated contractions in the stomach and small intestine, perhaps by facilitating neuronal ACh release. However, the major questions which now have to be answered are how does metoclopramide increase the cholinergic response and why is the drug selective for gut muscle? A receptor mechanism peculiar to the cholinergic nerves innervating the gut muscle (5HT-like?) may explain the selective actions of metoclopramide, although other reasons, such as pharmacokinetics, may also play a part.

Finally, it remains possible that metoclopramide could affect the motility of the gastrointestinal tract by affecting gut hormone release (which may be modulated by dopaminergic mechanisms in the central nervous system[53]), or by acting on the central nervous system or the peripheral ganglia. These are areas of metoclopramide research which have only occasionally been studied, but are necessary to further our understanding of the ways in which drugs can be used to control gastrointestinal motility.

REFERENCES

1. R. M. Pinder, R. N. Brogden, P. R. Sawyer, T. M. Speight, and G. S. Avery, Metoclopramide: A review of its pharmacological properties and clinical use, Drugs. 12:81 (1976).
2. R. A. Harrington, C. W. Hamilton, R. N. Brogden, J. A. Linkewich, J. A. Romankiewicz, and R. C. Heel, Metoclopramide, an updated review of its pharmacological properties and clinical use, Drugs. 25:451 (1983).
3. K. Schulze-Delrieu, Metoclopramide, Gastroenterol. 77:768 (1979).
4. B. Costall, S. J. Gunning, R. J. Naylor, and K. H. Simpson, A central site of action for benzamide facilitation of gastric emptying, Eur. J. Pharmac. 91:197 (1983).
5. O. P. W. Robinson, Metoclopramide - a new pharmacological approach? Postgrad. Med. J. 49, Suppl 4:9 (1973).
6. K. Kowalewski and A. Kolodej, Effect of metoclopramide on myoelectrical and mechanical activity of the isolated canine stomach perfused extracorporeally, Pharmacology. 13:549 (1975).

7.   R. D. N. Birtley and M. W. Baines, The effects of metoclopramide
     on some isolated intestinal preparations, Postgrad. Med. J.
     49 (Suppl. 4):13 (1973).
8.   F. K. Okwuasaba and J. T. Hamilton, The effect of metoclopramide
     in intestinal muscle responses and the peristaltic reflex in
     vitro, Can. J. Physiol. Pharmacol. 54:393 (1976).
9.   P. R. Blower, Some aspects of the pharmacology of metoclopramide,
     Ph.D. thesis, University of Aston in Birmingham, U.K. (1977).
10. M. Eisner, Gastro-intestinal effects of metoclopramide in man.
     In vitro experiments with human smooth muscle preparations,
     Br. Med. J. 4:679 (1968).
11. J. Fontaine and J. J. Reuse, Pharmacological analysis of the
     effects of metoclopramide on the guinea-pig ileum in vitro,
     Arch. int. Pharmacodyn. 204:293 (1973).
12. F. K. Okwuasaba and J. T. Hamilton, The effect of metoclopramide
     on inhibition induced by purine-mucleotides, noradrenaline and
     theophylline ethylenediamine on intestinal muscle and on peri-
     stalsis in vitro, Can. J. Physiol. Pharmacol. 53:972 (1975).
13. A. M. Hay, Pharmacological analysis of the effects of metoclo-
     pramide on the guinea-pig isolated stomach, Gastroenterol.
     72:864 (1977).
14. L. Beani, C. Bianchi, and C. Crema, Effects of metoclopramide
     on isolated guinea-pig colon. 1. Peripheral sensitization to
     acetylcholine, Eur. J. Pharmac. 12:320 (1970)
15. C. Bianchi, L. Beani, and C. Crema, Effects of metoclopramide on
     isolated guinea-pig colon. 2. Interference with ganglionic
     stimulant drugs, Eur. J. Pharmac. 12:332 (1970).
16. R. W. Bury and M. L. Mashford, The effects of metoclopramide in
     modifying the response of isolated guinea-pig ileum to
     various agonists, J. Pharmacol. Exp. Ther. 197:641 (1976).
17. J. D. Anderson, M. D. Day, and J. K. Watson, Potentiation by
     metoclopramide of responses to cholinergic nerve stimulation
     in the isolated gastric fundus preparation of the rat,
     J. Pharm. Pharmac. 29:53P (1977).
18. A. M. Hay and W. K. Man, Effect of metoclopramide on guinea-pig
     stomach: Critical dependence on intrinsic stores of acetyl-
     choline, Gastroenterol. 76:492 (1979).
19. C. M. McClelland and G. J. Sanger, Effects of metoclopramide and
     domperidone on cholinergic responses in rat isolated stomach,
     Br. J. Pharmac. 77, Proc. Suppl: 539P (1982).
20. C. M. McClelland and G. J. Sanger, Antagonism by metoclopramide
     of an inhibitory response to clonidine in rat isolated stomach
     muscle, Br. J. Pharmac. 77, Proc. Suppl: 484P (1982).
21. C. M. McClelland and G. J. Sanger, Increased cholinergic
     responses with BRL 20627 in rat isolated stomach: Comparison
     with metoclopramide, Br. J. Pharmac. 80, Proc. Suppl:
     568P (1983).
22. G. J. Sanger, unpublished.

23. C. M. McClelland, B. McRitchie, and D. H. Turner, BRL 20627 – A non-dopaminergic blocking stimulant of gastric motility, Br. J. Pharmac. 80, Proc. Suppl: 569P (1983).

24. B. McRitchie, C. M. McClelland, S. Cooper, D. H. Turner, and G. J. Sanger, Dopamine antagonists as anti-emetics and as stimulants of gastric motility, in: "This book".

25. M. A. Heazell, A non-adrenergic component to the inhibitory innervation of the fundus of the rat stomach, Br. J. Pharmac. 36:186P (1969).

26. W. B. Hunt, D. J. O'Hagan, and J. Wilkinson, Inhibition by perivascular nerve stimulation of the rebound contraction of the rat gastric corpus muscle to field stimulation, Br. J. Pharmac. 74:849P (1981).

27. W. B. Hunt, D. G. Parsons, A. Wahid, and J. Wilkinson, Influence of 2-2'-pyridylisatogen tosylate on responses produced by ATP and by neural stimulation of the rat gastric corpus, Br. J. Pharmac. 63:378P (1978).

28. T. Hongo and Y. Kasuya, Effects of various drugs and extrinsic denervation of the non-adrenergic inhibitory neurons in the rat stomach, J. Pharm. Dyn. 5:451 (1982).

29. A. Bennett and H. L. Stockley, The intrinsic innervation of the human alimentary tract and its relation to function, Gut. 16:443 (1975).

30. G. Huizing and A. J. Beckett, The acetylcholinesterase inhibitory activity of metoclopramide and some of its biotransformation products, Pharm. Weekblad Sci. Ed. 2:117 (1980).

31. B. Costall, R. J. Naylor, and C. C. W. Tan, On the mechanisms of contraction and relaxation of circular smooth muscle from guinea-pig stomach to field stimulation, Br. J. Pharmac. 78, Proc. Suppl: 175P (1983).

32. H. Kilbinger, R. Kruel, I. Pfeuffer-Friederich, and I. Wessler, The effects of metoclopramide on acetylcholine release and on smooth muscle response in the isolated guinea-pig ileum, Naunyn-Schmiedeberg's Arch. Pharmacol. 319:231 (1982).

33. M. A. Zar, O. O. Ebong, and D. N. Bateman, Effect of metoclopramide in guinea-pig ileum longitudinal muscle: Evidence against dopamine mediation, Gut. 23:66 (1982).

34. E. E. Daniel, Pharmacology of adrenergic, cholinergic, and drugs acting on other receptors in gastrointestinal muscle, in: "Handb. Exp. Pharmac, 59, Mediators and drugs in gastrointestinal motility II". G. Bertaccini, ed., Springer-Verlag, Berlin, Heidelberg, New York (1982).

35. L. I. Goldberg, P. H. Volkman, and J. D. Kohli, A comparison of the vascular dopamine receptors with other dopamine receptors, Ann. Rev. Pharmac. 18:57 (1978).

36. M. Spedding, Antagonism of the inhibitory effects of clonidine and dopamine in the guinea-pig ileum by metoclopramide, sultopride and sulpiride, Br. J. Pharmac. 73:279P (1981).

37. J. Fontaine and J. J. Reuse, Étude comparative de l'action de quelques benzamides substituées sur l'iléon isolé de cobaye, Arch. int. Pharmacodyn. 213:322 (1975).
38. J. Fontaine and J. J. Reuse, Pharmacological analysis of the effects of substituted benzamides on the isolated guinea-pig ileum. Study of metoclopramide, sulpiride, bromopride, tiapride, sultapride, Arch. int. Pharmacodyn. 235:51 (1978).
39. D. Wallis, Neuronal 5-hydroxytryptamine receptors outside the central nervous system, Life Sci. 29:2345 (1981).
40. P. Fosbraey, M. F. Hird and E. S. Johnson, The effects of some dopamine antagonists on cholinergic mechanisms in the guinea-pig ileum, J. Auton. Pharmac. 1:17 (1980).
41. R. J. Flower, Drugs which inhibit prostaglandin synthesis, Pharmac. Rev. 26:33 (1974).
42. R. A. Lefebvre, J. P. Blancquaert, J. L. Willems, and M. G. Bagaert, In vitro study of the inhibitory effects of dopamine on the rat gastric fundus, Naunyn-Schmiedeberg's Arch. Pharmacol. 322:228 (1983).
43. M. Costa and J. B. Furness, The sites of action of 5-hydroxy-tryptamine in nerve-muscle preparations from the guinea-pig small intestine and colon, Br. J. Pharmac. 65:237 (1979).
44. J. B. Furness and M. Costa, Identification of gastrointestinal neurotransmitters, in: "Handb. Exp. Pharmac, 59, Mediators and drugs in gastrointestinal motility I", G. Bertaccini, ed., Springer-Verlag, Berlin, Heidelberg, New York (1982).
45. D. J. De Carle and J. Christensen, A dopamine receptor in oesophageal smooth muscle of the opossum, Gastroenterol. 70:216 (1976).
46. J. M. Van Nueten, Is dopamine an inhibitory modulator of gastric motility? Trends in Pharmacological Sciences. May:233 (1980).
47. Y. Kamikawa, Y. Shimo, and K. Uchida, Inhibitory actions of catecholamines on electrically induced contractions of the submucous plexus-longitudinal muscularis mucosae preparation of the guinea-pig oesophagus, Br. J. Pharmac. 76:271 (1982).
48. B. Cox and C. Ennis, Mechanism of action of dopamine on the guinea-pig gastro-oesophageal junction in vitro, Br. J. Pharmac. 71:177 (1980).
49. H. A. Sahyoun, B. Costall, and R. J. Naylor, Catecholamine-induced relaxations and contraction of the lower oesophageal and pyloric sphincters of guinea-pig stomach: Modification by domperidone, J. Pharm. Pharmac. 34:318 (1982).
50. J. Wikberg, Differentiation between pre- and post-junctional α-adrenoceptors in guinea-pig ileum and rabbit aorta, Acta Physiol. Scand. 103:225 (1978).
51. R. Gorich, T. R. Weihrauch, and H. Kilbinger, The inhibition by dopamine of cholinergic transmission in the isolated guinea-pig ileum, Naunyn-Schmiedeberg's Arch. Pharmacol. 318:308 (1982).

52. B. K. Thompson and D. J. De Carle, The effect of dopamine on human gastric smooth muscle, Aust. J. Exp. Biol. Med. Sci. 60:123 (1982).

53. K. Uvnas-Wallensten and M. Goiny, Dopaminergic control of gastrointestinal hormones, in: "Apomorphine and other dopaminomimetics, 1: Basic Pharmacology", G. L. Gessa and G. U. Corsini, ed., Raven Press, New York (1981).

54. B. Costall, R. J. Naylor and H. A. Sahyoun, On the nature of the catecholamine receptor mechanisms mediating relaxation and contraction of circular smooth muscle of guinea-pig stomach, Br. J. Pharmac. 74:179P (1981).

55. R. Caldara, C. Ferrari, C. Barbieri, and M. Romussi, Effect of four dopamine receptor antagonists on gastrin secretion in healthy subjects, Scand. J. Gastroent. 15: 481 (1980).

56. R. G. Long, M. G. Bryant, P. M. Yuille, J. M. Polak, and S. R. Bloom, Mixed pancreatic apudoma with symptoms of excess vasoactive intestinal polypeptide and insulin: improvement of diarrhoea with metoclopramide, Gut, 22:505 (1981).

57. D. Byrnes, L. Henderson, and C. Meridith, Release of motilin by metoclopramide, Aust. N.Z. Med. J. 10:109 (1980).

58. T. J. Borody, D. J. Byrnes, and L. A. Henderson, In vitro release of motilin from human duodenal mucosa, Aust. N.Z. Med. J. 10:336 (1980).

59. I. M. Spitz, E. Zylber, D. Leroith, M. Shapiro, R. Luboshitsky, J. Jersky, and J. Hoffman, The human pancreatic polypeptide response to metoclopramide, Diabetes. 27, Suppl 2: 506 (1978).

60. S. Cohen and A. J. DiMarino, Mechanisms of action of metoclopramide on opossum lower oesophageal sphincter muscle, Gastroenterol. 71:996 (1976).

LAXATIVES: A REVIEW OF THEIR MECHANISMS OF ACTION

Paul Bass and Deborah A. Fox

School of Pharmcy
University of Wisconsin
425 N. Charter Street
Madison, Wisconsin 53706

Laxatives are a heterogeneous group of drugs used to increase the frequency of bowel movements. They have been associated with two distinct effects on the gastrointestinal tract: a laxative-induced smooth muscle electric and motor pattern in the small bowel and an accumulation of fluid in the lumen of both the small and large intestines. All laxatives tested may act by one or both of these mechanisms. In addition to these two distinct actions of quantitatively different responses in these two parameters for the small and large intestines. Reginal deiffrences within either of the intestinal organs probably also exists adding further complexity in the responses to laxative drugs.

There does not appear to be a relationship between the diversified chemical structure of laxatives and their similar effects on intestinal motility and fluid accumulation. The organic substances that are laxatives are, however, unified by possessing a common physical property, surfactant activity. Figure 1 depicts the structures of several of the common laxatives. All of these agents except magnesium sulfate, lactulose, and the dietary fibers (not shown) are capable of nonspecifically interacting with biological membranes by virtue of their surfactant activity. This property, as will be shown subsequently, accounts at least in part for laxatives' ability to cause net fluid accumulation in the lumen of the intestine.

The purpose of the present review is to present the current views on the mechanisms of action of laxative drugs. Our aim is not to elucidate the means by which each drug acts but to discuss

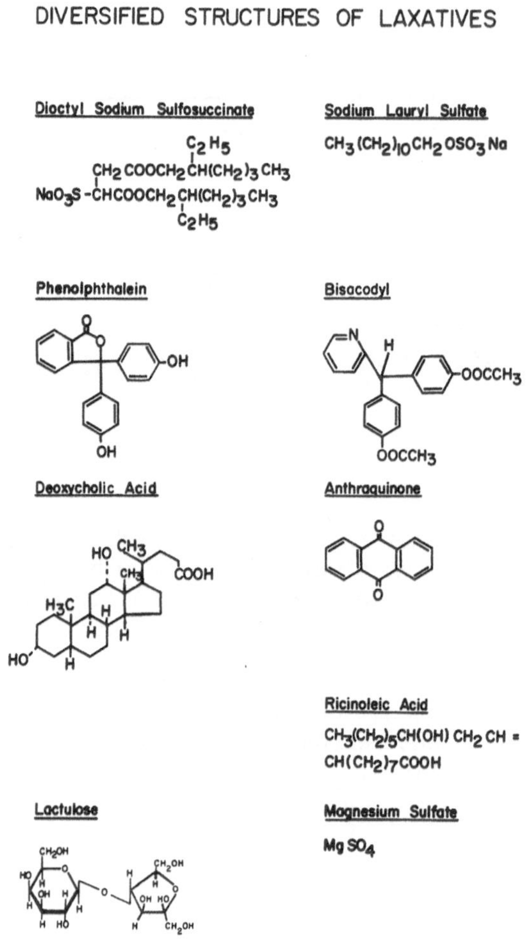

DIVERSIFIED STRUCTURES OF LAXATIVES

Dioctyl Sodium Sulfosuccinate

$$C_2H_5$$
$$CH_2COOCH_2CH(CH_2)_3CH_3$$
$$NaO_3S-CHCOOCH_2CH(CH_2)_3CH_3$$
$$C_2H_5$$

Sodium Lauryl Sulfate

$$CH_3(CH_2)_{10}CH_2OSO_3Na$$

Phenolphthalein

Bisacodyl

Deoxycholic Acid

Anthraquinone

Ricinoleic Acid

$$CH_3(CH_2)_5CH(OH)CH_2CH =$$
$$CH(CH_2)_7COOH$$

Lactulose

Magnesium Sulfate

$$MgSO_4$$

Fig. 1. Chemical structures of a select group of laxatives. Note
the range of diversified chemical compounds including an
inorganic salt, a dissacharide, a steroid, phenolic
derivatives, and an hydroxy fatty acid.

the general mechanisms whereby these agents alter the GI tract to produce laxation. (This area has been previously reviewed by Binder, 1977; Gaginella and Bass, 1978; Sund, 1982; and Gullikson and Bass, 1984.)

EFFECTS OF LAXATIVES ON INTESTINAL MOTILITY

Traditionally, several laxatives have been classified as "stimulants" of intestinal motility (Bonnycastle, 1965). Laxation was thought to be due to a stimulation of intestinal motility which increased the transit of intestinal content, and consequently decreased membrane contact time for the absorption of fluid. Also, laxatives can produce coordinated motility patterns in portions of the colon, referred to as mass movements (Ritchie, 1972). Recent evidence, however, indicates that these agents can depress smooth muscle contractility both in vivo and in vitro, rather than stimulate motility as originally thought. In addition, in vivo, laxatives elicit a distinct propulsive pattern of intestinal motility. The effect of laxatives on intestinal motility in vivo and in vitro is discussed in greater detail below.

Studies utilizing isolated intestinal smooth muscle verify that laxatives such as anthraquinones (Latven et al., 1952), sodium ricinoleate (active component of castor oil) (Stewart et al., 1975a), or other surfactants (Gaginella et al., 1975b) depress contractility. The structurally related abilities of fatty acid derivatives, such as sodium ricinoleate, to inhibit smooth muscle activity paralleled their abilities to alter fluid movement (Gaginella et al., 1975a). Dioctyl sodium sulfosuccinate (DSS), sodium dodecyl sulfate (SDS), and several bile acids can depress the electrically driven guinea pig ileum over the same narrow concentration range required for the depressant action of ricinoleate (Gaginella et al., 1975b). These agents also caused a corresponding increase in lumenal fluid accumulation. In addition to the above laxatives, the magnesium ion contained in several commercial laxative preparations has also been shown to depress smooth muscle activity (Beleslin, 1970). Therefore, it can be seen that in vitro, these laxatives are not "stimulants" of motility.

The smooth muscle of the normal untreated gastrointestinal tract in vivo, displays patterns associated with two physiological states: the interdigestive (fasted) state and the digestive (fed) state. In the interdigestive state, 40-60 minutes of quiescence (basal) is followed by intermittent activity (preburst) for 20 to 30 minutes which terminates in high amplitude maximal activity (burst) lasting for 10 to 20 minutes (Carlson et al., 1970). These three portions of the cycle have also been referred to as Phase I, II, and III, respectively (Code and Marlett, 1975). This cycle repeats itself every 2 hours in the fasted state in man and dogs.

This complex, which originates in the upper GI tract and migrates down the tract, is referred to as the migrating myoelectric complex (MMC) (for review, see Wingate, 1981). The digestive pattern is initiated by feeding and is characterized by an intermediate motor pattern (Carlson et al., 1970). (See Figure 3 in the chapter "Motility: Methods for In Vivo Measurement.")

Laxatives produce differing effects on smooth muscle activity depending on whether they are administered in the fed or fasted state. At a given dose, either castor oil or magnesium sulfate may decrease the contractile frequency when administered during the interdigestive (fasted) state and yet appear to exhibit no pharmacological response when given during the digestive (fed) state (Stewart et al., 1975b). If, however, we examine the laxatives in the fasted state only, there is a tendency toward a decrease in contractions (BER with spikes) when compared to the digestive state, while no change or an increase in contractions when compared to the interdigestive state (Table). Therefore, if one analyzes the data by a comparison of the number of laxative-induced contractions with contractions occurring during these two normal physiological states, the effect of laxatives on motility cannot be ascertained.

Table. The number of spikes produced during a 2 h interval: a comparison of fasted, fed, and drug states

Drug condition	Mean number of BER with spikes generated in 2 h postdosage* (± SEM)	Comparison of means of Duncan's range test†
Interdigestive (fasted)	413.6 ± 67.3	
Phenolphthalein	478.3 ± 85.2	
NaCl‡	565.4 ± 63.5	
Magnesium sulphate	623.0 ± 78.4	
Castor oil	707.8 ± 115.3	
Digestive (fed)	846.5 ± 72.4	

*Each mean represents the average of two replicates at two sites for four animals
†Any two means not paralleled by the same line are significantly different (p < 0.05)
‡ 0.9% w/v
(adapted from Atchison et al., 1978a)

The discrepancy in laxative-induced contractile activity led to the postulation that the _pattern_ of contractile activity rather than the absolute number of contractions may be important to the mechanism of laxation. A number of reports of migrating spike potential activity during intestinal secretion have been made (Mathias et al., 1976; Mathias et al., 1977; Mathias et al., 1978; Burns et al., 1978; Burns et al., 1980). This intestinal secretogogue-induced spiking pattern has been termed the migrating action potential complex (MAPC) by Mathias. The laxatives studied to date also demonstrate this unique electric pattern. As shown in Figure 2, magnesium sulfate elicits a spiking pattern consisting of

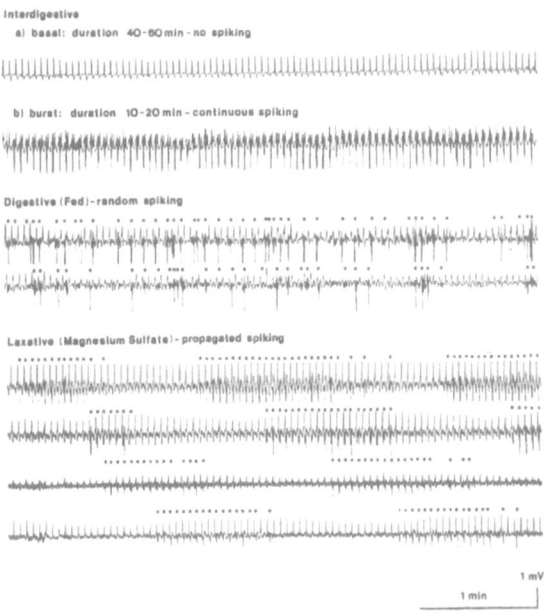

Fig. 2. Representative samples of electromyograms recorded during interdigestive (a) basal and (b) burst, digestive, and laxative-induced states. Dots (•) have been placed over each spike potential in the lower two panels for clarity. The time and voltage scale are shown; time constant = .3S. Note the distinct propagated spike pattern seen with the magnesium sulfate. This has been identified as a MAPC pattern. (Adapted from Atchison et al., 1978a.)

recurrent bursts of 3-15 spike potentials that presumably sweep the contents of the small bowel into the colon where the absorptive capacity is exceeded or fluid secretion may occur (Atchison et al., 1978a; Atchison et al., 1978b). A similar MAPC pattern has been demonstrated with phenolphthalein and castor oil. Shiff et al., 1982, suggest that deoxycholic acid-induced MAPCs may originate by a mucosal neuronal reflex. Thus, it can be seen that structurally differing laxatives produce a distinct propagating contractile pattern which is associated with intestinal secretion and hence laxation.

It has been possible to separate the secretogogue-induced motor pattern from the intestinal secretory activity. Sinar et al., 1982, have confirmed that cholera toxin is an intestinal se-cretogogue. However, by using only the B subunit of the molecule, they demonstrated that MAPCs could be initiated <u>without</u> intestinal secretions. In addition, Mathias et al., 1980, have shown that Shigella enterotoxin can elicit MAPCs without concomitant lumenal fluid production. These experiments illustrate that the motor and secretory events are two separate phenomenon or that the two are related but possess different sensitivities to various stimuli.

EFFECTS OF LAXATIVES ON FLUID AND ELECTROLYTE MOVEMENT

Lumenal fluid accumulation may result from effects on intes-tinal absorption or secretory processes. Ricinoleic and deoxy-cholic acids, DSS, bisacodyl, and other laxatives are capable of producing net inhibition of fluid absorption and even secretion in the jejunum, ileum, and colon in a number of animal models and man (Mekhjian and Phillips, 1970; Mekhjian et al., 1971; Teem and Phillips, 1972; Ammon and Phillips, 1974; Gaginella et al. 1975a; Gaginella et al., 1975b; Rachmilewitz et al., 1976; Saunders et al., 1977; Gaginella et al., 1977a; Gullikson et al., 1977). The mechanisms of intestinal fluid accumulation produced by laxatives are diverse. These include: cellular and mucosal damage, enhanced mucosal permeability, increases in c-AMP, inhibition of Na/K ATPase, and changes in hormone levels. Most of these actions appear to be intimately related to the abilities of these compounds to nonspecifically interact with biological membranes. Each of these mechanisms are discussed below.

Cellular and Mucosal Damage

Surfactants are compounds which have the ability to lower sur-face tension at an air and water or oil and water interface. This property is an indirect measure of nonspecific interactions with membranes. Most laxatives, except lactulose and the bulks, have surfactant activity and are able to interact with cell membranes. Gullikson et al. (1977) have shown that the order of potency of ricinoleic acid, dihydroxy bile acids, DSS, and SDS to inhibit water absorption paralleled their abilities to lower surface tension. These same diverse chemicals were also potent lytic agents on red blood cell membranes, while trihydroxy bile salts, which had little effect on water absorption, were not hemolytic. Ricinoleate, deoxycholate, and DSS have also produced dose-dependent cytotoxicity on isolated hamster and small intestinal cells (Gaginella et al., 1977b). In vivo, DSS, ricinoleate, and magnesium sulfate produced jejunal cell loss in man, which is coincident with intestinal fluid secretion (Bernier et al., 1979). Therefore, it can be seen that intestinal cytotoxicity produced by surfactant-type laxatives occurs over the same concentration ranges as the effects on water transport.

Laxatives considerably alter the integrity of the intestinal mucosa in vivo. Figure 3 illustrates the dramatic alteration in the villus tips after deoxycholate perfusion. Dihydroxy and unconjugated bile salts are more potent in producing histological alterations than trihydroxy and conjugated bile salts (Low-Beer et al., 1970; Teem and Phillips, 1972; Gullikson et al., 1977; Chadwich et al., 1979) reflecting a similar relationship for water transport effects. Ricinoleic acid, DSS, and bisacodyl also alter intestinal mucosal integrity and structure at concentrations which produce either net inhibition of fluid absorption or secretion (Saunders et al., 1975; Cline et al., 1976; Gaginella et al., 1977a; Saunders et al., 1977).

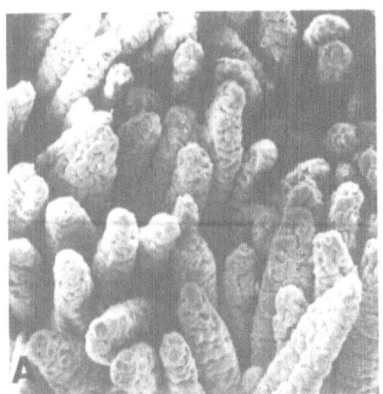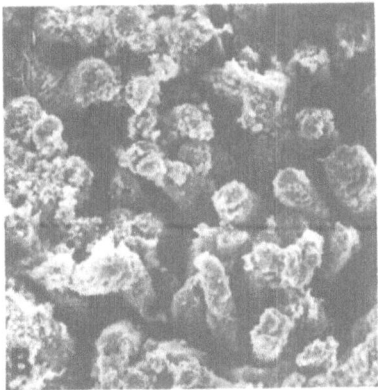

Fig. 3. Comparison of scanning images of small intestine after control (0.9% saline) perfusion, A, and perfusion with deoxycholate, B. The villus tips were drastically altered by deoxycholate perfusion, whereas perfusion with saline left almost all villus tips intact (x100). (Adapted from Gullikson et al., 1977.)

331

Enhanced Mucosal Permeability

Increases in mucosal permeability have been produced by anti-absorptive concentrations of ricinoleate and deoxycholic acids. Blood to lumen clearance of inulin (MW-6000) and dextran (MW-16,000) in the small intestine were markedly enhanced by ricinoleic acid. Deoxycholate even produced a leakage of albumin (MW-60,000) into the gut lumen (Cline et al., 1976; Gullikson et al., 1977). Substances with low colonic permeability, such as urea, creatinine, and polyethylene glycol (average MW-400), were found to be readily permeable either in the blood to lumen or lumen to blood direction following exposure of the colon in a dose-related manner to ricinoleic acid (Gaginella et al., 1977a). Notably, the alteration in small intestinal permeability did not occur in the response to either cholera toxin (Cline et al., 1976) or taurocholate (Gullikson et al., 1977). Cholera toxin acts via a c-AMP mechanism whereas taurocholate was not able to induce altered histological or secretory effects. Further evidence of altered mucosal integrity in these studies were the loss of sucrase, a brush-border-marked enzyme, and DNA from exfoliated cells. Similarly, bile acid-induced changes in the permeability of the small intestine and colon reflect the differential abilities of di- and tri-hydroxy bile acids to produce net fluid secretion (Chadwick et al., 1979; Caspary and Meyne, 1980). Thus, the changes in mucosal permeability occur within the same concentration range for antiabsorptive effects.

c-AMP and Laxatives

Stimulation of adenylate cyclase and corresponding rises in c-AMP are believed to be responsible for the intestinal water secretion elicited by cholera toxin (Sharp and Hynie, 1971; Kimberg et al., 1971; Kimberg, 1974), certain prostaglandins (Kimberg et al., 1971; Kimberg, 1974), and vasoactive intestinal peptide (VIP) (Schwartz et al., 1974; Waldman et al., 1977). Calcium may be the mediator between elevated c-AMP and fluid secretion. Calcium is released by c-AMP (Berridge, 1975) and produces active anion secretion (Bolton and Field, 1977).

Adenylate cyclase and c-AMP have also been implicated in laxative-induced fluid and electrolyte effects. Bile salts can alter ion permeabilities and increase short-circuit current in both the small and large intestine (Binder et al., 1975) in a manner similar to cholera toxin. The dihydroxy salts were more effective than the trihydroxy bile salts reflecting the potency relationship for water secretory effects. Furthermore, agents such as DSS, bile acids, and ricinoleic acid, which increase short circuit current, also significantly increase c-AMP levels in the rat colon (Donowitz and Binder, 1975).

The mechanism by which laxatives increase c-AMP is unknown. Deoxycholate and SDS have been shown to stimulate adenylate cyclase in vitro in a nonspecific manner (Perkins and Moore, 1971; Helenius and Simons, 1975). This is in contrast to the specificity of activation of adenylate cyclase by cholera toxin, VIP, and prostaglandins. RMI 12330A, an inhibitor of c-AMP formation, was able to block ileal adenylate cyclase activity and intestinal secretion after exposure to cholera toxin (Tai et al., 1978; Farack and Nell, 1979) but not deoxycholate or bisacodyl (Farack and Nell, 1979). Alternatively, laxatives by their damaging effects may release prostaglandins which could alter adenylate cyclase activity (Beubler and Juan, 1978; Rachmilewitz et al., 1980). It appears that laxative-induced c-AMP changes may be quantitatively different from those elicited by bacterial toxins and endogenous secretogogues.

Effects of Laxatives on Na/K ATPase and Energy Metabolism

Na/K ATPase is located on the basolateral membrane of the villus cells and is responsible for the active extrusion of Na^+ in the serosal direction. The creation of an electrochemical gradient results in the passive absorption of water through transcellular and intercellular pathways. Inhibition of this enzyme would consequently result in inhibition of water absorption. Several studies have shown that laxatives have an inhibitory effect on Na/K ATPase (Parkinson et al., 1964; Phillips et al., 1965; Chignell, 1968; Faust and Wu, 1967; Guiraldes et al. 1975; Powell et al., 1980; Rachmilewitz et al., 1980; Wanitscke, 1980).

In addition to the inhibition of the enzyme Na/K ATPase, laxatives may reduce absorptive function by inhibiting cellular metabolic functions involved in ATP production. Reduced tissue levels of ATP have been correlated with impaired intestinal fluid absorption after treatment with taurocholate and glycocholate (Faust and Wu, 1965). Also, agents such as ricinoleate, deoxycholic and oleic acids and sodium dodecyl sulfate, which elicit intestinal fluid accumulation, inhibit adenine nucleotide translocase (ANT) (Gaginella et al., 1975c; Wojtczak and Zaluska, 1967; Duszynski and Wojtczak, 1974). ANT transports ADP across the mitochondrial membrane in exchange for ATP which may be used as a substrate for Na/K ATPase. These metabolic effects of laxatives are reflected in a generalized inhibition of transport processes rather than of electrolyte transport in particular (Parkinson and Olsen, 1964).

Hormones as Mediators of Laxative Action

A number of hormones found in the gastrointestinal tract are capable of altering intestinal motility (Parker and Beneventano, 1970; Dinoso et al., 1973; Stewart and Bass, 1976) and inducing net fluid secretion in the small or large intestines (Gardner et al., 1967; Barbezat and Grossman, 1971 a and b; Moritz et al., 1973;

Waldman et al., 1977). Because of these dual actions, a role for these substances in the effects of laxatives has been evoked.

Cholecystokinin (CCK) has been implicated in the actions of at least two laxative drugs, ricinoleic acid and magnesium sulfate. Similar effects on intestinal motility were obtained by ricinoleate and CCK in the small intestine of the dog (Stewart and Bass, 1976). The mechanism of action of the magnesium ion in the intra-lumenal fluid accumulation and altered motility has also been attributed to CCK release (Stewart and Bass, 1976; Harvey and Read, 1973).

Elevated plasma levels of vasoactive intestinal peptide (VIP) are associated with clinically observed types of diarrhea (Bloom et al., 1973; Said and Faloona, 1975; Krejs et al., 1977). VIP, which may be released after intestinal exposure to cholera toxin (Bloom et al., 1976) has been shown to be depleted from isolated enterocytes by ricinoleic acid (Kerzner et al., 1979). However, determination of plasma levels of VIP after exposure to laxatives would be needed to verify its involvement in laxative-induced fluid secretion.

Prostaglandins may mediate the effects of laxatives on motor and secretory activities of the gastrointestinal tract. Prostaglandin $F_2\alpha$ infusion produces an electrical pattern associated with fluid secretion similar to that observed with the laxatives (Atchison et al., 1978a, Atchison et al., 1978b; Mathias et al., 1978). Tissue prostaglandin levels have been observed to be elevated in diseases characterized by diarrhea (Sandler et al., 1968; Gould, 1975), and prostaglandin cyclooxygenase inhibitors have been effective in the treatment of various types of diarrhea (Dupont et al., 1977; Mennie et al., 1975). Laxative agents such as aloe and phenolphthalein (Collier et al., 1976) stimulate the formation of E and F prostaglandins from arachodonic acid. Bisacodyl increases jejunal and colonic levels of PGE_2 (Rachmilewitz and Karmeli, 1979; Rachmilewitz et al., 1980). It has further been shown that laxatives such as bisacodyl and phenolphthalein lead to enhanced release of PGE activity in the rat colon which could be blocked by indomethacin pretreatment (Beubler and Juan, 1978).

The above studies suggest that laxatives cause a direct release of various secretogogue hormones. It must be considered, however, that it is the surfactant property of the various laxatives which initiate membrane alterations which may cause the release of these hormones.

BULK LAXATIVES AND DIETARY FIBERS

A major group of laxatives consist of a heterogeneous group of polysaccharides (glycans). These agents also exert effects on fluid movement and motor activity on the intestinal tract, but the mechanism by which they act are different than those previously described in this review. While they have been thought to act entirely by hydration and swelling, the simple property of in vitro water imbibition does not directly correlate with their pharmacological effects (Stephen and Cummings, 1979). As a group, these chemicals have a wide variety of biological actions which may account for their laxative properties. (This area has been recently reviewed by Connell, 1981.)

Bacteria have been shown to have a role in the action of bulk laxatives. It is well established that bacteria in the cecum and stomach of ruminents readily break down plant constuents. Complex carbohydrates when broken down can produce increases in the total amount of volatile fatty acids (Spiller et al, 1980). The kinetics of colonic and rectal absorption of short chain fatty acids, such as those released by fiber digestion, have been reported in man (McNeil et al., 1978; Ruppin et al., 1980). At concentrations up to 90 mM, these substances are readily absorbed along with water. Though it is unlikely that an increase in colonic fatty acids alone will lead to laxation, the effect of fiber products on the bacteria may be a factor.

The idea that certain types of indigestible matter in the colon fosters the growth of bacteria was made by Hoppert and Clark (1945). This increase in bacterial population was quantified by Fuchs et al. 1976). Subjects on wheat bran obtained the expected laxative effect which was accompanied by a significant increase in the fecal anaerobic bacterial population. A clinical comparison between relatively indigestible (wheat) and digestible (cabbage) fiber has lead to a hypothesis that dietary fibers may have two distinct actions on the colon - hydration of undigested fiber and stimulation of bacterial growth (Stephens and Cummings, 1980). The increases in bacteria lead to increases in fecal weight accompanied by a greater fecal output.

Bacteria may also be the causative agent of gas production in the colon, a further action related to laxation. As demonstrated by Steggerta (1968) and Hellendoorn (1978) with bean diets and in certain grain cereals (Hickey et al., 1972), one can markedly increase flatus output. The increases in gas production was attributed to the presence of sugars which were not digested in the small bowel. These substances appear to be substrate for the bacteria in the colon and lead to formation of carbon dioxide, hydrogen, and possibly methane. This colonic gas accumulation may contribute to defecation (Hoppert and Clark, 1945).

SUMMARY

Despite their use since ancient times, the mechanisms by which laxatives act are only currently being clarified. Laxatives can either alter intestinal motility or cause a net accumulation of lumenal fluid. Both of these mechanisms, acting alone or in concert, lead to intestinal secretion and eventual laxation.

Regarding motility, laxatives depress contractile activity in vitro and in vivo, defying the earlier term "stimulants" of motility. In addition in vivo, laxatives elicit a distinct migratory pattern of intestinal contractions. This may sweep the contents of the small bowel into the colon where the absorptive capacity is exceeded or fluid secretion may occur.

The ability of laxatives to exert a net fluid accumulation is due to a multitude of actions. Laxatives can enhance mucosal permeability, stimulate c-AMP, inhibit Na/K ATPase, and elicit release of several secretogogue hormones. These diverse actions of laxatives are probably due to their nonspecific interaction with the mucosal membranes because of their surfactant activity.

The dietary fibers or bulk laxatives produce laxation through a different mechanism. They appear to act through an interrelated process which is dependent upon the action of colonic bacteria on the complex carbohydrate material of the fiber. The bacteria reduce the fibers to short chain fatty acids which then become substrate for the bacteria. Therefore, bulk laxatives lead to an increased fecal output by increasing the amount of bacteria in the feces. Thus with all laxatives, current studies have lead to new ideas for their mechanisms of action.

REFERENCES

Ammon, H. V. and Phillips, S. F., 1974, Inhibition of ileal water absorption by intraluminal fatty acids, J. Clin. Invest., 53:205-210.

Atchison, W. D., Klasek, G. J., and Bass, P., 1978a, Laxative effects on small intestinal electric activity of the conscious dog, in: "Gastrointestinal motility in health and disease," Duthie HL ed., 6th international symposium on gastrointestinal motility, MTP Press Ltd, Lancaster England, p 73-81.

Atchison, W. D., Stewart. J. J., and Bass, P., 1978b, A Unique distribution of laxative-induced spike potentials from the small intestine of the dog, Am. J. Dig. Dis., 23:513-520.

Barbezat, G. O. and Grossman, M. I., 1971a, Intestinal secretion: stimulation by peptides, Science, 174:422-424.

Barbezat, G. O. and Grossman, M. I., 1971b, Cholera-like diarrhea induced by glucagon plus gastrin, Lancet., 1:1025-1026.

Beleslin, D. B., 1970, Nature of the peristaltic block produced by magnesium, Nature, 225:383-384.

Bernier, J-J, L'Hirondel, C., and Bretagne, J-F, 1979, Cell loss under laxatives in human jejunum, Gastroenterology, 76:1099.

Berridge, 1975, The interaction of cyclic nucleotides and calcium in the control of cellular activity, Adv. Cyclic. Nucleotide. Res., 6:1-98.

Beubler, E. and Juan, H., 1978, PGE-mediated laxative effects of diphenolic laxatives, Naunyn-Schmiedeberg's Arch. Pharmacol., 305:241-246.

Binder, H. J., Filburn, C., and Volpe, B. T., 1975, Bile salt alteration of colonic electrolyte transport: role of cyclic adenosine monophosphate, Gastroenterology, 68:503-508.

Binder, H. J., 1977, Pharmacology of laxatives, Ann. Rev. Pharmacol. Toxicol., 17:355-367.

Bloom, S. R., Polak, J. M., and Pearse, A. G. E., 1973, Vasoactive intestinal polypeptide and watery diarrhea syndrome, Lancet, 2:14-16.

Bloom, S. R., Nalin, D. R., Mitchell, S. J., and Bryant, M. G., 1976, Proceedings of the 1st International Symposium on Gastrointestinal Hormones, Asilomar, Ca.

Bolton, J. E. and Field, M., 1977, Ca ionophore-stimulated ion secretion in rabbit ileal mucosa; relation to actions of cyclic 3', 5' AMP and carbamylcholine, J. Memb. Biol., 35:159-173.

Bonnycastle, D. D., 1965, Cathartics and laxatives, in: "Drill's pharmacology in medicine," Di Palma JR ed. 3rd edn. McGraw-Hill, New York, p 747.

Burns, T. W., Mathias, J. R., Carlson, G. M., Martin, J. L., and Shields, R. P., 1978, Effect of toxigenic Escherichia coli on myoelectric activity of small intestine, Am. J. Physiol., 235:E311-E315.

Burns, T. W., Mathias, J. R., Martin, J. L., Carlson, G. M., and Shields, R. P., 1980, Alteration of myoelectric activity of small intestine by invasive Escherichia coli, Am. J. Physiol., 238:G57-G62.

Carlson, G. M., Ruddon, R. W., Hug, C. C. Jr., and Bass, P., 1970, Effects of nicotine on gastric antral and duodenal contractile activity in the dog, J. Pharmacol. Exp. Ther., 172:367-376.

Caspary, W. F. and Meyne, K., 1980, Effects of chenodeoxy- and ursodeoxycholic acid on absorption, secretion and permeability in rat colon and small intestine, Digestion, 20:168-174.

Chadwick, V. S., Gaginella, T. S., Carlson, G. L., Debongnie, J-C, Phillips, S. F., and Hofmann, A. F., 1979, Effect of molecular structure on bile acid-induced alterations in absorptive function, permeability, and morphology in the perfused rabbit colon, J. Lab. Clin. Med., 94:661-674.

Chignell, C. F., 1968, The effect of phenolphthalein and other purgative drugs on rat intestinal (Na$^+$ + K$^+$) adenosine triphosphatase, Biochem. Pharmacol., 17:1207-1212.

Cline, W. S., Lorenzsonn, V., Benz, L., Bass, P., and Olsen, W. A., 1976, The effects of sodium ricinoleate on small intestinal function and structure, J. Clin. Invest., 58:380-390.

Code, C. F. and Marlett, J. A., 1975, The interdigestive myoelectric complex of the stomach and small bowel of dogs, J. Physiol., 246:289-309.

Collier, H. O. J., McDonald-Gibson, W. J., and Saeed, S. A., 1976, Stimulation of prostaglandin biosynthesis by drugs: effects in vitro of some drugs affecting gut function, Br. J. Pharmacol., 58:193-199.

Connel, A. M., 1981, Dietary Fiber, in: "Physiology of the Gastrointestinal Tract," Johnson, LR ed. Raven Press, NY, p 1291-1299.

Dinoso, V. P., Meshkinpour, H., Lorber, S. H., Gutierrex, J. G., and Chey, W. Y., 1973, Motor responses of the sigmoid colon and rectum to exogenous cholecystokinin and secretion, Gastroenterology, 65:438-444.

Donowitz, M. and Binder, J. H., 1975, Effect of dioctyl sodium sulfosuccinate on colonic fluid and electrolyte movement, Gastroenterology, 69:941-950.

Dupont, H. L., Sullivan, P., Pickering, L. K., Haynes, G., and Ackerman, P. B., 1977, Symptomatic treatment of diarrhea with bismuth subsalicylate among students attending a Mexican university, Gastroenterology, 73:715-718.

Duszynski, J., Wojtczak, L., 1974, Effect of detergents on ADP translocation on mitochondria, FEBS Lett., 40:72-76.

Farack, U. M. and Nell, G., 1979, The influence of an adenylcyclase inhibitor on the cholera toxin-desoxycholic acid- and bisacodyl-induced intestinal secretion in the rat, Naunyn Schmiedebergs Arch. Pharmacol., 308(suppl):R27.

Faust, R. G. and Wu, S. L., 1967, The effect of bile salts on oxygen consumption, oxidate phosphorylation and ATPase activity of mucosal homogenates from rat jejunum and ileum, J. Cell Physiol., 67:149-158.

Faust, R. G. and Wu, S. L., 1965, The action of bile salts on fluid and glucose movement by rat and hamster jejunum in vitro, J. Cell. Comp. Physiol., 65:435-448.

Fuchs, H. M., Dorfman, S., and Flock, M. H., 1976, The effect of dietary fiber supplementation in man: II. Alteration in fecal physiology and bacterial flora, Am. J. Clin. Nutr., 29:1443-1447.

Gaginella, T. S., Stewart, J. J., Olsen, W. A., and Bass, P., 1975a, Actions of ricinoleic acid and structurally related fatty acids on the gastrointestinal tract. II. Effects on water and electrolyte absorption in vitro, J. Pharmacol. Exp. Ther., 195:355-361.

Gaginella, T. S., Stewart, J. J., Gullikson, G. W., Olsen, W. A., and Bass, P., 1975b, Inhibition of small intestinal mucosal and smooth muscle cell function by ricinoleic acid and other surfactants, Life Sci., 16:1595-1606.

Gaginella, T. S., Bass, P., Olsen, W., Shug, A., 1975c, Fatty acid inhibition of water absorption and energy production in the hamster jejunum, FEBS Lett., 53:347-350.

Gaginella, T. S., Chadwick, V. S., Debongnie, J. C., Lewis, J. C., and Phillips, S. F., 1977a, Perfusion of rabbit colon with ricinoleic acid: dose related mucosal injury, fluid secretion and increased permeability, Gastroenterology, 73:95-101.

Gaginella, T. S., Haddad, A. C., Go, V. L. W., and Phillips, S. F., 1977b, Cytotoxicity of ricinoleic acid (castor oil) and other intestinal secretagogues on isolated intestinal epithelial cells, J. Pharmacol. Exp. Ther., 201:259-266.

Gaginella, T. S. and Bass, P., 1978, Laxatives: an update on mechanism of action, Life Sci., 23:1001-1010.

Gardner, J. D., Peskin, G. W., Cerda, J. J, and Brooks, F. P., 1967, Alterations of in vitro fluid and electrolyte absorption by gastrointestinal hormones, Am. J. Surg., 113:57-64.

Gould, S. R., 1975, Prostaglandins, ulcerative colitis and sulphasalazine, Lancet., 2:988.

Guiraldes, E., Lamabadusuriya, S. P., Oyesiku, J. E., Whitfield, T. E., and Harries, J. T., 1975, A comparative study on the effects of different bile salts on mucosal ATPase and transport in the rat jejunum in vivo, Biochem. Biophys. Acta, 389:495-505.

Gullikson, G. W., Cline, W. S., Lorenzsonn, V., Benz, L., Olsen, W. A., and Bass, P., 1977, Effects of anionic surfactants on hamster small intestinal membrane structure and function: relationship to surface activity, Gastroenterology, 73:501-511.

Gullikson, G. W. and Bass, P., 1984, Mechanisms of action of laxative drugs, in: Handbook of Pharmacology. In press.

Harvey, R. F. and Read, A. E., 1973, Saline purgatives act by releasing cholecystokinin, Lancet, 2:185-187.

Helenius, A. and Simons, K., 1975, Solubilization of membranes by detergents. Biochem. Biophys. Acta, 415:29-79.

Hellendoorn, E. W., 1978, Fermentation as the principal cause of the physiological activity of indigestible food residue, in: "Topics in dietary fiber research," Spiller Ga, Amen RJ eds., Plenum Press, NY, p 127.

Hickey, C. A., Murphy, E. L., Calloway, D. H., 1972, Intestinal gas production following ingestion of commercial wheat cereals and milling fractions, Cereal Chem., 49:276-281.

Hoppert, C. A. and Clark, A. J., 1945, Digestibility and effect on laxation of crude fiber and cellulose in certain common foods, J. Am. Dietet. Assn., 21:157-160.

Kerzner, B., O'Dorisio, T., Gaginella, T., Mechjian, H., Super, D.,

Frye, T., Ailabouni, A., and McClung, H. J., 1979,
Ricinoleic acid: mechanism of action in isolated
enterocytes, Gastroenterology, 76:1168.

Kimberg, D. V., Field, M., Johnson, J., Henderson, A., and Gershan,
E., 1971, Stimulation of intestinal mucosal adenyl cyclase
by cholera enterotoxin and prostaglandin, J. Clin. Invest.,
50:1218-1230.

Kimberg, D. V., 1974, Cyclic nucleotides and their role in
gastrointestinal secretion, Gastroenterology, 67:1023-1064.

Krejs, G. J., Walsh, J. H., Morawski, S. G., and Fordtran, J. S.,
1977, Intractable diarrhea. Intestinal perfursion studies
and plasma VIP concentrations in patients with pancreatic
cholera syndrome and surreptitious ingestion of laxative and
diuretics, Am. J. Dig. Dis. 22:280-292.

Latven, A. R., Sloane, A. B., and Munch, J. C., 1952, Bioassay of
cathartics I. Emodin type, J. Am. Pharm. Assoc., 41:548-552.

Low-Beer, T. S., Schneider, R. E., and Dobbins, W. O., 1970,
Morphological changes of the small intestinal mucosa of
guinea pig and hamster following incubation in vitro and
perfusion in vivo with unconjugated bile salts, Gut,
11:486-492.

Mathias, J. R., Carlson, G. M., DiMarino, A. J., Bertiger, G.,
Morton, H. E., and Cohen, S., 1976, Intestinal myoelectric
activity in response to live vibrio cholerae and cholera
enterotoxin, J. Clin. Invest., 58:91-96.

Mathias, J. R., Carlson, G. M., Bertiger, G., Martin, J. L., and
Cohen, S., 1977, Migrating action potential complex of
cholera: a possible prostaglandin-induced response, Am. J.
Physiol., 232:E529-E534.

Mathias, J. R., Martin, J. L., Burns, T. W., Carlson, G. M., and
Shields, R., 1978, Ricinoleic acid effect on the electrical
activity of the small intestine in rabbits, J. Clin.
Invest., 61:640-644.

Mathias, J. R., Carlson, G. M., Martin, J. L., Shields, R. P., and
Formal, S., 1980, Shigella dysenteriae I enterotoxin: proposed role in pathogenesis of shigellosis, Am. J. Physiol.,
239:G382-G386.

McNeil, N. I., Cummings, J. H., James, W. P. T., 1978, Short chain
fatty acid absorption by the human large intestine, Gut,
19:819-822.

Mekhjian, H. S. and Phillips, S. F., 1970, Perfusion of the canine
colon with unconjugated bile acids, Gastroenterology,
59:120-129.

Mekhjian, H. S., Phillips, S. F., and Hofmann, A., 1971, Colonic
secretion of water and electrolytes induced by bile acids:
perfusion studies in man, J. Clin. Invest., 50:1569-1577.

Mennie, A. T., Dalley, V. M., Dinneen, L. C., Collier, H. O. J.,
1975, Treatment of radioation-induced gastrointestinal
distress with acetyl salicylate, Lancet, 2:942-943.

Moritz, M., Finkelstein, G., Meshkinpour, H., Fingerut, J., and

Lorber, S. H., 1973, Effect of secretin and cholecystokinin on the transport of electrolyte and water in human jejunum, Gastroenterology, 64:76-80.

Parker, J. G. and Beneventano, T. C., 1970, Acceleration of small bowel contrast study by cholecystokinin, Gastroenterology, 58:679-684.

Parkinson, T. M. and Olsen, J. A., 1964, Inhibitory effects of bile acids on adenosine triphosphatase oxygen consumption, and the transport and diffusion of water soluble substances in the small intestine of the rat, Life Sciences, 3:107-112.

Perkins, J. P. and Moore, M. M., 1971, Adenyl cyclase of rat cerebral cortex. J. Biol. Chem., 246:62-68.

Phillips, R. A., Love, A. H. G., Mitchell, T. G., and Neptune, E. M., 1965, Cathartics and the sodium pump, Nature, 206:1367-1368.

Powell, D. W., Lawrence, B. A., Morris, S. M., and Etheridge, D. R., 1980, Effect of phenolphthalein on in vitro rabbit ileal electrolyte transport, Gastroenterology, 78:454-463.

Rachmilewitz, D., Saunders, D. R., Rulein, C. E., and Tytgat, G. N., 1976, Pharmacology of laxatives: effects of bisacodyl (BIS) on structure and function of intestinal mucosa, Gastroenterology, 70:928.

Rachmilewitz, D. and Karmeli, F., 1979, Effect of bisacodyl (BIS) and dioctyl sodium sulfosuccinate on rat intestinal prostaglandin E_2 (PGE_2) content, Na-K ATPase and adenyl cyclase activity, Gastroenterology, 76:1221.

Rachmilewitz, D., Karmeli, F., Okon, E., 1980, Effects of bisacodyl on c-AMP and prostaglandin E_2 contents, (Na + K) ATPase, adenyl cyclase, and phosphodiesterase activities of rat intestine, Dig. Dis. Sci., 25:602-608.

Ritchie, J., 1972, Mass peristalsis in the human colon after contact with oxyphenisatin, Gut, 13:211-219.

Ruppin, H., Bar-Meir, S., Soergel, K. H., Wood, C. M., and Schmitt, M. G. Jr., 1980, Absorption of short-chain fatty acid by the colon, Gastroenterology, 78:1500-1507.

Said, S. I. and Faloona, G. R., 1975, Elevated plasma and tissue levels of vasoactive intestinal polypeptide in watery diarrhea syndrome due to pancreatic, bronchogenic and other tumors, N. Eng. J. Med., 293:155-160.

Sandler, M., Karim, S.M.M., and Williams, E.D., 1968, Prosta-glandins in amine-peptide-secretory tumor, Lancet, 2:1053-1054.

Saunders, D. R., Sillery, J., and Rachmilewitz, D., 1975, Effect of dioctyl sodium sulfosuccinate on structure and function of rodent and human intestine, Gastroenterology, 69:380-386.

Saunders, D. R., Sillery, J., Rachmilewitz, D., Rubin, C. E., and Tytgat, G. N., 1977, Effect of bisacodyl on the structure and function of rodent and human intestine, Gastroenterology, 72:849-856.

Schwartz, C. J., Kimberg, D. V., Sheerin, H. E., Field, M., and
    Said, S. I., 1974, Vasoactive intestinal peptide stimulation
    of adenylate cyclase and active electrolyte secretion in
    intestinal mucosa, J. Clin. Invest., 54:536-544.
Sharp, G. W. G. and Hynie, S., 1971, Stimulation of intestinal
    adenyl cyclase by cholera toxin, Nature (London),
    229:266-268.
Shiff, S. J., Soloway, R. D., and Shape, W. J., 1982, Mechanism of
    deoxycholic acid stimulation of the rabbit colon, J. Clin.
    Invest., 69:985-992.
Sinar, D. R., Charles, L. G., and Burns, T. W., 1982, Migrating
    action-potential complex in absence of fluid production is
    produced by B subunit of cholera enterotoxin, Am. J.
    Physiol., 242:G47-51.
Spiller, G. A., Chernoff, M. C., Hill, R. A., Gates, J. E., Nassar,
    J. J., and Shipley, E. A., 1980, Effect of purified cellu-
    lose, pectin and a low-residue diet on fecal volatile fatty
    acids, transit time and fecal weight in humans, Am. J. Clin.
    Nutr., 33:754-579.
Steggerta, F. R., 1968, Gastrointestinal gas following food
    consumption, Ann. NY. Acad. Sci., 150:57-66.
Stephen, A. M. and Cummings, J. H., 1980, Mechanisms of action of
    dietary fiber in the human colon, Nature, 284:283-284.
Stewart, J. J., Gaginella, T. S., and Bass, P., 1975a, Actions of
    ricinoleic acid and structurally related fatty acids on the
    gastrointestinal tract. I. Effects on smooth muscle
    contractility in vitro, J. Pharmacol. Exp. Ther.,
    195:347-354.
Stewart, J. J., Gaginella, T. S., Olsen, W. A., Bass, P., 1975b,
    Inhibitory actions of laxatives on motility and water and
    electrolyte transport in the gastrointestinal tract, J.
    Pharmacol. Exp. Ther., 192:458-467.
Stewart, J. J. and Bass, P., 1976, Effect of intravenous C-terminal
    octapeptide of cholecystokinin and intraduodenal ricinoleic
    acid on contractile activity of the dog intestine, Proc.
    Soc. Exp. Biol. Med., 152:213-217.
Sund, R. B., 1982, Aspects of the pharmacology of diphenylmethane
    laxatives (Bisacodyl, oxyphenisatin and phenolphthalein
    derivatives), University of Oslo, Oslo, Norway.
Tai, Y. H., Wong, R., Decker, R. A., Wright, J. A., and Marnane, W.
    G., 1978, Inhibitory effects of RMI 12330A on ileal total
    ionic transport and mucosal adenylate cyclase and Na-K-
    ATPase activities in normal tissues and tissues treated with
    purified cholera toxin from the rabbit, Gastroenterology,
    74:1101.
Teem, M. V. and Phillips, S. F., 1972, Perfusion of the hamster
    jejunum with conjugated and unconjugated bile acids:
    inhibition of water absorption and effects on morphology,
    Gastroenterology, 62:261-267.
Waldman, D. B., Gardner, J. D., Zfass, A. M., and Makhlouf, G. M.,

1977, Effects of vasoactive intestinal peptide, secretin, and related peptides on rat colonic transport and adenylate cyclase activity, Gastroenterology, 73:518-523.

Wanitschke, R., 1980, Influence of rhein on electrolyte and water transfer in the isolated rat colonic mucosa, Pharmacology, 20:(suppl. 1)21-26.

Wingate, D. L., 1981, Backwards and forwards with the migrating complex, Dig. Dis. Sci., 26:641-666.

Wojtczak, L. and Zaluska, H., 1967, The inhibition of translocation of adenine nucleotides through mitochondrial membranes by oleate, Biochem. Biophys. Res. Comm., 28:76-81.

LECTURERS

Adrian Allen
The University of Newcastle
upon Tyne
Department of Physiological
Sciences
The Medical School
Newcastle-upon-Tyne NE1 7RU, UK

Paul Bass
University of Wisconsin
Center for Health Sciences
School of Pharmacy
425 North Charter Street
Madison
Wisconsin 53706, USA

Giulio Bertaccini
Istituto di Farmacologia
Universita di Parma
Ospedale Maggiore
Italy

Henry J Binder
Yale University
333 Cedar Street
New Haven
CT06510, USA

Jeremy Jass
Westminster Medical School
London, UK

S J Konturek
Academia Medyczna W Krakowie
Instytut Fizjologi
Krakow
UL Grzegorzecka 16, Poland

Sidney F Phillips
Mayo Foundation Gastroenterology
Unit
Saint Mary's Hospital
Rochester
Minnesota 55905, USA

Gareth Sanger
Beecham Pharmaceuticals
Medical Research Centre
The Pinnacles
Harlow, Essex

Manfred V Singer
Universitatsklinikum der
Gesamthochschule Essen
Medizinische Klinik und Polik-
linik
Abteilung für Gastroenterologie
Hufelandstr 55
4300 Essen 1, West Germany

Joseph H Szurszewski
Mayo Foundation
Rochester
Minnesota 55905, USA

Gaston Vantrappen
Academisch Ziekenhuis
Sint-Rafael
3000 Leuven
Kapucijnenvoer 33, Belgium

John R Wood
Glaxo Pharmaceuticals Ltd
Greenford, Middlesex, UK

Sue Wood
Department of Endocrinology
Royal Postgraduate Medical
School
Hammersmith Hospital
London, UK

PARTICIPANTS

Bruno Annibale
Cattedra di Gastroenterologia
Policlinico Umberto I
00161 Rome, Italy

Michael Barer
Department of Medical Micro-
biology
London School of Hygiene and
Tropical Medicine
London WC1E 7HT, UK

Karsten Bech
Biomedical Laboratory
Odense University Hospital
DK-5000
Odense C-, Denmark

Alberto Bianchetti
Sanofi
MIDY SPA
38 via Piranesi
20137 Milan, Italy

R Bocchini
Medicina Generale
Ospedali GB Morgagni-L
Pierantoni
Forli, Italy

A Bonabello
Bayer Italia S.p.A
Reparto di Farmacologia
20024 Garbagnate, Milan, Italy

Francesco Borrelli
Istituto Farmacologico Serono
Rome, Italy

Giorgio Castelli
Direzione Ricerche Cliniche
GLAXO S.p.A
Via A Fleming 2
37135 Verona, Italy

P Cazzulani
Recordati Industria Chimica E
Farmaceutica SPA
20148 Milan, Italy

R Ceserani
Farmitilia Carlo Erba
20159 Milan, Italy

S Daniotti
Instituto de Angeli SpA
20139 Milan, Italy

Ricardo Migaes de Campos
Rua Ilha de S Tome 6- 30 Dto
1 100 Lisbon, Portugal

P W Dettmar
Department of Pharmacology
Pharmaceutical Division
Reckett & Colman
Kingston-upon-Hull HU8 7DS UK

Francesco Di Mario
Clinica Medica I
Policlinico Universitario
35100 Padova, Italy

John Gaffen
Department of Surgery
King's College School of
Medicine and Dentistry
London SE5 8RX, UK

Zoe Gaffen
Department of Pharmacology
Chelsea College
London, SW3, UK

Miss F Gokan
Bardacik sokak 69/4 Defne apt
Kucukesat
Ankara, Turkey

Miss B Greenwood
University of Sheffield
Department of Physiology
Sheffield S10 2TN, UK

Giovanni Gurrieri
Cattedra di Gastroenterologia
Clinica Medica I
Policlinico Universitario
35100 Padova, Italy

M Hanani
Head, Laboratory of Experimental
Surgery
Hadassah Medical Organisation
Hadassah University Hospital
Mount Scopus
POB 24035
il-91240 Jerusalem, Israel

David J Holt
School of Natural Sciences
Hatfield, Hertfordshire, UK

C Kalayci
Kaveklidere
Buklum sokak 48/7
Ankara, Turkey

K Kraglund
Surgical Gastroenterological
Department
Arhus Kommunehospital
8000 Arhus C, Denmark

Ivan M Lang
Department of Surgery
Medical College of Wisconsin
Wisconsin 53193, USA

Dr Lavezzo
Sanofi
Direction des Recherches
Midy SpA
20137 Milan, Italy

Otto Lawaetz
Vandrevej 10
DK 2900 Hellerup, Denmark

Bruno Lumachi
Camillo Corvi SpA
Stradone Farnese
118 Piacenza
Zip Code 29100, Italy

S Manzini
Pharmacology Department
A Menarini Pharmaceuticals
50131 Florence, Italy

Leonardo Marzio
Istituto di Patologia Medica
Ospedale "SS Annunziata"
University of Chieti
Chieti, Italy

G Mastropaolo
Department of Medicine
Clinical Sciences Building
Hope Hospital
Salford, UK

L McLeay
Department of Biological
Sciences
University of Waikato
Hamilton
New Zealand

Matteo Neri
Istituo di Patologia Medica
Ospedale "SS Annunziata"
University of Chieti
Chieti, Italy

N Ozturk
Hacettepe University
Institute of Biophysics
Ankara, Turkey

Michael Parsons
Department of Pharmacology
Smith, Kline & French
Welwyn, Hertfordshire, UK

Miss Louise E Peacock
Department of Surgery
King's College School of
Medicine and Dentistry
London SE5 8RX, UK

Ulrich Pohl
Clinical Research
Kali-Chemie Pharma GmbH
D-3000 Hannover 1, West Germany

Carolyn Price
Department of Pharmacology
Smith, Kline & French
Welwyn, Hertfordshire, UK

Antonio Schiavone
De Angeli
20139 Milan, Italy

Carola Severi
II Clinica Medica - Policlinico
00161 Rome, Italy

P Del Soldato
De Angeli
20139 Milan, Italy

Giuseppe Spina
Gruppo Lepetit
20158 Milan, Italy

Jan Thomassen
Department of Biochemistry
University of Bergen
N-5000 Bergen, Norway

Giancarlo Toson
Department of Pharmacology
Glaxo
37100 Verona, Italy

Luisa Varin
De Angeli
20139 Milan, Italy

Jill Williams
Duphar
1381 cp Weesp, Hooland

John Wilkinson
Hatfield Polytechnic
Hertfordshire A110 9AB, UK

Erdal Yilmaz
10 Sokak 38/12
Bahcelievler
Ankara, Turkey

INDEX

Absorption modifications, exper-
    imental observations,
    243-244
Acetylcholine, 3, 87, 88
  effect on
    electromechanical coupling of
      circular antral muscle,
      65, 66
    gallbladder, 164
  intra-arterial, 113
  ionophoretic application, 81
Acetylcholine esterase, 74
Achalasia, 178
Adenine nucleotide translocase
    (ANT), 333
Adenosine triphosphate (ATP), 88,
    97
Adrenaline, 88
Alcohol, see Ethanol
Alcoholic beverages, 282
Alcoholism, chronic
  gastrointestinal hormones
      plasma concentrations,
      282
  interdigestive pancreatic
      secretion, 282
Aloe, 332
y-Aminobutyric acid, 88
Angiotensin, 88
  effect on
    colonic motility, 96
    lower oesophageal sphincter,
      91
    small intestine motility, 94
Anthraquinones, 327
Anticholecystokinin peptide (ACP,
    pancreatone), 279

Antidiarrhoeals, 246
Anti-gastrin-releasing peptide
    antibodies, 266
Antihistamines, 190
Antral-duodenal motor co-
    ordination, 46
Antrum
  postprandial myoelectric
      activity, 48
  prostaglandin effect on
      motility, 138
Arachidonate, 129
Argentaffinoma, 182
ATP, 16
Atropine, 193, 197
Autonomic nerves, electrical
      stimulation, 24-27
  extrinsic nerves, 26-27
  intrinsic nerves, 25
  gastrointestinal nerves, 25

Bacteria, intestinal, 334-335
  bulk laxatives and gas pro-
      duction, 335
Basic electrical rhythm (BER,
    "slow waves"), 241
Bethanecol, gastric response to,
    197
Bile salts, 331, 332
Biliary reflux, 138
Bisacodyl, 330, 331, 333
Blood vessel endothelium, PGI_2
      production, 130
Bombesin, 88, 90
  distribution in neurons,
      endocrine cells, plasma,
      111

Bombesin (continued)
  effect on
    colonic activity, 96
    gallbladder, 166
    gastric motility, 92
    insulin secretion, 265
    lower oesophageal motility,
      91
    small intestine motility, 94
Bombesin-like peptides, 266-267
Bradykinin
  effect on
    colonic motility, 96
    gastric motility, 92
    muscularis mucosae, 249
    small intestine motility, 94
Breath hydrogen excretion, 244
BRL 20627, 298
Burimamide, 190

Calcitonin, 90
  effect on lower oesophageal
      sphincter motility, 91
  tumor produced, 143
Calcium
  activation of contractile
      proteins, 57-58
  entry blockers, 120
  pump, 58
Carbachol
  gastric response to, 197
  stimulation of nicotinic
      receptors, 197
Castor oil, 327, 328, 330
Cell population in columnar
      epithelium, 4-8
Cerulein (caerulin)
  effect on
    colonic motility, 96
    gallbladder, 160, 161
    gastric motility, 92
    lower oesophageal sphincter,
      91
    small intestine motility, 94
Cerulitide, 121
Chaga's disease, 178
Chloride absorption model, 224
  potential-dependent, 223
Chloride pump, electrogenic, 56

Chloride secretion
  active, 223
  cyclic AMP-mediated, 225
Cholecystokinin, 88, 90, 265
  cholera toxin and, 334
  different active forms, 110
  distribution in neurons,
      endocrine cells, plasma,
      111
  effect on
    colonic motility, 96
    gallbladder, 160-162
    gallbladder fluid, 232
    gastric motility, 92
    lower oesophageal sphincter,
      91
    pancreatic enzyme secretion,
      277
    small intestine motility, 94
    sphincter of Oddi, 167
  as incretin, 261
  magnesium sulphate and, 334
  riconoleic acid and, 334
Cholecystokinin fragments, 88
Cholera toxin, 330, 332
  VIP release, 332
Cigarette smokers, mucosal
      histamine content, 198
Cimetidine, 190
  effect on
    gastric acid secretion, 119
      191
    gastric emptying, 89
    pancreatic exocrine sec-
      retion, 121
Citrate equiosmolar meals, 46-47
Clebopride, 287
Colon,
  metaplastic polyps, 184-185
  motility, 20-21
    prostaglandin effect on, 140
  mucosa, 7-8
Congenital pyloric stenosis, 178,
      179
Coupled sodium chloride cotrans-
      port, 221
Cyclic AMP, 119, 120
  calcium release by, 332
  chloride secretion mediated,
      225

350

Cyclic AMP (continued)
  cholecystokin-produced fall,
      161
  effect on intestinal
      electrolyte transport,
      225
  gastric acid secretion, 131
  increased mucosal, 225
  laxatives and, 332-333
Cyclic GMP, 161-162, 225
Cyclo-oxygenase inhibition, 135

Deoxycholate, 332
Deoxycholic acids, 330, 332, 333
Differentiation disorders,
      secretory activity
      changes associated,
      182-185
6,7-Dihydroxyaminotetralin
      (6,7-ADTN), 293
Dihydroxybile acids, 330
Dimaprit, 190
  effect on
      gastric emptying, 89
      gastric secretion, 120
      pancreatic exocrine sec-
      retion, 121
Dioctyl sodium sulfosuccinate
      (DSS), 327, 330, 331
Diverticular disease, 181
Domperidone, 287
  anti-emetic effect, 288,
      288-289
  central nervous system pen-
      etration, 295
  effect on
      stomach motility and
      emptying, 289-295
      mouse climbing behavior, 295,
      296
  prolactin plasma concentration,
      287
  side effects, 294
Dopamine, 88, 89
  antagonism by metoclopramide,
      318
  neurotransmission in gut, 318
Dopamine antagonists, 287
  anti-emetic effects, 288-289
  effect on gastric motility and
      emptying, 289

Dopamine antagonists (continued)
  side effects, 295
Drug interactions with receptors,
      13
Dual ion exchange, 221
Duodenum
  contractions, 35
  postprandial myoelectric ac-
      tivity, 48
  receptors, 246

Eicosanoids, 88
Electrical activity in vitro,
      62-67
Electrical activity in vivo
  smooth muscle of corpus and
      antrum, 59-61
      pacemaker of action potent-
      ial, 61
  smooth muscle of fundus, 59
  smooth muscle of large intes-
      tine, 62
  smooth muscle of small intes-
      tine, 61-62
  slow wave pacemaker, 61
Electrical correlates of motor
      activity in smooth
      muscle, 59-69
Electrical signals for gastro-
      intestinal tract, 39-41
Electrophysiology of smooth
      muscle, 55-72
Emesis, 288
  apomorphine-induced, inhibition
      of, 289-290
Endocrine cells of gut, 110-111
Endocrine tumors, 181-182
Endoperoxide analogues (throm-
      boxane mimetics), 135
Endorphin, 267
Enkephalins, 74, 88, 266
  distribution in neurons,
      endocrine cells, plasma,
      111
  effect on
      colonic motility, 96
      myenteric neurons, 80
  release by electrical
      stimulation, 25
  in vagus, 112

Eneteric-coated drugs, 46
Enteric nervous system, 73
  sensory cells, 78
Enteric neurons, *see* myenteric
    neurons
Enterochromaffin tumors, 181
Enterogastrone, 88
Enteroglucagon
  distribution in neurons,
      endocrine cells, plasma,
      111
  release by gastrin, 260
Entero-insular axis, 259-276
Enteropancreatic cholinergic
      vagovagal reflexes, 279
Ethanol
  effect on
    gastrointestinal hormones,
      281
    pancreatic exocrine sec-
      retion, 281-286
  intragastric-intraduodenal
      effects, 281-282
  intravenous administration
      effects, 281, 282-283
Excretin, 260

Fibers, dietary, 335, 336
Fluid and electrolytes,
      intestinal absorption and
      secretion, 219-228
FMRFamide, 268

Gallbladder
  anatomy, 159
  innervation, 160, 233-234
  neurohumeral control of filling
      and emptying, 166-167
Gallbladder fluid transport,
      229-238
  autonomic nervous system influ-
      ence, 233-234
  fluid absorption, 230-231
  fluid secretion, 231
  gastrointestinal peptides
      effects, 232-233
  humoral and neural regulation,
      231
  physiological changes, 229
  sodium and chloride transport,
      230

Gamma-aminobutyric acid (GABA),
      74
Gamma-camera scintigraphy, 244
Gastric inhibitory peptide (GIP),
      88, 90
  distribution in neurons, endo-
      crine cells, plasma, 111
  effect on gallbladder, 163
Gastrin, 88, 90, 109
  different active forms, 110
  distribution in neurons, endo-
      crine, cells, plasma,
      111
  effect on
    colonic motility, 96
    electromechanical coupling of
      antral muscle, 65, 66
    gallbladder, 160
    lower oesophageal sphincter,
      91
    small intestine motility, 94
  endogenous, 260
  exogenous, 260
  isolation and synthesis, 190
  metoclopramide effect on re-
      lease, 319
  parietal cells (canine) stimu-
      lated, 193
Gastrin-like peptides, 266
Gastrin receptors, 194
Gastrin-releasing peptide,
      266-267
  distribution in neurons, endo-
      crine cells, plasma, 111
Gastro-intestinal innervation and
      motility, relationships
      between, 97-98
Gastro-intestinal motility
  bathing solutions, 14
  distension effects, 21-23
  electrical stimulation of
      autonomic nerves, 24-27
    extrinsic nerves, 26-27
    intrinsic nerves, 25-26
    gastro-intestinal nerves, 25
  gastric, 17-19
  intestinal peristalsis, 19-21
    colon, 20-21
    ileum, 19-20
  methodology, general, 14

Gastro-intestinal motility
(continued)
muscle segment and strip preparation, 14–17
circular fibres, 15–16
drug action, 16
longitudinal fibres, 15–16
oxygenation, 14
perfusion of isolated gut,
16–17
storage of smooth muscle, 14
temperature, 14
tissue baths, 14
transducers, muscle-activity
detecting, 14
Gastro-intestinal motility in
vitro techniques, 13–33
Glucagon
distribution in neurons, endocrine
cells, plasma, 111
effects on
colonic motility, 96
gallbladder, 162
gastric motility, 92
lower oesophageal sphincter,
91–92
small intestine motility, 95
secretion, 264
Glucagonoma, 182
Glucose-dependent insulinotropic
peptide (GIP), 260, 261
Gut non-peptides affecting
gastrointestinal muscle,
88
Gut peptides affecting gastrointestinal muscle, 88

Hexamethonium
bursting activity suppression,
77
electrical field stimulation of
acid secretion inhibited
by, 197
Hirschsprung's disease, 178–180
Histamine, 16, 88, 89, 117–118
calcium ions interference, 120
gastric acid secretion,
118–120, 189–203
gastric mucosa content, 198
gastro-intestinal motility,
122–124

Histamine (continued)
H1, 190
H1 receptor, 117, 118
excitation, 122–124
relaxation post-excitation,
122
H1-receptor agonists, 190
H2, 190
H2 antagonist, 119
H2-antagonist insensitive, 196
H2 receptor, 117–118, 120
in gastric acid secretion,
190–195
stimulation, 122–124
H2-receptor agonists, 190
H3 receptor, 120
mediator/final common chemostimulator concept,
191–192, 193
multi-messenger concept,
192–195
pancreatic exocrine secretion,
120–122
presynaptic receptors, 123
release by gastrin and vagal
stimulation, 195–197
role in peptic ulcer disease,
198
vagotomy effect, 198
Histamine cells, hormonal
receptors, 197
Histamine methyltransferase, 191
Histaminocytes, 196
Histidine decarboxylase, 189,
190–191
Hormones as mediators of laxative
action, 333–334
5-hydroxytryptamine, 3, 88, 89
antagonists, 24
effect on gut muscle, 15
release, 136–137
tachyphylaxis, 315, 316, 317
5-Hyrdoxytryptamine-induced
nerve-mediated responses,
metoclopramide antag-
onism, 315
Hypogangliosis, 180

Ileocaecal sphincter, 247–249
Ileum, peristalsis, 19–20

Immunocytochemistry, 109
Impromidine, 120, 121
  + burimamide, 120
  synthesis, 190
Incretin, 260–261
Indomethacin, 136
  effect on
    cyclic GMP concentration, 161
    small intestine, 139
Innervation of gut, 2–3
Insulin
  distribution in neurons,
        endocrine cells, plasma,
        111
  effects on
    colonic motility, 96
    gastric motility, 93
    lower oesophageal sphincter,
        91
  small intestine motility, 95
Intestinal chloride absorption
        mechanisms, 233
Intestinal motility-transit-
        absorption relationships,
        239–258
  chronobiological rhythms, 239
Intestinal muscle
  ring contractions, 240
  sleeve contractions, 240
Intestinal neuronal dysplasia,
        180
Intestinal peristalsis, 19–21
Intestinal villi movement,
        248–249
Intubation-perfusion techniques,
        261
In vivo measurements methods,
        35–54
  balloons, small, 37–39
  catheter sleeve, 38–39
  electrodes, 40–41
  electrogastrogram, 43–44, 45
  historical, 36–37
  intraluminal pressure record-
        ing, 37–39
  opaque markers, 43
  open-tip catheter, 37–39
  pressure recording probe, 39
  radiotelemetering capsule, 39
  serosal recordings, 39
  transducers, 40, 41–43

In vivo vs. in vitro monitoring,
        49–50
Islets of Langerhans
  intraportal transplantation,
        262
  neural regulation, 262
  parasympathetic influence on,
        262–263
  peptidergic influence on, 265
  sympathetic influence on,
        264–265

KSCN, 119

Lactulose, for oral-colon transit
        time, 46
Lanthanum, 162
Laxatives, 325–345
  bulk, 334–335
  cellular and mucosal damage,
        330–331
  chemical structure, 326
  cyclic-AMP and, 332–333
  effects on
    energy metabolism, 333
    fluid and electrolyte
        movement, 330–331
    intestinal motility, 327–330
    Na/K ATpase, 333
  enhanced mucosal permeability,
        332
  hormones as mediator, 333–334
  prostaglandins released by, 334
Leu-enkephalin, 267–268
Leukotrienes, 89–90
Leuteinizing hormone-releasing
        factor, 268

Magnesium sulfate, 328, 329
Malabsorption, effect on
        intestinal function, 239
Met-enkephalin, 267
Methysergide, 89
Metiamide, 190
Metoclopramide, 19, 89, 287
  α_2-adrenoceptor-mediated
        inhibition of gastro-
        intestinal motility,
        antagonism of, 318
  antagonism of dopamine, 318

Metoclopramide (continued)
  anti-emetic effect, 288,
      288–289
  central nervous system effects,
      303
  clinical uses, 288
  companion of in vitro/in vivo
      effects (rat), 309–311
  effects on acetylcholine and
      carbachol induced con-
      tractions, 308, 314
  effects on cholinergic-mediated
      contractions, 304–319
    human stomach, 311–313
    rat stomach, 304–311
  effects on gastric motility and
      emptying, 289–295
  effects on gastro-intestinal
      hormones and peptide
      release, 319
  effects on mouse climbing
      behavior, 296
  effects on nerve-mediated
      responses (rat), 304–308
    corpus longitudinal muscle,
        307–308
    forestomach circular muscle,
        306
    forestomach longitudinal
        muscle, 305–306
  mechanisms of increasing neural
      acetycholine release,
      315–316
  miscellaneous actions, 319–320
  reflux oesophagitis treated by,
      291
  side effects, 295
Migrating action potential com-
      plex (MAPC), 329, 330
Migrating myoelectrical complex
      (MMC), 241, 328
  diarrheogenic conditions, 243
  "interdigestive housekeeper",
      241–242
  transit and, 242–243
Monoamine oxidase, 74
Morphine
  effect on gut muscle, 16
  spasm of colonic circular
      muscle, 137

Motilin, 88
  distribution in neurons, endo-
      crine cells, plasma, 111
  effect on
    colonic motility, 96
    gallbladder, 163
    gastric motility, 93
    lower oesophageal sphincter,
        91
    small intestine motility, 95
  metoclopramide effect on
      release, 319
Motility
  "clusters" of contractions,
      243
  chronobiological, 243
  definition of, 240
  drug effects, 246
  markers, 244
  measurement-transit relations,
      449
  paradoxical, 241
  "propulsive/retropulsive
      events", 243
  transit and, 240–242
Motility disorders, 177–181
Motility-intestinal absorption,
      integrated patterns,
      246–248
Motor nerves, intramural, 87–89
Muscosa, anatomy of, 2
Mucus, gastro-intestinal, 205–218
  bicarbonate barrier against
      luminal acid, 215
  cancer of head of pancreas, 212
  carbachol action on, 214
  contents, 207
  functions, 205–206
  gel cover measurement, 212–213
  glycoproteins, 207–211
    carbohydrates, 208
    disulphide bridges, 211
    negative charge, 208
    in vivo 211–213
  peptic ulceration, 212
  prostaglandin action on, 214
  protection by, 213–215
  resistance to ulcerogenic
      agents, 215
  soluble, 206
  structure, 206–211

Muscarinic cholinergic agonists, 164
Muscarinic cholinergic receptors, 192
Muscular effetor unit, 55-56
Muscularis mucosae, 249-250
Myenteric neurons, 3
  cultured, pharmacology of, 80-83
  electrophysiological characterization, 75-78
  electrophysiological studies, in tissue culture, 73-85
  "erratic bursters", 77
  nicotinic cholinergic synapses, 77-78
  pacemaker cells, 78
  Stage 4 culture, 74-75
  tissue culture, 74
    Stage 4, 74-75
  type AH (type 2), 76-77
  type S (type 1), 75-76, 77
Myenteric (Auerbach's) plexus, 1, 2

Neuron
  excitatory (cholinergic), 2-3
  inhibitory (non-cholinergic), 2, 3
Neurotensin, 88, 267
  distribution in neurons, endocrine cells, plasma, 111
  effect on
    colonic motility, 96
    gastric motility, 93
    lower oesophageal sphincter, 91
    small intestine motility, 95
Nitrosamines, carcinogenic, 183
Non-adrenergic-non-cholinergic inhibitory nerves, transmitter at, 97
Non-enterochromaffin tumors, 181, 182
Noradrenaline, 3, 87, 88
  abnormal overflow, 98
Nutmeg treatment of diarrhoea, 144

Oesophagus, mucosa, 4
Oleic acid, 333
Omeprazole, 119
Opiates, action on myenteric neurons, 80
Opioid peptides, 267-268
  effect on gallbladder, 165-166
Oral-anal transit time, 45-46
Oxmetidine, 119, 121

Pancreatic exocrine secretion, 278
  cephalic phase, 278
  gastric phase, 278
  intestinal phase, 278, 279
  neuro-hormonal control, 277-280
Pancreatic polypeptide (PP), 88
  distribution in neurons, endocrine cells, plasma, 111
  effect on gallbladder contraction, 163-164
  metoclopramide effect on release, 319
  secretion, 261, 263
  tumor produced, 143
Pancreatone (anticholecystokinin peptide), 279
Paracrine mechanisms, 113-114
Paralytic ileus, adrenergic activity in, 98
Parasympathetic nerve supply of gut, 2
Parietal cell stimulants, potenitatin interactions, 195
Pentagastrin
  effects on
    colonic motility, 96
    gastric motility, 92
    parietal cells, 195-196
    small intestine motility, 94
Peptide(s), 90-97
  cerebral, 110
  molecular heterogeneity, 110
  PHI, *see* Peptide histidine isoleucine
  PYY, *see* Peptide tyrosine tyrosine precursor, 110
Peptidergic nerves of gut, 112-113

Peptide histidine isoleucine
(PHI), 268
  distribution in neurons,
      endocrine cells, plasma,
      111
  effect on
    gallbladder, 165
    gallbladder fluid, 232
Peptide tyrosine tyrosine (PYY),
    268
  distribution in neurons,
      endocrine cells, plasma,
      111
  effect on gallbladder
      contraction, 164
Peristaltic reflex, 19
Phenophthalein, 330, 334
Physalaemin, 88
Platelets, thromboxane pro-
    duction, 130
Polyethylene glycol, 332
Potassium
  colonic secretion, 227
  intestinal transport, 225
Presynaptic adrenergic receptors,
    123
Presynaptic histamine receptors,
    123–124
Prostaglandin(s), 89–90, 129–157
  adenylaye cyclase stimulation,
      332
  antagonists, 137
  bacterial endotoxins, 142
  cholera, 142
  cytoprotection, 133
  diarrhoea, 141–142
  dysmenorrhoea, 144
  formation by gastro-intestinal
      tissues, 129–131
  gastric anti-ulcer effect,
      132–134
  gastric secretion, 131–132
  gastric ulcers, 140
  gastro-intestinal diseases,
      140–144
  gastro-intestinal disturbances,
      141
  gastro-intestinal food
      intolerance, 143–144

Prostaglandin(s) (continued)
  gastro-intestinal muscle,
      134–140
    in vitro, 134–136
    in vivo, 138–140
  gastro-oesophageal reflux, 141
  idiopathic postural hypo-
      tension, 144
  inactivation by human gastric
      mucosa, 131
  inflammatory bowel disease,
      140–141
  intestinal motility, 139
  intestinal secretion, 132
  irritable colon syndrome, 143
  laxatives and, 334
  menstruation, 144
  mucosal protection, 133–134
  post-irradiation of cancer of
      cervix, 143
  receptors, 136–137
  as secretagogues, 225
  sites of action, 136–137
  small bowel pseudo-obstruction,
      142
Prostaglandin analogues, 131
  anti-ulcer effect, 132
Prostaglandin cyclo-oxygenase
    inhibitors, 334
Prostaglandin-like material
  release by electrical
      stimulation, 25
  tumor synthesized, 143
Prostaglandin-metabolising en-
    zymes, 131
Prostanoids, 89–90
  gastro-intestinal motility
      disorders, 144–145
  gastro-intestinal muscle, 135
  motility roles, 137–138
Pseudo-Hirschsprung's disease,
    180

^{3}H-Quinuclidinyl benzilate, 197

Radioimmunoassay, 109
Ranitidine, 119, 190, 191
  cerulitide potentiation, 121
  cholinergic-like effect, 122
Rectoanal reflexes (cat), 26

357

Rectum
  metaplastic polyps, 184–185
  mucosa, 7–8
Ricinoleate, 332, 333
Ricinoleic acid, 330, 332
RMI12330A, 333

Secretagogues
  potentiating interactions, 194
Secretin, 88, 109
  discovery, 259–260
  distribution in neurons,
        endocrine cells, plasma,
        111
  effect on
    colonic motility, 96
    gallbladder, 162
    gallbladder fluid, 232
    lower oesophageal sphincter,
        91
    small intestine motility, 95
  insulin response to, 261
Sensory cells, 78
Serotonin, 81–82
Shigella enterotoxin, 330
Sigmoid motility, prostaglandin
        effect, 140
Small intestine, mucosa, 6–7
Small/large intestine comparison,
        219–220
Smooth muscle, gastro-intestinal,
        3
  electrophysiology, 55–72
  ionic basis for electrical
        activity, 56–58
  structure, 55–56
Sodium absorption
  chloride-dependent, 221
  glucose-stimulated, 221
  mechanisms, 220–221
  model, 224
Sodium chloride absorption
        neutral, 223
Sodium dodecyl sulfate (SDS),
        327, 330
  adenine nucleotide translocase
        inhibition, 333
  adenylate cyclase stimulation,
        333
Sodium pump, electrogenic, 56,
        220–221

Sodium ricinoleate, 328
Solvent drag, 222
Somatostatin, 88, 90, 267
  in adrenergic ganglion cells,
        112
  circulating hormone, 114
  different active forms, 110
  distribution in neurons, endo-
        crine cells, plasma, 111
  effect on gallbladder, 165
  release by nerves, 114
Somatostatinoma, 182
Splanchic nerve stimulation,
        effects on
  gallbladder, 164
  pancreatic slucagon, 264
  pancreatic polypeptide, 265
  sphincter of Oddi, 164
  somatostatin, 265
Stomach
  electrical pacemaker, 62–64
  emptying, 46–49
    prostaglandin effect, 139
  intestinal metaphasia, 182–183,
        184
  intracellular electrical
        activity regional differ-
        ences, 63, 64
  motility, 289–295
  in vitro study, 17–19
  mucosa, 4–6
  spike-free region, 65
Stool weight, total, 244
Submucous (Meissner's) plexus, 1,
        2
Substance P, 3, 74, 88
  distribution in neurons,
        endocrine cells, plasma,
        111
  effect on
    central neurons, 82
    colonic activity, 96
    gallbladder, 165
    gastric motility, 93
    islet peptide secretion, 268
    muscularis mucosae, 251, 253
    myenteric neurons, 80, 81–88
    small intestine motility, 95
  in vagus, 112

Sulfasalazine (Sulphasalazine),
        134
    enteric-coated, 46
Sulphomucins, 182, 183
Surface potentials from muscle,
        40
    basic electric rhythm (BER,
        slow wave), 40
    cyclic potential, 40
Sympathetic nerve supply of gut,
        2

Taenia coli preparation, 64
Taurocholate, 332
Tetrodotoxin, 197
    resistance to, 25
Thromboxane mimetics (endo-
        peroxide analogues), 135
Thyrotropin releasing hormone
        (TRH), 97, 268
    effect on human gastric
        motility, 93
Transducers, strain gage force,
        40, 41-43
Transit
    measurement techniques, 45-46
    migrating myoelectrical complex
        (MMC), 242-243
    modifications: experimental
        observations, 243-244
    retrograde pacing, 244-245
Transmembrane potentials, 40
Transmucosal potentials, 39-40

Urea, 332

Vagotomy, pancreatic response to,
        263, 279
Vagus nerve
    cholinergic reflex, 262
    electrical stimulation effects
        (ferrets), 25
    pancreatic polypeptide
        secretion regulator, 263
Vasoactive intestinal polypeptide
        (VIP), 3, 74, 88, 265-266
    diarrhoea and, 334
    distribution in neurons, endo-
        crine cells, plasma, 111

Vasoactive intestinal polypeptide
        (VIP) (continued)
    effect on
        adenylate cyclase, 332
        colonic motility, 96
        gallbladder, 165
        gallbladder fluid, 232
        gastric motility, 93
        muscularis mucosae, 251, 252
    in gallbladder wall nerves, 166
    intra-arterial infusion, 113
    metoclopramide effect on, 319
    as neurotransmitter in gut, 113
    release by vagal stimulation,
        263
    tumor produced, 143
    in vagus, 112
Vasopressin
    effects on
        colonic motility, 96
        lower oesophageal sphincter,
            91
        small intestine motility, 95
Villikinin, 248
VIPOMA, 182
Voltage-tension relationship of
        gastric smooth muscle,
        67-69

Wall of alimentary canal, 1-2

Zollinger-Ellison syndrome, 182